Integrative Environmen ...ie

Integrative Medicine Library

Published and Forthcoming Volumes

SERIES EDITOR

Andrew Weil, MD

Donald I. Abrams and Andrew Weil: *Integrative Oncology*

Robert Bonakdar and Andrew W. Sukiennik: *Integrative Pain Management*

Richard Carmona and Mark Liponis: *Integrative Preventive Medicine*

Timothy P. Culbert and Karen Olness: *Integrative Pediatrics*

Stephen DeVries and James Dalen: *Integrative Cardiology*

Randy Horwitz and Daniel Muller: *Integrative Rheumatology, Allergy, and Immunology*

Mary Jo Kreitzer and Mary Koithan: *Integrative Nursing*

Daniel A. Monti and Bernard D. Beitman: *Integrative Psychiatry*

Gerard Mullin: *Integrative Gastroenterology*

Robert Norman, Philip D. Shenefelt, and Reena N. Rupani: *Integrative Dermatology*

Myles D. Spar and George E. Munoz: *Integrative Men's Health*

Victoria Maizes and Tieraona Low Dog: *Integrative Women's Health*

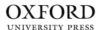

OXFORD
UNIVERSITY PRESS

Oxford University Press is a department of the University of Oxford. It furthers
the University's objective of excellence in research, scholarship, and education
by publishing worldwide. Oxford is a registered trade mark of Oxford University
Press in the UK and certain other countries.

Published in the United States of America by Oxford University Press
198 Madison Avenue, New York, NY 10016, United States of America.

CIP data is on file at the Library of Congress
ISBN 978-0-19-049091-1

Integrative Environmental Medicine

EDITED BY

Aly Cohen, MD, FACR

Founder & Medical Director, Integrative Rheumatology Associates, PC
Founder & Medical Director, The Smart Human LLC
Faculty, Academy of Integrative Health & Medicine (AIHM)
Jones/Lovell Fellow, Arizona Center for Integrative Medicine
Monroe Township, NJ

Frederick S. vom Saal, PhD

Curators' Distinguished Professor
Division of Biological Sciences
University of Missouri—Columbia
Columbia, MO

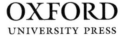

OXFORD
UNIVERSITY PRESS

CONTENTS

Foreword   *vii*

Preface   *ix*

Contributors   *xiii*

Section 1   History and Overview of Environmental Chemicals

1. The Age of Chemicals in the 21st Century: New Inventions,
   New Problems   3
   Carol F. Kwiatkowski

2. The Plastic Age: Worldwide Contamination, Sources of Exposure,
   and Human Health Consequences   23
   Charles Moore and Sarah S. Mosko

3. Environmental Chemicals and their Effects on Human Physiology   51
   Joel A. Maruniak

Section 2   Sources and Clinical Aspects of Environmental Exposures

4. Sources of Contaminants in the Home: Indoor Air Quality and
   Human Health   67
   James S. Denninghoff and Frederick S. vom Saal

5. Chemical Water Pollution and Human Health   87
   Christopher P. Weis and Donald E. Tillitt

6. Diet, Environmental Chemicals, and the Gut Microbiome   115
   Marvin M. Singh and Gerard E. Mullin

7. Interaction of Pharmaceuticals with Environmental Chemicals   141
   Anderson J. Martino-Andrade and Shanna H. Swan

8. Pesticides and Neurodegenerative Disorders   175
   John W. McBurney

9. Disinfection in the 21st Century: Is There Harm in Being Clean?   197
   Patricia A. Hunt, Terry C. Hrubec, and Vanessa E. Melin

10. Microwave/Radiofrequency Radiation and Human Health:
Clinical Management in the Digital Age   223
Devra Davis, Margaret E. Sears, Anthony B. Miller, and Riina Bray

Section 3   Regulatory Issues, Exposure Mitigation, and Resources for Clinicians and Patients

11. Food Additives: Health Consequences of Regulatory
Oversight Failure   255
Maricel V. Maffini and Sarah Vogel

12. Classic Toxicology vs. New Science: Unique Issues of
Endocrine-Disrupting Chemicals   279
Laura N. Vandenberg

13. Sustainable Chemistry: Addressing Low-Dose Adverse Effects
Through Contaminant Remediation and Design of Safe Products
for Our Future   305
Genoa R. Warner and Terrence J. Collins

14. Proactive Approaches to Reduce Environmental Exposures:
Avoidance, Lifestyle Changes, and Practical Resources   339
Aly Cohen

Index   383

FOREWORD

ANDREW WEIL, M.D.

An English surgeon, Sir Percivall Pott, was the first scientist to demonstrate that cancer could be caused by exposure to an environmental carcinogen. That occurred in London in 1775. Chimney sweeps of the period developed "soot wart" on the skin of the inferior surface of the scrotum; if these growths were not removed, they turned into squamous cell carcinomas that metastasized and killed. Pott correctly identified the cause as irritation from soot particles. Chimney sweeps often started work as children and therefore were in contact with soot for years. Sweat running down the body caused it to accumulate in the folds of scrotal skin. English chimney sweeps wore minimal or no clothing. German chimney sweeps wore protective garments and did not develop scrotal cancers. Pott's hypothesis was confirmed in 1922, when a carcinogen in coal soot was isolated.

One would think that environmental influences on health would have been a major focus of medical research, teaching, and practice over the years since Pott's discovery, but that has not been the case. Except for a lecture on the carcinogenic effects of tobacco smoking, my medical school education in the late 1960s included little information about environmental causation of cancer or any other diseases. Even as public concerns about air and water pollution grew in the late 20th century and scientists began to document the endocrine-disrupting, neurotoxic, teratogenic, carcinogenic, and other harmful effects of the many man-made chemicals in the environment, clinicians remained poorly informed about them, unable to respond to patients' fears and questions.

Lack of education about environmental medicine has also left physicians and allied health professionals unable to take effective political action. Too often, the lobbying efforts of polluting industries have had much greater influence on legislators and regulatory agencies than the voices of concerned citizens.

My colleagues and I at the University of Arizona Center for Integrative Medicine have made environmental health a core subject of our curriculums. As a result, a growing number of physicians, medical residents and students, and other health care professionals now have basic knowledge of the field. The publication of this newest volume in the Oxford University Press Integrative Medicine Library makes this information available to many more clinicians. Drs. Aly Cohen and Fred vom Saal have put together a thorough text that covers the main environmental chemicals that threaten human health, the sources and clinical consequences of environmental exposures, and ways to mitigate exposures. They also discuss regulatory and legislative issues surrounding these issues. I consider *Integrative Environmental Medicine* a landmark in the evolution of a field that is critically important to understanding health and illness.

PREFACE

Our environment has changed profoundly over the past 100 years. More than 87,000 new chemicals have been developed and integrated into our way of living without adequate testing to ensure safety for adults and particularly for fetuses, infants and children. Although modern materials have afforded us many advantages, we are now seeing the human health and environmental drawbacks to these conveniences. Indoor air pollution is associated with a variety of diseases, water contamination is a regular story on the evening news, and processed food contains thousands of chemicals that have never been tested for their effects on human health. Other sources for potential chemical exposure include cleaning products, food and beverage packaging, new pharmaceuticals and supplements, and personal care products that contain undisclosed, proprietary ingredients. Radiation sources are also a health concern, along with ever-expanding forms of technology and growing populations of users.

As the number and quantities of chemicals in the environment have dramatically increased since World War II, the incidence of many chronic health problems, such as type 2 diabetes, obesity, thyroid disease, asthma, allergy, autoimmune disease, autism, attention deficit hyperactivity disorder, and several cancers, have also increased. Evidence reveals that exposure to chemicals in the environment and in everyday products may increase the risk of these conditions. Add to this picture the lack of mandated chemical safety testing prior to their use in products, unknown synergistic effects of these individual chemicals mixed together or in combination with pharmaceuticals, and ineffective chemical regulation reform, and the level of concern increases dramatically. Chemicals are wrongly assumed to have the same regulatory oversight and testing as pharmaceuticals, with most consumers believing that "if it's on the shelf, it must be safe." Public ignorance about ineffective regulation and oversight exposes them to thousands of untested and unregulated chemicals on a daily basis.

Evidence presented in this book shows that contaminants are implicated in the rise in incidence of many illnesses, and there is concern that they could dismantle the infrastructure of our health care system if the disease trends are not altered. As the burden of chronic preventable diseases continues to overwhelm health care systems around the world, clinicians and the general public need accurate information about environmental risk factors that can impact human health.

Here is the good news: There is no better time to inform and help patients make lifestyle changes and better choices. Several medical and scientific societies, led by The Endocrine Society, are working to bring the issues addressed in this book to the attention of regulatory agencies, the U.S. Congress, and EU Parliament. Health care practitioners are in a unique position to be able to convey to patients important tenets: It is possible to mitigate chemical exposures, to make healthier lifestyle changes, and to choose safer consumer products, food, and water. This information can have profound effects on the health of the population, of our offspring, and of future generations.

This book provides the latest information about environmental exposures to humans and the tools and proactive recommendations to limit adverse health effects due to exposures. It highlights the vulnerability of fetuses, infants, and children when exposures occur during critical periods of growth and development. To offer a complete picture, we describe the history of the chemical revolution in the 20th century, legislative issues related to modern chemicals, the unique toxicologic problems related to exposure to chemicals known as endocrine disruptors, and the current diseases linked by epidemiologic and experimental animal studies to various exposures. Throughout the text and especially in Chapter 14, we share important tools, resources, and practical information to empower clinicians to inform their patients about making practical lifestyle changes to reduce exposures to environmental hazards.

In keeping with the philosophy of integrative medicine, which is healing-oriented medicine that takes account of the whole person (i.e., body, mind, spirit) and all aspects of lifestyle, our focus is on prevention rather than management of symptoms. In line with this philosophy, we embrace the "precautionary principle," which states that when an activity raises threats of harm to the environment or human health, precautionary measures should be taken even if some cause-and-effect relationships are not fully established.

As co-editors of this text, we have chosen authors who are leaders in their respective areas, share a common interest in experimental and clinical research, and have a strong desire to educate health practitioners and the public. This book represents a unique collaboration of researchers and clinicians who have joined together to provide the most up-to-date information for clinicians and those seeking a deeper knowledge of their diseases.

We have divided the text into three sections: (1) history and overview of chemicals, (2) sources and clinical aspects of environmental exposures to chemicals and radiation, and (3) regulatory and legislative issues, exposure mitigation, and resources for clinicians and patients.

In Section 1, Chapter 1 begins with an overview of the chemical revolution that occurred over the 20th century, leading to the development of tens of thousands of chemicals currently in commercial use without adequate pre-market testing. Chapter 2 discusses our love affair with plastics since World War II. An astounding approximately one trillion pounds of plastics are produced globally every year. We describe the lifecycle of plastics, including invention, manufacture, use, and disposal by consumers and industry, highlighting the environmental and human health consequences. Chapter 3 describes how common environmental chemicals can hijack the endocrine system to disrupt normal physiology and homeostasis, particularly during critical periods of human development.

In Section 2, Chapters 4 and 5 focus on sources of pollution and the importance of clean indoor air, water, and food for optimal health. Chapter 4 focuses on the relationship between dust and mold in the home and respiratory diseases, including the consequences of exposure to toxic chemicals that bind to dust. Chapter 5 covers chemical pollutants in water and water contamination events that have unveiled serious problems with drinking water systems in the United States. Chapter 6 shows that diet and the chemicals in processed food and the environment need to be considered in order to maintain a healthy gut microbiome and reduce inflammatory diseases. Chapter 7 discusses commonly used medications, including acetaminophen and antidepressants, that have the unexpected capacity to exacerbate the harmful effects of chemicals that leach our of products found in virtually every home. Chapter 8 describes the pervasiveness of pesticides and their effects on the development of neurodegenerative disease, such as Parkinson's disease, Alzheimer's disease, and amyotrophic lateral sclerosis (ALS). Chapter 9 describes the precipitous rise in antimicrobial cleaning chemicals used in households, schools, and workspaces, including medical offices and hospitals, as well as the consequences of antimicrobial resistance. Chapter 10 explains the health risks associated with electromagnetic radiofrequencies, WiFi, cell phone, and tablet use, with an important focus on childhood exposures.

In Section 3, Chapter 11 focuses on the failure of regulatory bodies to properly vet food additives that affect the safety of all processed food, the health effects that have been elucidated, and the need for a rational approach to identifying and regulating these chemicals. Chapter 12 describes the unique properties and health hazards of endocrine-disrupting chemicals found in a wide range of common household products. This class of environmental toxicants disrupts hormones whose actions are mediated by receptors in specific target tissues that respond to very low concentrations, rather than being acute systemic toxicants that are hazards only at high doses. Chapter 13 brings to light innovations for remediation of existing polluted environments and the "green chemistry" strategy for developing chemicals that are not a risk to human health. Chapter 14 outlines best practices for clinicians to screen for chemical exposure in patients and describes tools, practical tips, online resources, and proactive lifestyle recommendations for reducing exposure and increasing elimination of harmful chemicals found in everyday life.

We hope this book affords clinicians and the public an increased awareness of environmental medicine and its critical contribution to disease prevention and management. By providing helpful resources such as smart phone apps, links to websites, and printable clinician and patient information (see Chapter 14), our aim is to facilitate a change in health outcomes for patients, their families, and the global population. We hope you will feel enlightened and empowered and possibly respond with a call to arms, no matter where on the path you may be starting your journey.

Aly Cohen and Fred vom Saal

CONTRIBUTORS

Riina Bray, BASc, MSc, MD, FCFP, MHSc
Assistant Professor, Department of
    Family and Community Medicine
Dalla Lana School of Public Health
University of Toronto
Medical Director, Environmental
    Health Clinic
Women's College Hospital
Toronto, Canada

Aly Cohen, MD, FACR
Founder & Medical Director,
    Integrative Rheumatology
    Associates, PC
Founder & Medical Director
The Smart Human LLC
Faculty, Academy of Integrative
    Health & Medicine (AIHM)
Jones/Lovell Fellow, Arizona Center
    for Integrative Medicine
Monroe Township, NJ

Terrence J. Collins, PhD
Teresa Heinz Professor of Green
    Chemistry and Director, Institute
    for Green Science
Department of Chemistry
Carnegie Mellon University
Pittsburgh, PA

Devra Davis, PhD, MPH, FACE
Visiting Professor of Medicine, The
    Hebrew University
Environmental Health Trust

James S. Denninghoff, MD
Midwest Sinus Allergy
Columbia, MO

Terry C. Hrubec, DVM, PhD
Department of Biomedical Sciences
    and Pathobiology
VA-MD College of Veterinary
    Medicine
E. Via College of Osteopathic
    Medicine–Virginia Campus
Blacksburg, VA

Patricia A. Hunt, PhD
School of Molecular Biosciences
Center for Reproductive Biology
Washington State University
Pullman, WA

Carol F. Kwiatkowski, PhD
Executive Director, The Endocrine
  Disruption Exchange
Paonia, CO
Assistant Professor Adjunct,
  Department of Integrative
  Physiology
University of Colorado
Boulder, CO

Maricel V. Maffini, PhD
Independent Consultant
Germantown, MD

Anderson J. Martino-Andrade, PhD
Department of Preventive Medicine
Icahn School of Medicine at Mount
  Sinai
New York, NY
Department of Physiology
Universidade Federal do Paraná
Curitiba, Brazil

Joel A. Maruniak, PhD
Associate Professor, Emeritus
Biological Sciences
University of Missouri
Columbia, MO

John W. McBurney, MD
McBurney Integrative Neurology, LLC
Contributing Instructor, Arizona
  Center for Integrative Medicine
Portland, OR

Vanessa E. Melin, PhD
Department of Biomedical Sciences
  and Pathobiology
VA-MD College of Veterinary
  Medicine
Blacksburg, VA

Anthony B. Miller, MD, FACE
Professor Emeritus
Dalla Lana School of Public Health
University of Toronto
Toronto, Canada

Capt. Charles Moore, PhD (hon)
Research Director, Algalita Marine
  Research and Education
Long Beach, CA

Sarah S. Mosko, PhD
Research Associate, Algalita Marine
  Research and Education
Long Beach, CA

Gerard E. Mullin, MD
Associate Professor, Division of
  Gastroenterology/Hepatology
Johns Hopkins Hospital
Baltimore, MD

Margaret E. Sears, PhD
Prevent Cancer Now
Ottawa, Canada
Environmental Health Trust
Teton Village, WY

Marvin M. Singh, MD
Assistant Clinical Professor of
  Medicine, Division of Digestive
  Diseases
UCLA Health
Los Angeles, CA

Shanna H. Swan, PhD
Department of Preventive Medicine
Icahn School of Medicine
New York, NY

Donald E. Tillitt, PhD
Biochemistry & Physiology Branch
   Chief
Columbia Environmental Research
   Center
U.S. Geological Survey, Department
   of Interior
Columbia, MO

Laura N. Vandenberg, PhD
University of Massachusetts–Amherst
School of Public Health & Health
   Sciences
Department of Environmental Health
   Sciences
Amherst, MA

Sarah Vogel, PhD, MPH, MEM
Vice President, Health.
   Environmental Defense Fund
Washington, DC

Frederick S. vom Saal, PhD
Curators' Distinguished Professor
Division of Biological Sciences
University of Missouri–Columbia
Columbia, MO

Genoa R. Warner, MS
Presidential Fellow, Institute for
   Green Science
Department of Chemistry
Carnegie Mellon University
Pittsburgh, PA

Christopher P. Weis, PhD, DABT
Toxicology Liaison/Senior Advisor
Office of the Director
National Institute of Environmental
   Health Science
National Institutes of Health
Bethesda, MD

History and Overview of Environmental Chemicals

1

The Age of Chemicals in the 21st Century: New Inventions, New Problems

CAROL F. KWIATKOWSKI

Key Concepts

- Humans are exposed on a regular basis to many types of chemicals, including pesticides, metals, industrial products and byproducts, plastics, and antimicrobials.
- Exposure to very low concentrations of chemicals, particularly endocrine disruptors, can have detrimental and lasting effects that may not manifest for years.
- The effects of exposure during prenatal and childhood development can be permanent and can persist for multiple generations.
- Several medical societies recommend avoiding or reducing exposure to chemicals implicated in adverse health conditions, even in the absence of definitive scientific evidence proving cause and effect.
- Governments should correct deficiencies in safety testing protocols, require that chemicals be tested before use in consumer products or at least prohibit substitution of a harmful chemical with one that is untested, and promote the development of safer alternatives and green chemistry.

Introduction

The 20th century was filled with tragic incidents of chemical exposures that killed or sickened hundreds of human and animal victims. These events capture the attention of the media and the public and may be addressed by swift government action. However, behind each major news event is a little-known story of damage that erodes the health of millions who are exposed in a less dramatic manner, day in and day out, to the same chemicals that led to the newsworthy tragedies. These and similar chemicals are present in our air, water, and soil, and we are exposed in our homes, work places, and play areas. We eat, drink, and breathe them; we rub them on our skin.

The warning signs of chemical exposures are not posted on office or bathroom walls; they are not even listed on the containers that hold the chemicals. For the most part, evidence of the existence of these chemicals and their potential damage to our health and that of future generations lies buried in the annals of academic libraries. Although public awareness is growing, government response has been too slow, and generation after generation continues to be exposed.

This chapter provides examples of pesticides, metals, air pollutants, flame retardants, plastics, antimicrobials, and other common contaminants encountered by most humans in the developed world on a daily basis. Exposure to these chemicals has been documented in numerous academic studies[54] and in data collected through the U.S. Centers for Disease Control and Prevention (CDC) National Biomonitoring Program. The program assesses more than 300 environmental chemicals by sampling blood, urine, breast milk, and other biologic specimens in the general population. Most people have numerous detectable chemicals in their bodies, and some have hundreds. Socioeconomically stressed communities have higher levels of exposure to many environmental chemicals. Even people living in remote areas where chemicals are not used or manufactured can have high levels due to transport of chemicals by wind and water and through the food web.

Children typically have higher levels of chemicals in their bodies than adults because children spend more time closer to the ground, where chemicals settle; they have more hand-to-mouth behavior than adults; they have greater food and water intake per unit of body weight; and their immature immune and metabolic systems do not process chemicals as well as adult systems do. They are also born "prepolluted" with chemicals that cross the placenta. One biomonitoring report identified as many as 232 chemicals in the umbilical cord blood of minority newborns.[21] Breast milk and baby formula are other early sources of contaminants in young children.

Chemical impacts on the endocrine system are of particular concern because many synthetic chemicals can disrupt hormone function at very low concentrations, within the range of human exposure.[55] Adverse effects from exposure that occurs in utero can be permanent. Laboratory research on the effects of prenatal and early postnatal exposure to low concentrations of chemicals can be seen in an online learning tool developed by The Endocrine Disruption Exchange (TEDX).[4,52] The timing of chemical exposure in each rodent study is mapped to a timeline of events in human prenatal development, showing adverse effects on the central nervous system, the male and female reproductive systems, and the endocrine and immune systems.

Despite these facts, the toxicologic tests used by government regulatory agencies do not routinely assess sensitive end points related to the endocrine system; they do not include the effects of exposure to low chemical concentrations; and they do not include examination of immediate or long-term effects due to exposure during critical periods in development. Therefore, we cannot rely on safe exposure levels set by the government to protect people from harm, particularly fetuses, infants, and children. This is alarming given the dramatic growth in synthetic chemical production in the United States over the past century, as shown in Figure 1.1.

Mirroring this growth is an increase in the prevalence and/or incidence of many diseases in which environmental chemicals are implicated. Examples include infertility, hypospadias, cryptorchidism, childhood cancer, autism, attention deficit hyperactivity disorder (ADHD), diabetes, and obesity. Birth rates and sex ratios have also been affected. In one heavily polluted First Nation community living along the Great Lakes in eastern Canada, the proportion of male births over a 5-year period declined from 0.54 to 0.35.[33] Many population statistics attest to major changes in chronic disease rates over the past century. It is time for individuals to become aware of changes they can make to avoid harmful chemical exposures and

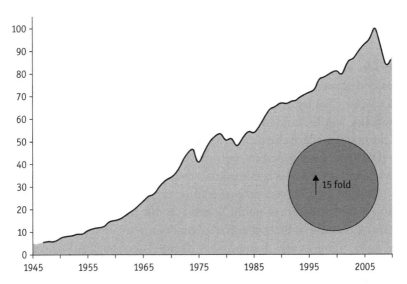

FIGURE 1.1. Chemical production in the United States, 1945–2007. Federal reserve data on chemical production is only offered as relative production, which is unit-less. A specific reference year is chosen and values are calculated relative to that year's production. In this particular data set 2007 is the reference year and is assigned a value of 100. Data from: U.S. Federal Reserve Board, Division of Research and Statistics. Reprinted with permission from the University of California San Francisco Program on Reproductive Health and the Environment.

for governments to take a precautionary approach to regulating chemicals in order to protect the public health.

Chemicals of Concern

After World War II, chemists, having excelled at developing agents of chemical warfare, began synthesizing compounds (e.g., polymers, resins, plastics, lubricants, solvents, surfactants) for the purpose of improving modern living. The conveniences offered by these products were welcomed by consumers, and it did not take long before these chemical compounds pervaded almost every aspect of daily life. Man-made chemicals are found in clothing, cosmetics, fragrances, furniture, building materials, electronics, cleaning products, and toys, as well as food and water.

Table 1.1 provides a categorization scheme designed to organize chemicals according to their use (e.g., household chemicals, personal care products), function (e.g., flame retardant, solvent, antimicrobial), and type of chemical (e.g., metal, biogenic compound). In the following sections, selected chemicals are described to illustrate the history, exposure routes, and health effects of several chemical categories.

PESTICIDES

Pesticides are unique in the chemical pollution realm because they are specifically designed to kill living organisms, usually by means of acute neurotoxicity (see Chapter 8). Unfortunately, their use results in collateral damage to humans, wildlife, and the ecosystem.

Like many modern chemicals, the pesticide dichlorodiphenyltrichloroethane (DDT) was developed in the early 20th century. Initially used to fight insect-borne diseases such as malaria, it was quickly adopted in agricultural and household use for general pest control. Rachel Carson's 1962 book, *Silent Spring*, raised widespread public concern about the use of DDT and other pesticides because of their effects on the nervous system and liver and their roles as carcinogens and mutagens.[8] A decade later, the U.S. Environmental Protection Agency (EPA) cancelled the use of DDT in the United States, although it is still used in other countries to fight malaria and other insect-borne diseases.[18]

Today, hundreds of pesticides are registered by the EPA to kill weeds, insects, rodents, mites, fungus, and more. A common insecticide is chlorpyrifos, which the EPA cancelled for all home uses in 2000 and recently proposed

Table 1.1. Chemical Categories

Category	Description
Household Product Ingredient	Chemicals found in items such as appliances, vehicles, building materials, electronics, crafts, textiles, furniture, and household cleaning products.
Personal Care Product/ Cosmetic Ingredient	Chemicals found in products such as cosmetics, shampoos, lotions, soaps, deodorants, fragrances, and shaving products.
Food Additive	Antioxidants, dyes, and compounds used in food processing, and as components in food packaging.
Flame retardant	Chemicals used to prevent fires.
Plastic/Rubber	Components, reactants, or additives used in the manufacturing of rubbers or plastics.
Pesticide Ingredient	Insecticides/acaricides (miticides), herbicides, fungicides, rodenticides, and other biocides, including chemicals described as 'inert'.
Antimicrobial	Chemicals that prevent the growth of and/or destroy microorganisms.
Biogenic compound	Naturally occurring or biologically derived chemicals such as phytoestrogens, flavonoids, monophenols, mycochemicals and phenolic acids.
Industrial Additive	Chemicals such as preservatives, antioxidants and surfactants used in such things as glue, plastic, rubber, paint, and wood products.
Solvent	Chemicals used to dissolve other chemicals.
Metal/Metallurgy	Elements or chemicals used in the extraction, processing, or manufacturing of a metal or metal-containing product, including welding.
Byproduct/Intermediate/ Reactant	Chemicals used in the synthesis of other compounds, and/or unwanted byproducts such as impurities and contaminants, including combustion byproducts.
Medical/Veterinary/Research	Chemicals used in hospitals, medical supplies, and equipment, in laboratories or as reagents, and pharmaceuticals.
Metabolite/Degradate	Breakdown products of other chemicals.

to cancel for all food-related uses.[20] Chlorpyrifos is an example of a pesticide that can have numerous effects on brain development and function and to which almost everyone is exposed.[12]

People are often exposed to several pesticides at once. A graphic example of the neurodevelopmental effects of exposure to pesticides can be seen in Figure 1.2, in which artwork created by exposed children clearly demonstrates an impaired ability to draw a person.[25] Wildlife is also exposed to mixtures of pesticides, such as from sewage effluent or agricultural runoff in rivers and lakes. Intersex fish (e.g., males with testicular oocytes) have been found in numerous water bodies in the United States.[30] Alligators living in lakes that are highly polluted by pesticides have been shown to have smaller gonads and reduced testosterone levels compared with alligators living in unpolluted water.[26] Wildlife share the same water, air, and soil as humans, and the effects of chemical exposure on animals may serve as harbingers of the health effects in humans.

Pesticides have transgenerational effects. When exposure occurs during pregnancy, three generations are exposed at once: the mother, the fetus, and the fetal germ cells. Furthermore, research on laboratory animals has demonstrated effects of pesticides on subsequent generations that were not directly exposed. The effects were most strikingly shown in studies of vinclozolin (a fungicide). Three generations after exposure, descendants

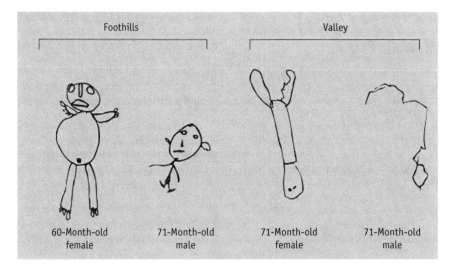

FIGURE 1.2. Representative drawings of a person by 5-year-old children who were unexposed (i.e., in the foothills) or exposed (i.e., in the valley) to pesticides.
From Guillette, E.A., Meza, M.M., Aquilar, M.G., Soto, A.D., & Garcia, I.E. 1998. An anthropological approach to the evaluation of preschool children exposed to pesticides in Mexico. *Environ Health Perspect.* 106:347–353.

displayed effects on metabolic activity, brain development, and behavior, including altered responses to stressful environments in adolescence.[13] These effects would be extremely difficult to study in humans.

Pesticide exposure can lead to effects that do not manifest until years later. Laboratory research on early life exposure to several different pesticides has revealed links to Parkinson's disease through alterations in the neurochemicals that affect locomotor activity.[46,53]

Despite growing interest in organic practices, pesticides are considered to be essential to modern agriculture. It is unlikely that the use of chemicals in large-scale farming will be eliminated in the near future. It is therefore imperative that governments develop ways of identifying the safest alternatives and continue to raise public awareness about the best ways to reduce exposure.

METALS: LEAD

Exposure to lead has been known since ancient times to have adverse health effects. Nevertheless, people have used it in everything from water pipes to paints to cosmetics. In the early 1970s, the EPA began phasing lead out of gasoline, in which it was used as an additive to boost octane levels; this process took more than 25 years to complete. In an effort to reduce childhood exposures, lead was also removed from household paint, although exposure is still a problem in older houses. Aging infrastructure can create new public health emergencies, as was shown in Flint, Michigan, where a switch to a more corrosive water source (i.e., a river) in 2014 caused lead to leach from pipes into drinking water. The incidence of elevated blood lead levels in children doubled as a result.[27]

Although regulatory efforts have been successful at lowering the levels of lead in blood, continued scientific research has made it clear that there are no safe levels of lead exposure. Even minute amounts encountered during development can cause devastating and permanent damage to the growing child. Although some of the effects of this *legacy chemical* are fairly well known, others are not. The CDC's Agency for Toxic Substances and Disease Registry (ATSDR) provides a long list of adverse outcomes in numerous physiologic systems as a result of acute and chronic exposures.[2]

SOLVENTS: BTEX

BTEX is an acronym for the aromatic hydrocarbons benzene, toluene, ethylbenzene, and the xylene isomers. BTEX are acquired during the extraction of fossil fuels and then refined and used as feedstock for the synthesis of thousands of other chemicals. When lead was banned as a fuel additive, BTEX hydrocarbons were the chosen replacement chemicals, and today they comprise up to 28% of high-octane gasoline.[39] They are also used in the production of numerous consumer and industrial products, including adhesives, detergents, solvents, paints, and pesticides. They are in such items as cleaning products, wall paint, glue, nail polish, and air fresheners.

According to the EPA, toluene is among the top 10 chemicals used in consumer products, and ethylbenzene is among the top 10 for children's products, including toys, furniture, playground equipment, and plastic and rubber products.[19] As a result, indoor air has become polluted, and concentrations of BTEX indoors can be four to six times higher than in outdoor air due to the off-gassing of household products and building materials. Although BTEX chemicals can be controlled by limiting their use as gasoline additives, there is currently little awareness of the issue and few regulatory approaches for cleaning up indoor air.

A review of BTEX exposure in humans at ambient (low) concentrations found effects in the respiratory, immune, cardiovascular, and reproductive systems.[6] Many of the studies were conducted in children exposed prenatally or during early childhood.

New sources of exposure are potentially affecting millions of people in the United States and other countries. A relatively new approach to extracting fossil fuels called hydraulic fracturing (i.e., fracking) has brought raw and refined petrochemicals into people's neighborhoods and backyards. During hydraulic fracturing, complex mixtures of chemicals combined with water and sand are pumped into the ground at high pressure to release the desired methane. BTEX and other toxic chemicals come up with the methane and are released into the air near homes, schools, and urban centers. They can also contaminate ground, surface, and drinking water sources. Research is beginning to emerge, and epidemiologic studies have reported adverse developmental outcomes (e.g., congenital heart failure, increased preterm births) associated with living in close proximity to hydraulic fracturing sites.[9,34,47]

INDUSTRIAL BYPRODUCTS: DIOXINS

Dioxins are the byproducts of numerous industrial operations. 2,3,7,8-Tetrachlorodibenzo-p-dioxin (TCDD) is the most toxic and best-studied form of dioxin. Although dioxins are not intentionally produced, they enter the air from thousands of sources, including incinerators that burn medical, municipal, and hazardous wastes; chemical processing facilities that use chlorine to make products such as pesticides and plastics; and metal refining and smelting operations.

Before industrialization and the introduction of chlorine, dioxins existed naturally only in very small amounts, but they are now found everywhere in the world. Transported through the air, they do not react with oxygen or water and are not broken down by bacteria. They are among a list of chemicals known as *persistent organic pollutants* (POPs).

When dairy cows and beef cattle eat feed crops containing settled airborne dioxins or are given feed that contains dioxins from other animal fats, these chemicals become concentrated in the fat of the animals. Humans ingest dioxins primarily in fatty foods such as beef, dairy products, and fish, but they also occur in lesser concentrations in other foods. Dioxins accumulate in human fatty tissue, with a half-life of 7 to 12 years. Children, nursing infants, workers exposed occupationally, people who eat fish as a main staple of their diet, and people who live near industrial sites where dioxins are released may be highly exposed.

Perhaps the most famous dioxin incident occurred in 1976, when a chemical plant in Seveso, Italy, exploded, releasing a cloud of dioxins that quickly settled over the town and surrounding areas. Animals began to die immediately. A 2010 *TIME* magazine article,[14] which listed the incident as one of its top 10 environmental disasters, described a man's cat dying and the tail falling off. Two days later, there was nothing left but the skull. People quickly began to get sick, many with the signature symptom of dioxin poisoning, a skin disease known as chloracne. It was weeks before the town was evacuated and the area quarantined. Long-term health studies have found evidence of cardiovascular and respiratory disease, diabetes, and cancer among affected individuals.[5]

The EPA has studied dioxins at length and recognizes that they can cause cancer, interfere with the endocrine system, lead to reproductive and developmental problems, and damage the immune system. Because they alter the fundamental ways in which cells develop and grow, they can lead to a broad spectrum of physiologic effects. Importantly, effects can occur within the range of exposures in the general population. Children are particularly susceptible, and human perinatal exposure has been associated with impaired brain development; endocrine, liver, and lung dysfunction; and other adverse outcomes.[51]

PERFLUORINATED COMPOUNDS

Perfluorinated compounds (PFCs) are a group of chemicals that have been made since the 1950s for specific uses in industrial and consumer products.

They also occur as byproducts and breakdown products of other fluorinated chemicals. The two most widely studied PFCs are perfluorooctanoic acid (PFOA) and perfluorooctane sulfonic acid (PFOS), which have been used in many applications. PFOS has been used in nonstick cookware; stains and water repellants for apparel, carpets, and furniture; food packaging; paints, cosmetics; shampoos; and denture cleaners. PFOA has been used in breathable waterproof fabrics, insulations for electrical wiring, and foam-based fire extinguishers.

PFCs are found ubiquitously in human populations and other species, even in remote locations far from manufacturing or use of PFCs. This widespread detection has been attributed to their resistance to biodegradation and their bioaccumulative properties. It is thought that most human exposure occurs through food and drinking water. Crops grown in PFC-contaminated soil can take up and accumulate these compounds. Exposure to PFC-contaminated air or house dust and direct contact with PFC-containing consumer products are other potential sources of exposure.

PFCs are primarily found in the kidney and liver. PFOA and PFOS have long half-lives in humans, ranging from 2 to 9 years for PFOA and up to 21 years for PFOS. They cross the placenta and have been measured in maternal and cord blood and in breast milk. Laboratory studies indicate that PFCs interfere with reproduction and development and may cause cancer.[1,32,57] Despite the known toxicities of PFCs, enactment of regulations to control their production and use has been difficult, and voluntary action by industry to remove them from consumer products has led to substitution with other harmful chemicals.

FLAME RETARDANTS

California's fire safety regulation TB117, enacted in 1975, led to the use of large quantities of flame-retardant chemicals in consumer products across the United States. These products include furniture foam, carpet padding, electronics, and building insulation. Many products used for babies and children are made with foam that contains flame retardants, including car seats, crib mattresses, and nursing pillows. The chemicals migrate out of the foam and are a common component in house dust[62] (see Chapter 4).

Although some may consider flame retardants a necessary evil, their purpose of delaying or preventing the ignition and spread of fire has been challenged, and their toxicity to the health of firefighters who inhale toxic gases is a serious concern.[45] Further, they have been associated with numerous adverse effects in humans and laboratory animals, including decreased fertility, altered neurodevelopment, lowered IQ, hyperactivity, and hormone disruption.[29,35,43]

Some flame retardants have been banned due to their toxicity, but because they are extremely long lasting in the environment and bio accumulate, the risks of exposure remain. Laboratory research into one common replacement chemical identified it as an endocrine disruptor and an obesogen at low, environmentally relevant levels.[36] In a bit of good news, the flammability standard for TB117 was revised in 2013 in a manner that allows many products to meet the standard without the use of harmful chemicals.

PLASTICS: BISPHENOL A

In contrast to legacy chemicals such as lead and PFCs, bisphenol A (BPA) is perhaps the most widely studied *emerging chemical*, a term used to describe chemicals of emerging concern. Manufacturers began using BPA in industrial and commercial products in the 1950s, although it had been shown in the 1930s to have the efficacy of an endogenous estrogen in animals. Its hardness and clarity made it appear to be the ideal plastic for everything from baby bottles and eyeglass lenses to airplanes and automobiles. It is used as an epoxy resin in food and beverage can linings, water pipes, dental sealants and fillings, and adhesives. It is speculated that the widest source of human exposure may come from its use as a coating on thermal receipt paper, from which it readily migrates onto hands and into mouths. BPA is metabolized and excreted quickly, but exposure is so prevalent that it is found in almost everyone tested and in many different bodily fluids.[10]

BPA has become an iconic chemical to demonstrate the issue of endocrine disruption, particularly with regard to prenatal exposure. Millions of dollars in government research funds have been spent studying BPA alone. Hundreds of studies have been published identifying adverse health effects, including effects at low, environmentally relevant levels.[38,40,56,59] Outcomes include impaired male and female reproduction, metabolic disease, altered immune function, and adverse effects on brain development and behavior.

Despite these findings, industry pushback has stalled national regulations that would reduce the production or use of BPA (see Chapters 11 and 12). Worldwide BPA production is almost 5 million tons, and its functional and economic qualities make industry reluctant to replace it. Cities and states in the United States have been more proactive than the federal government, and public concern has been perhaps the most effective at motivating industry to create BPA-free products. Unfortunately, replacement of BPA with chemicals such as bisphenol S (BPS), bisphenol F (BPF), and 4-hydroxyphenyl

4-isoprooxyphenylsulfone (BPSIP) may not be any better in terms of health. However, the replacements are so new that little is known about their potential health effects. This is an example of the pervasive issue of *regrettable substitution*, in which chemicals with health concerns are replaced by chemicals we know nothing about.

PLASTICS: PHTHALATES

Phthalates are plasticizers added to make plastics such as polyvinyl chloride (PVC) softer and more flexible. They are also commonly used to make fragrances last longer. Several types of phthalates are used, and many are produced in volumes of tens of millions of pounds. Common uses are in food packaging, fragrances, personal care products (e.g., soap, shampoo), and numerous household products such as garden hoses, detergents, shower curtains, and toys. They are also in building materials, paints, and adhesives.

Because phthalates are not bound to the plastics in which they are mixed, they are readily released by leaching or evaporation. As plastics age and break down, the release of phthalates accelerates. Leaching also increases from contact with fatty foods and oily substances. Some phthalates are detected in almost every person tested, and sometimes they are found at very high levels.[10]

Diet is the primary route of exposure for phthalates, likely because the FDA has approved 30 phthalates for use as food additives (including in packaging), although some of the approved phthalates are now regulated in children's products. Skin absorption is an important route of exposure that has not been well studied. Absorption can occur through the use of men's and women's personal care products, sunscreens, and insecticides. Potential sources of inhalation include breathing fragrances and hair sprays and baking modeling clay. A major concern about phthalates is their use in medical devices such as fluid bags and tubing, particularly in neonatal care units.

Like BPA, phthalates are commonly recognized by the scientific community as endocrine disruptors. Prenatal phthalate exposure in humans has been correlated with effects in baby boys including incomplete testicular descent, increased risk of hypospadias, and shorter anogenital distance, which is a marker for androgenic effects.[50] There is also evidence for effects on neurodevelopment, pointing to cognitive and behavioral outcomes including ADHD-like behaviors.[17] In adult men, altered sperm, increased abdominal obesity, and insulin resistance have been shown.[28,48]

Worldwide, various phthalates have been banned by countries, states, and cities for specific uses (e.g., in children's toys that can be placed in the mouth), but they are typically replaced by other phthalates that have undergone little scientific research on their health effects. An expert panel was convened by the U.S. Consumer Product Safety Commission to review the full range of phthalates in children's products. Their 2014 report concluded that eight phthalates had sufficient data to confirm they should be banned from children's products at levels greater than 0.1%.[11]

Although we are continuously exposed to mixtures of many different phthalates, regulations typically focus on individual chemicals. Further, although phthalates have been shown to be harmful during prenatal development, regulations have focused on children's products, ignoring the potential effects of fetal exposure through the maternal diet. More effective regulations are needed to reduce phthalate exposure.

ANTIMICROBIALS: TRICLOSAN

Triclosan is one of the most commonly used synthetic broad-spectrum antimicrobial agents. It is used primarily to prevent the growth of bacteria (see Chapter 9). It is widely used in hospitals and in many consumer products such as liquid soap, deodorant, cosmetics, toothpaste, and clothing. It is also used in durable items such as toys, cutting boards, and fitness mats. Although the FDA requires over-the-counter drugs and cosmetics to be labeled if they contain triclosan, this does not apply to other items. Triclosan is registered with the EPA as a pesticide and is used as a preservative to prevent bacterial deterioration in many commercial and consumer products (e.g., adhesives, fabrics, vinyl, plastics, sealants).

Triclosan is readily absorbed through the skin and has been found in serum, in breast milk, and as metabolites in the urine of 75% of Americans.[7] Although it is not generally regarded as toxic, numerous laboratory studies attest to its endocrine-disrupting properties, which affect the estrogen, androgen, and thyroid systems.[23,31,37,41,49] Triclosan is also thought to be adding to the increase in antibiotic-resistant bacteria. For many consumer products containing triclosan (e.g., soaps, body washes), there does not appear to be any added health benefit compared with regular soap and water. Triclosan is a common pollutant in surface water (i.e., rivers and streams), sewage sludge, and sediment, potentially affecting aquatic ecosystems and wildlife.

Summary

The recitation of adverse environmental effects of chemicals could continue for many pages, describing the exposure routes and health impacts of fragrance ingredients, food additives, mercury, arsenic, and much more. However, the point has been made that we live in a world infused with man-made chemicals. Exposure at very low concentrations can have detrimental and lasting impacts that may not manifest for years, making it very difficult to connect cause and effect. Moreover, the effects of exposure during prenatal and childhood development can be permanent and can persist for multiple generations. The urgency with which we must begin to address these problems cannot be overstated.

Looking Forward

Scientists are beginning to weave together research to explain the unacceptable prevalence of chronic conditions that are disabling society. They are telling the story in terms such as *adverse outcome pathways*. These are models that attempt to connect events at the molecular level (e.g., hormonal changes) through the subsequent cellular and organ responses to adverse outcomes for the whole being.[58] New, high-volume in vitro test methods and in silico computational models are being developed, and many more chemicals are being screened and identified as having endocrine activity.[22] Methods are being advanced to systematically review animal and human epidemiologic data to definitively identify the hazards associated with environmental chemicals[42] (see Chapter 13).

New approaches are being developed to estimate exposure to chemical mixtures that attempt to reflect real-world chemical body burdens.[16] They include characterization of the *exposome*, the totality of exposures humans experience throughout their lives.[60] Green chemistry approaches, in which chemicals are "benign by design," may provide incentives for industry to create products without harmful chemicals.[44] However, we are many years away from positive health impacts of these new scientific developments in the real world.

For most chemicals, no information about health effects exists. For those that have proved harmful, protective health measures continue to be delayed by arguments that regulatory and other preventive actions should not be initiated until definitive proof of cause and effect is demonstrated. However, the standard of proof—randomized clinical trials—is unethical in environmental health research. There is already enough evidence that the chemicals of concern are toxic, thus they cannot be administered to humans. However, if they are unethical to administer in a clinical trial, why are we allowing them to be released into the environment? The current U.S. approach of allowing chemicals to be brought to market without appropriate safety testing is untenable. Europe is one step ahead in that legislation has been passed to require chemicals to be tested for adverse health effects before market entry.

Health care professionals in the 21st century who treat patients with cancer, diabetes, obesity, reproductive problems, thyroid conditions, and developmental and behavioral disorders must become educated about indoor and outdoor environments and the potential sources of chronic and long-term chemical exposures that affect their patients.

Medical professionals can provide a tremendous service to improve public health by educating patients about how to reduce exposures to potentially harmful chemicals. Numerous professional societies have issued statements advocating for preventive measures even in the absence of scientifically established cause and effect (i.e., the *precautionary approach*). They include The Endocrine Society,[24,61] the American College of Obstetricians and Gynecologists,[3] the American Society for Reproductive Medicine,[3] and the International Federation of Gynecology and Obstetrics.[15] Health care professionals are encouraged to incorporate these recommendations into patient care practices for children and adults. In the face of uncertainty, preventive action should be the norm, and the medical community has a critical role to play in helping patients learn how to avoid unnecessary chemical exposure.

Acknowledgments

I am extremely grateful to the staff of TEDX, who work diligently every day to advance the scientific study and public awareness of environmental chemical exposure, and whose work was used extensively in this chapter; and to Kristina Thayer and Ashley Bolden for providing feedback on an earlier draft.

REFERENCES

1. Environmental Protection Agency. 2014. Emerging Contaminants—Perfluorooctane Sulfonate (PFOS) and Perfluorooctanoic Acid (PFOA). EPA 505-F-14-001.
2. Agency for Toxic Substances and Disease Registry. Lead Toxicity. http://www.atsdr.cdc.gov/csem/csem.asp?csem=7&po=10.
3. American College of Obstetricians and Gynecologists. 2013. Exposure to toxic environmental agents. *Fertil Steril.* 100:931–934.
4. Barrett, J.R. 2009. Endocrine disruption: Developmental picture window. *Environ Health Perspect.* 117:A101.

5. Bertazzi, P.A., Bernucci, I., Brambilla, G., Consonni, D., & Pesatori, A.C. 1998. The Seveso studies on early and long-term effects of dioxin exposure: A review. *Environ Health Perspect.* 106:625–633.

6. Bolden, A.L., Kwiatkowski, C.F., & Colborn, T. 2015. New look at BTEX: Are ambient levels a problem? *Environ Sci Technol* 49:5261–5276.

7. Calafat, A.M., Ye, X., Wong, L.Y., Reidy, J.A., & Needham, L.L. 2008. Urinary concentrations of triclosan in the U.S. population: 2003-2004. *Environ Health Perspect.* 116:303–307.

8. Carson, R. 1962. *Silent Spring.* Boston, MA: Houghton Mifflin.

9. Casey, J.A., Savitz, D.A., Rasmussen, S.G., et al. 2016. Unconventional natural gas development and birth outcomes in Pennsylvania, USA. *Epidemiology.* 27:163–172.

10. Centers for Disease Control and Prevention. 2009. Fourth Report on Human Exposure to Environmental Chemicals. http://www.cdc.gov/exposurereport/.

11. Chronic Hazard Advisory Panel on Phthalates and Phthalate Alternatives. 2014. Final Report of the Chronic Hazard Advisory Panel on Phthalates and Phthalate Alternatives. https://www.cpsc.gov/PageFiles/169902/CHAP-REPORT-With-Appendices.pdf.

12. Colborn, T. 2006. A case for revisiting the safety of pesticides: A closer look at neurodevelopment. *Environ Health Perspect.* 114:10–17.

13. Crews, D., Gillette, R., Scarpino, S.V., Manikkam, M., Savenkova, M.I., & Skinner, M.K. 2012. Epigenetic transgenerational inheritance of altered stress responses. *Proc Natl Acad Sci U S A.* 109:9143–9148.

14. Cruz, G. Top 10 Environmental Disasters. http://content.time.com/time/specials/packages/article/0,28804,1986457_1986501_1986449,00.html.

15. Di Renzo, G.C., Conry, J.A., Blake, J., et al. 2015. International Federation of Gynecology and Obstetrics opinion on reproductive health impacts of exposure to toxic environmental chemicals. *Int J Gynaecol Obstet.* 131:219–225.

16. EDC-MixRisk. Effects of Mixtures of Endocrine Disruptive Chemicals. http://edcmixrisk.ki.se/aboutedcmixrisk/.

17. Ejaredar, M., Nyanza, E.C., Ten Eycke, K., & Dewey, D. 2015. Phthalate exposure and childrens neurodevelopment: A systematic review. *Environ Res.* 142:51–60.

18. Environmental Protection Agency. DDT–A Brief History and Status. http://www.epa.gov/ingredients-used-pesticide-products/ddt-brief-history-and-status.

19. Environmental Protection Agency. 2013. Chemical Data Reporting Under the Toxic Substances Control Act. http://epa.gov/cdr/pubs/guidance/2nd_CDR_snapshot 5_19_14.pdf.

20. Environmental Protection Agency. 2016. Registration Review of Chlorpyrifos. Docket ID EPA-HQ-OPP-2008-0850. https://archive.epa.gov/oppsrrd1/registration_review/web/html/index-299.html

21. Environmental Working Group. 2009. Pollution in People: Cord Blood Contaminants in Minority Newborns. http://static.ewg.org/reports/2009/minority_cord_blood/2009-Minority-Cord-Blood-Report.pdf?_ga=1.7967410.10135877 61.1439587253

22. Filer, D., Patisaul, H.B., Schug, T., Reif, D., & Thayer, K. 2014. Test driving ToxCast: Endocrine profiling for 1858 chemicals included in phase II. *Curr Opin Pharmacol.* 19:145–152.
23. Gee, R.H., Charles, A., Taylor, N., & Darbre, P.D. 2008. Oestrogenic and androgenic activity of triclosan in breast cancer cells. *J Appl Toxicol.* 28:78–91.
24. Gore, A.C., Chappell, V.A., Fenton, S.E., et al. 2015. EDC-2: The Endocrine Society's second scientific statement on endocrine-disrupting chemicals. *Endocr Rev.* 36:E1-E150.
25. Guillette, E.A., Meza, M.M., Aquilar, M.G., Soto, A.D., & Garcia, I.E. 1998. An anthropological approach to the evaluation of preschool children exposed to pesticides in Mexico. *Environ Health Perspect.* 106:347–353.
26. Guillette, L.J.J., Pickford, D.B., Crain, D.A., Rooney, A.A., & Percival, H.F. 1996. Reduction in penis size and plasma testosterone concentrations in juvenile alligators living in a contaminated environment. *Gen Comp Endocrinol.* 101:32–42.
27. Hanna-Attisha, M., LaChance, J., Sadler, R.C., & Champney Schnepp, A. 2015. Elevated blood lead levels in children associated with the Flint drinking water crisis: A spatial analysis of risk and public health response. *Am J Public Health.* 106:283–290.
28. Hauser, R., Meeker, J.D., Singh, N.P., et al. 2007. DNA damage in human sperm is related to urinary levels of phthalate monoester and oxidative metabolites. *Hum Reprod.* 22:688–695.
29. Herbstman, J.B., Sjodin, A., Kurzon, M., et al. 2009. Prenatal exposure to PBDEs and neurodevelopment. *Environ Health Perspect.* 118:712–719.
30. Iwanowicz, L.R., Blazer, V.S., Pinkney, A.E., et al. 2016. Evidence of estrogenic endocrine disruption in smallmouth and largemouth bass inhabiting Northeast U.S. national wildlife refuge waters: A reconnaissance study. *Ecotoxicol Environ Saf.* 124:50–59.
31. Kumar, V., Chakraborty, A., Kural, M.R., & Roy, P. 2009. Alteration of testicular steroidogenesis and histopathology of reproductive system in male rats treated with triclosan. *Reprod Toxicol.* 27:177–185.
32. Lam, J., Koustas, E., Sutton, P., et al. 2014. The Navigation Guide—evidence-based medicine meets environmental health: integration of animal and human evidence for PFOA effects on fetal growth. *Environ Health Perspect.* 122:1040–1051.
33. Mackenzie, C.A., Lockridge, A., & Keith, M. 2005. Declining sex ratio in a First Nation community. *Environ Health Perspect.* 113:1295–1298.
34. McKenzie, L.M., Witter, R.Z., Newman, L.S., & Adgate, J.L. 2012. Human health risk assessment of air emissions from development of unconventional natural gas resources. *Sci Total Environ.* 424:79–87.
35. Meeker, J.D., Johnson, P.I., Camann, D., & Hauser, R. 2009. Polybrominated diphenyl ether (PBDE) concentrations in house dust are related to hormone levels in men. *Sci Total Environ.* 407:3425–3429.
36. Patisaul, H.B., Roberts, S.C., Mabrey, N., et al. 2013. Accumulation and endocrine disrupting effects of the flame retardant mixture Firemaster(R) 550 in rats: An exploratory assessment. *J Biochem Mol Toxicol.* 27:124–136.

37. Paul, K.B., Hedge, J.M., Bansal, R., et al. 2012. Developmental triclosan exposure decreases maternal, fetal, and early neonatal thyroxine: A dynamic and kinetic evaluation of a putative mode-of-action. *Toxicology.* 300:31–45.

38. Peretz, J., Vrooman, L., Ricke, W.A., et al. 2014. Bisphenol A and reproductive health: update of experimental and human evidence, 2007-2013. *Environ Health Perspect.* 122:775–786.

39. Potter, T.L., & Simmons, K.E. (eds.). 1998. *Composition of Petroleum Mixtures,* vol. 2. Amherst, MA: Amherst Scientific Publishers.

40. Rochester, J.R. 2013. Bisphenol A and human health: A review of the literature. *Reprod Toxicol.* 42:132–155.

41. Rodriguez, P.E., & Sanchez, M.S. 2010. Maternal exposure to triclosan impairs thyroid homeostasis and female pubertal development in Wistar rat offspring. *J Toxicol Environ Health A.* 73:1678–1688.

42. Rooney, A.A., Boyles, A.L., Wolfe, M.S., Bucher, J.R., & Thayer, K.A. 2014. Systematic review and evidence integration for literature-based environmental health science assessments. *Environ Health Perspect.* 122:711–718.

43. Roze, E., Meijer, L., Bakker, A., Van Braeckel, K.N., Sauer, P.J., & Bos, A.F. 2009. Prenatal exposure to organohalogens, including brominated flame retardants, influences motor, cognitive, and behavioral performance at school age. *Environ Health Perspect.* 117:1953–1958.

44. Schug, T.T., Abagyan, R., Blumberg, B., et al. 2013. Designing endocrine disruption out of the next generation of chemicals. *Green Chem.* 15:181–198.

45. Shaw, S.D., Berger, M.L., Harris, J.H., et al. 2013. Persistent organic pollutants including polychlorinated and polybrominated dibenzo-*p*-dioxins and dibenzo-furans in firefighters from Northern California. *Chemosphere.* 91:1386–1394.

46. Singh, A.K., Tiwari, M.N., Upadhyay, G., et al. 2012. Long term exposure to cypermethrin induces nigrostriatal dopaminergic neurodegeneration in adult rats: Postnatal exposure enhances the susceptibility during adulthood. *Neurobiol Aging.* 33:404–415.

47. Stacy, S.L., Brink, L.L., Larkin, J.C., et al. 2015. Perinatal outcomes and unconventional natural gas operations in southwest Pennsylvania. *PLoS One.* 10:e0126425.

48. Stahlhut, R.W., van Wijngaarden, E., Dye, T.D., Cook, S., & Swan, S.H. 2007. Concentrations of urinary phthalate metabolites are associated with increased waist circumference and insulin resistance in adult U.S. males. *Environ Health Perspect.* 115:876–882.

49. Stoker, T.E., Gibson, E.K., & Zorrilla, L.M. 2010. Triclosan exposure modulates estrogen-dependent responses in the female Wistar rat. *Toxicol Sci.* 117:45–53.

50. Swan, S.H. 2008. Environmental phthalate exposure in relation to reproductive outcomes and other health endpoints in humans. *Environ Res.* 108:177–184.

51. ten Tusscher, G.W., & Koppe, J.G. 2004. Perinatal dioxin exposure and later effects. A review. *Chemosphere.* 54:1329–1336.

52. The Endocrine Disruption Exchange. http://endocrinedisruption.org/prenatal-origins-of-endocrine-disruption/critical-windows-of-development/timeline-test/.

53. Thiruchelvam, M., McCormack, A., Richfield, E.K., et al. 2003. Age-related irreversible progressive nigrostriatal dopaminergic neurotoxicity in the paraquat and maneb model of the Parkinson's disease phenotype. *Eur J Neurosci.* 18:589–600.

54. Thornton, J.W., McCally, M., & Houlihan, J. 2002. Biomonitoring of industrial pollutants: Health and policy implications of the chemical body burden. *Public Health Rep.* 117:315–323.

55. Vandenberg, L.N., Colborn, T., Hayes, T.B., et al. 2012. Hormones and endocrine-disrupting chemicals: Low-dose effects and nonmonotonic dose responses. *Endocr Rev.* 33:378–455.

56. Vandenberg, L.N., Ehrlich, S., Belcher, S.M., et al. 2013. Low dose effects of bisphenol A. *Endocr Disruptors.* 1:e26490.

57. Vested, A., Ramlau-Hansen, C.H., Olsen, S.F., et al. 2013. Associations of in utero exposure to perfluorinated alkyl acids with human semen quality and reproductive hormones in adult men. *Environ Health Perspect.* 121:453–458.

58. Vinken, M. 2013. The adverse outcome pathway concept: A pragmatic tool in toxicology. *Toxicology.* 312:158–165.

59. vom Saal, F.S., Akingbemi, B.T., Belcher, S.M., et al. 2007. Chapel Hill Bisphenol A Expert Panel consensus statement: Integration of mechanisms, effects in animals and potential to impact human health at current levels of exposure. *Reprod Toxicol.* 24:131–138.

60. Vrijheid, M., Slama, R., Robinson, O., et al. 2014. The human early-life exposome (HELIX): Project rationale and design. *Environ Health Perspect.* 122:535–544.

61. Zoeller, R.T., Brown, T.R., Doan, L.L., et al. 2012. Endocrine-disrupting chemicals and public health protection: A statement of principles from The Endocrine Society. *Endocrinology.* 153:4097–4110.

62. Zota, A.R., Rudel, R.A., Morello-Frosch, R.A., & Brody, J.G. 2008. Elevated house dust and serum concentrations of PBDEs in California: unintended consequences of furniture flammability standards? *Environ Sci Technol.* 42:8158–8164.

2

The Plastic Age: Worldwide Contamination, Sources of Exposure, and Human Health Consequences

CHARLES MOORE AND SARAH S. MOSKO

Key Concepts

- We live in the plastic age, but most people are ignorant about the material that they use most in their daily lives.
- Manufacturers of plastic products divorce themselves from the issue of recovery of the material after its useful life, which can be as brief as a few minutes, resulting in vagrant plastic waste.
- Plastics often are made from harmful chemicals, a percentage of which are still free monomers after polymerization. Many chemicals are added to convert plastic resin feedstocks into useful products and can leach into the things they contact.
- All shapes, sizes, and colors of plastic debris have amassed in the world's oceans, where they adsorb and absorb harmful chemicals from seawater due to their lipophilic and hydrophobic qualities, providing a vehicle for the entry of toxic chemicals into the ocean food web.
- Increasing numbers of animal studies in the past decade have documented developmental derailments, including endocrine disruption and cancers, that are attributable to fetal and postnatal exposure to certain plastic monomers (e.g., bisphenol A, styrene) and plastic additives (e.g., phthalates, brominated flame retardants) at environmentally relevant doses.
- Human studies have revealed that fetuses and infants are exposed to an alarming number of industrial chemicals in utero and through breast milk and that some of these chemicals are associated with ubiquitous plastics.
- The list of human health problems that correlate with exposure to chemicals in plastics reads like a catalog of modern Western diseases.

Introduction

Natural polymers are molecules formed with repeating constituent units; examples include lignin, rubber, and silk. Although they are abundant, most of nature's natural plastics have not been implicated in environmental or health issues, principally because they biodegrade rather than persist. The post-World War II (WWII) era has been increasingly dominated by man-made plastic materials designed to defeat oxidation and other natural decay processes by sealing them off from contact with the atmosphere.

During WWII, the warring nations were cut off from traditional supply routes for raw materials. This created an urgent need for increased production of important synthetic replacements that had been invented in the 1930s, such as nylon, polyvinyl chloride (PVC), and acrylic (polycarbonate). This mass-production technology served as an addition to the postwar economy of Keynesian consumerism and was ushered in with a *Life Magazine* article from August 1955, entitled "Throw Away Living." The article included the famous photo by Peter Stackpole of a nuclear family—mom, dad, and two kids—throwing disposable food service items into the air next to a trash can. It claimed that the modern housewife would soon be liberated from the chore of doing dishes; she would simply throw them away and buy more. In 1967, the father figure in the movie *The Graduate* famously exhorted the young protagonist, Benjamin Braddock (Dustin Hoffman), "There's a great future in plastics." This scene is often invoked by those concerned with plastic's dark side as an example of prophecy fulfilled but with unforeseen consequences.

We live in the plastic age, and about one half of the world's chemists are polymer chemists at some point in their careers.[1] Plastic is what we drive and sit on, wear, carpet our homes with, and use as part of the delivery system for most foods and virtually every other product we consume. The average consumer in the developed world contacts manufactured plastic polymers daily. As of 2014, annual plastic production and the weight of the entire human population were about equal at 311 million metric tons.[10] An average person in the developed world consumes his or her weight in a variety of plastic products every year.

Between 1960 and 2000, the world production of plastic resins increased 25-fold, but recovery of the material remained below 5%[31] (Fig. 2.1). Glass, metal, and paper are recovered and recycled at much higher rates than plastic. Only senior citizens remember a world not dominated by plastics. For such a major economic player, the plastic industry has largely been off the radar screen of environmental regulation and even critical thinking.

We have yet to draw back the "plastic curtain" and discuss the problem. This conversation is desperately needed on a global scale because less than a century after the introduction of plastic materials into world commerce, they have been found to be persistent polluters of most environmental niches. Numerous objects orbit the earth as space debris; the slopes of Mount Everest display much of the gear and consumables needed to reach the summit; and the bottom of the sea is the resting place for polyester fibers and other plastics that sink. The surface of the ocean teams with an estimated 18,000 plastic particles per square kilometer according to a panel of experts assembled by the United Nations.[50] Double this amount has been found in the surface waters of the Great Lakes in the United States.[11] According to a 2016 report by the Ellen MacArthur Foundation, there will be as much plastic in the ocean as fish by 2050.[10]

Plastic Polymers: Constituents and Characteristics

Modern synthetic polymers are mainly materials made from petroleum products that can be molded, cast, spun, or applied as a coating. Because synthetic plastics are largely nonbiodegradable or at best biodegrade very slowly, they tend to persist in natural environments.

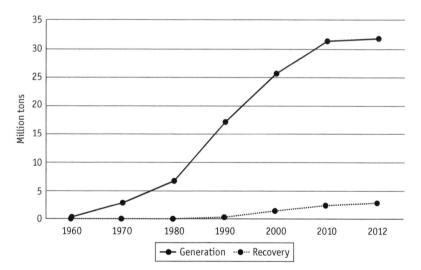

FIGURE 2.1. U.S. plastic waste generation from the municipal waste stream and recovery.
Data from the U.S. Environmental Protection Agency.

Thermoplastics are the main type of consumer plastics. They are formed by melting the raw material of solid plastic resin and forming it into products, which theoretically can be recovered and melted again. They are distinguished from *thermoset plastics*, which are liquids that are set (i.e., solidified) by the use of a catalyst. The solid forms (e.g., computer casings, synthetic rubber tires, fiberglass boats, surfboards) scorch rather than remelt when exposed to heat. Thermoset plastics, like thermoplastics, can break into small bits and persist in the environment. Although they are produced in less quantity than thermoplastics, thermoset plastics are recovered or recycled at an even lower rate.

Thermoplastics and thermoset plastics are mainly derived from petroleum and natural gas feedstocks, although they can be derived from coal.[2] Increasingly, renewable resources such as row crops (e.g., corn, soy, sugar cane) are being used. Among several factors, the price of the feedstock is the main determinant.

Plastics are the fastest growing component of waste, and vagrant plastics litter the landscape. Because the ocean is downhill from almost everywhere humans live, a key characteristic that makes plastic useful—its light weight—also allows inappropriately handled waste plastics to easily blow or run off into the sea, where they have become a major threat to the world's oceans. When exposed to the ultraviolet B (UVB) radiation in sunlight, the oxidative properties of the atmosphere, and the hydrolytic properties of seawater, synthetic polymers become brittle and break into smaller and smaller pieces, eventually becoming individual polymer molecules that must undergo further degradation before becoming bioavailable.[49]

The eventual biodegradation of plastics in the marine environment consumes an unknown amount of time, but estimates on the order of centuries have been made. However, because of the lack of experimental data, these estimates are only educated guesses (A.L. Andrady, personal communication). The idea that the evolution of plastic-eating bacteria can somehow deal with the waste is tempered by the fact, based on the fossil record, that the first natural polymer, lignin, existed for 10 million years before bacteria evolved to degrade it (C. Calver, personal communication).

Slow biodegradation rates do not mean that plastic polymers and their additives are not bioactive. The process of polymerization of the monomers that form plastics is never 100% complete, and the remaining monomer building blocks of the polymer, along with residual catalysts, can migrate from the polymer matrix into compounds with which they come in contact. Many plastic polymers in commercial use have high concentrations of bioactive monomer additives, which leach out at faster or slower rates based on environmental conditions.

Concern about the body burden of synthetic chemicals is heightened by the fact that the trillions of plastic products produced and consumed every year each contain the plastic manufacturer's chemical suite of additives based on the qualities needed for a specific product. Many of these additives do not strongly bond with the polymer and leach out on contact with foods or the human body. In the marine environment, polycarbonate plastics, when exposed to the salts in seawater near pH 8, show accelerated leaching of the bioactive bisphenol A monomer.[41,46]

The largest market sector for plastic resins is plastic packaging. These materials are designed for immediate disposal,[19] earning the *throw-away society* descriptor in the modern era. The quantity of plastic waste improperly disposed of each year worldwide by population centers with an ocean coastline has been estimated at 31.9 million metric tons (Fig. 2.2).

The consequences of not recovering waste plastics have been observed most extensively in the ocean, which receives an average of 8 million tons per year.[19] A paper by Gall and Thompson in 2015 found that "340 original publications reported encounters between marine debris and 693 species. Plastic debris accounted for 92% of encounters between debris and individuals. Numerous direct and indirect consequences were recorded, with the potential for sublethal effects of ingestion, an area of considerable uncertainty and concern."[12]

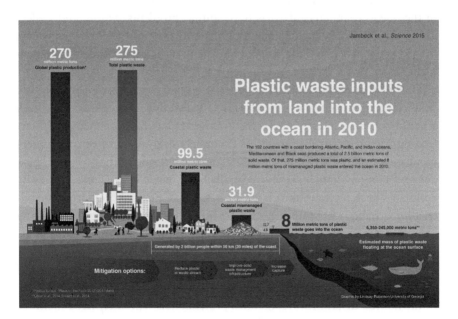

FIGURE 2.2. Plastic waste inputs from the land into the ocean in 2010. Data from Jambeck, J.R., Geyer R, Wilcox C, et al. 2015. Plastic waste inputs from land into the ocean. *Science.* 347:768–771.

Entanglement in the debris is also a serious issue, with an estimated 100,000 marine mammals dying each year entrapped in plastic trash.[58]

Because human activity influences essential planetary systems, it is important to understand certain basic facts about the earth. Although the earth's two poles are very cold, the southern and northern hemispheres both have deserts that are very hot. The earth's surface has twice as much ocean as land, and 40% of the ocean consists of depauperate areas centered in ocean basins known as subtropical gyres.[34] They are poor in fish resources and are not on major shipping routes.

In 2001, Moore and colleagues[33] published the first study showing that plastics in the ocean tended to accumulate in a subtropical gyre in the central North Pacific. Since then, all five subtropical gyres, which are located similar to the major terrestrial deserts at between 20 and 40 degrees latitude north and south of the equator, have been found to accumulate floating plastics.[11]

Gyre is a Greek word that means "to turn," and each gyre's circular current has a distinct period of rotation.[10] As these regions accumulate the plastic detritus of civilization over time, the materials become brittle.[3] The plastic breaks into tiny particles, and they begin to compete with the sparse planktonic life forms there. In the North Pacific, such particles have been found to outweigh the associated zooplankton near the surface by a factor of 6 to 1.

Although the gyres contain the highest levels of plastic waste pollution in the open ocean, coastal areas have similar problems. Moore and Zellers found that ratios of plastic to plankton in Southern California coastal waters ranged between 1.4 to 1 and 2.5 to 1, and some individual samples had much higher levels.[25]

One form of plastic found in all oceans is fibers, which are derived mostly from clothing, woven lines, and fabrics.[4] The fact that coastal areas have high amounts of small plastic fibers and fragments has consequences for filter-feeding organisms in these areas. For example, a study of European consumers of mussels and oysters found that they might eat 11,000 of these plastic fibers per year along with their shellfish.[5] Small plastic particles can concentrate oily pollutants such as polychlorinated biphenyls (PCBs) and dichlorodiphenyl-trichloroethane (DDT) up to 1 million times their level in the surrounding seawater.[27] Consumption of these plastic particles by fish transfers the pollutants to their tissues and has been shown to cause pathologic changes to their livers, including cancer.[39] Areas as distant from one another as Indonesia and California have been found to be selling fish with plastic in their stomachs.[40] In the not too distant future, medical professionals will likely need methods for assessing the plastic load in their patients.

DIFFICULTY OF RECYCLING AND PROPER DISPOSAL

Given the ominous proliferation of plastic in the biosphere and beyond, why are more plastics not recovered for reuse and recycling? The principal reason is that the cost to recover, clean, and reprocess used plastics exceeds in most cases the cost of virgin plastic resin. When melted together, mixed plastic resin types are essentially without value to manufacturers who need to chemically tailor a plastic's characteristics for a given application. Even formulas for the same generic polymer are different enough to cause similar problems.

Plastics are hydrophobic or lipophilic molecules that readily adsorb or absorb oily contaminants that are not easily washed off. Plastics melt at low temperatures that fail to oxidize these contaminants during production of new plastic feedstocks. For this reason, recycled plastics cannot be used in food-contact applications, which would require an expensive process of lining a recycled plastic container with a protective layer of virgin plastic. Furthermore, almost all plastic products fashioned from recovered waste plastics require a significant percentage of virgin resin to meet specification requirements. Only crude, artisanal construction components (e.g., building blocks) and often-impressive works of art are made entirely with plastic recovered from the environment. Nevertheless, these efforts are often successful in recycling at least some plastic waste and raising public awareness about the problem of plastic pollution.

All of these challenges to recycling are compounded by the proliferation of new polymers, which are patented at the rate of 15 per week in the United States alone.[32] The only plastics that have a large enough production and reuse market to be profitably recyclable in a widespread way are #1 polyethylene terephthalate (PET) and #2 high-density polyethylene (HDPE). Even these items may need subsidies by government or industry to be profitable. State bottle bills that require a deposit are one example. The lack of takeback infrastructure for unprofitable plastics is a contributing factor in the proliferation of plastic waste in the environment (see Fig.2.1).

The sad state of plastics recycling stands in sharp contrast to inherent promises by the American Chemistry Council in its flagship public relations program entitled Responsible Care Guiding Principles. The principles were proposed "to design and develop products that can be manufactured, transported, used, and disposed of or recycled safely" and "to promote pollution prevention, minimization of waste, and conservation of energy and other critical resources at every stage of the life cycle of products."

Feasibility of Cleanup Schemes. Because of vagrant plastic's visibility, solidity, and light weight, the impulse to pick it up for proper disposal is widespread. Since the Ocean Conservancy started its annual International Coastal Cleanup in 1986, beach cleanups in coastal communities have become routine throughout the year. From the Boy Scouts to the Surfrider Foundation, regular beach cleanups have become a way of life. Most of these beaches are sandy, not rocky. Removing plastic objects lodged in rocks is difficult and dangerous.

Cleanup of ocean plastics is even more problematic. Beaches act like sieves, filtering out plastics from the ocean and leaving them on a relatively narrow space. In the ocean, plastics are disbursed, and although there are accumulation zones, the five major gyre areas have a huge spatial extent—approximately 145 million square kilometers.[32] These areas lie outside the exclusive economic zone of any country, creating a disincentive to expend scarce resources on open ocean cleanup. Only floating plastics accumulate there. Heavier plastics sink to the bottom, and neutrally buoyant plastics travel in slabs of ocean water that serpentine throughout the water column.[9]

Even if ambitious schemes to clean up plastic waste from the ocean were to materialize and capture large quantities, the average input of 8 million tons per year would cancel the effort. For a clinical perspective, consider the frustration in treating a diabetic whose diet consists of sugary sodas and doughnuts. Preventing the disease from progressing would be challenging. Solutions to the plague of plastic waste in the ocean lie not in high-tech cleanup methods but in drastic reduction of the many sources. For the ocean, prevention is the answer because cure is impossible. Movements are legion to reduce problem plastics (e.g., bags, cups, straws) through legislation and consumer pressure. Redesigns to eliminate throw-away plastics also are an important part of the solution. In the most extreme formulation of the problem of ocean plastic pollution, one might say that we are turning a liquid into a solid.

RISKY CHEMICALS INTRINSIC TO PLASTICS

Toothbrushes, medical tubing, bicycles, eyeglasses, food packaging, car upholstery, garden hoses, and electronics casings are just a small sample of products created out of synthetic plastics. Given their endless applications, plastic materials appear nothing short of marvelous. However, a grasp of the complicated chemistry that makes these applications possible reveals a rarely mentioned dark underbelly of potential health threats to humans and wildlife.

Storing spaghetti sauce in some plastic containers or brewing tea in expanded polystyrene cups can leave stains not easily removed with soap and water. This suggests that plastics are more permeable materials than glass and metals. However, from a health perspective, it is the substances that migrate out of plastics that merit concern. The foundation polymer used and the plethora of additives that imbue plastics with diverse properties are potential sources of chemical migrants.

For the purpose of this overview, only the more troubling known migrants and their better-documented health effects are discussed. The volume of research in this area is growing exponentially, with new revelations of worrisome effects every year. This adds to the urgency to fully understand how plastics threaten health, coupled with the staggering and continually escalating quantity of plastic materials being manufactured and the degree to which humans in industrialized societies interact intimately with plastics all day long.

Plastic Monomers. Thousands of monomer molecules are linked together to produce a single giant molecule of synthetic plastic polymer. However, unlike most other chemicals with a definite structure and molecular weight, plastic monomers can link up at various sites and orientations so that the resulting polymer molecules are not uniform in structure or molecular weight. The polymerization process is never complete, leaving individual monomers chemically unbonded and free to migrate into whatever the plastic contacts. There is also the potential for polymers to release monomers as the material ages, and the health safety of the monomers therefore comes into question.

Three plastics in particular have been singled out because of the toxicity of their monomers: polycarbonates, PVC, and polystyrene. The monomers of all three are ranked among the highest-volume chemicals produced worldwide. Each is produced in billions of pounds annually.

Bisphenol A. Probably no single plastic constituent has been studied as extensively or generated as much debate among scientists, industry, and regulatory agencies as bisphenol A (BPA), the key monomer in the synthesis of polycarbonate plastics (including food packaging) and the resin lining of many food and beverage cans and water pipes. Although BPA was never used as a drug, it was once considered for use as a synthetic estrogen. This came well before the discovery that reacting BPA with phosgene (i.e., chemical warfare gas used in WWII) created polycarbonate, a clear material that is so shatter-proof that is used as windshield material in aircraft. This welcome finding led to widespread use of polycarbonates in common nonbreakable items such as baby bottles, sippy cups, 5-gallon water bottles, dinnerware, medical devices, eyeglass lenses, CDs, and DVDs.

BPA's high production volume, estrogen mimicry, and widespread infant exposure triggered an avalanche of research, starting with the 1997 publication of a ground-breaking finding by developmental biologist Frederick vom Saal (an editor of this textbook). He discovered that feeding very low doses of BPA to pregnant mice produced prostate enlargement in male offspring.[35,55] Since then, industry-funded studies have consistently reported no harm to laboratory animals exposed to low levels early in life, in sharp contrast to most independently funded studies reporting permanent harm to many developmental health end points.[53] That BPA is also widely used in thermal paper receipts, where it is free (i.e., nonpolymerized) and directly adsorbed dermally during handling,[17] has intensified concerns about the risks of exposure in adults. As a result, the European Union has banned the use of BPA in thermal paper.

The National Institute of Environmental Health Sciences defines endocrine disruptors (EDs) as chemicals that "may interfere with the body's endocrine system and produce adverse developmental, reproductive, neurologic, and immune effects in humans and wildlife." Like natural hormones, EDs can act at receptors in the cell membrane and cytosol, where they affect protein synthesis, or in the cell nucleus, where they directly affect gene activity. Some EDs act as hormone mimics, whereas others affect the production, metabolism, uptake, or release of hormones (see Chapter 12). BPA's affinity for nuclear estrogen receptors is weaker than that of 17β-estradiol, but it is equipotent at nonnuclear estrogen receptors.

Unraveling the ED properties of BPA has helped overturn two traditional notions in toxicology: that the dose makes the poison and that the relationship between dose and toxicity is monotonic. It is now known that the response to low-dose (physiologic) exposure cannot be predicted by what happens at high (toxicologic) doses, and detrimental effects seen at low doses can be absent at high doses. Low-dose exposure effects are seen in the picomolar and nanomolar ranges at which natural hormones are active. Hormonal systems are designed so that even modest changes in hormone concentrations within the low-dose range can trigger significant biologic effects.[52]

BPA was among the EDs selected by The Endocrine Society in a detailed 2012 explanation of how EDs exploit these sensitively engineered hormone systems. In essence, BPA and some similar molecules derail normal cellular function, organ development, and behaviors, especially during the fetal and neonatal periods, which are specifically sensitive to chemicals that alter endocrine signaling.[52,60] Consequently, exposure levels that have profound effects at critical points in early development can have negligible impacts in exposed adults.

In addition to binding the nuclear and membrane estrogen receptors, BPA binds to the thyroid hormone and androgen receptors. This likely explains its many affected end points in animal studies, which include effects on the prostate, mammary gland, brain development, behavior, reproduction, immune system, cardiovascular system, and metabolism. In less than 2 decades, there have been hundreds of laboratory studies, and a complete review of all the reports of harm is not possible here.[53] However, the changes seen in mammary gland histology and the rise in mammary cancer incidence are viewed as conclusive effects of BPA, and there is ample evidence that the development of the prostate gland also is affected by fetal or perinatal low-dose exposure.[44] Additional impacts of early exposure include aneuploidy in oocytes during meiosis, changes in sexually dimorphic regions of the brain and behaviors, and alterations in social behaviors, learning, and maternal-neonatal interactions. In numerous studies of vertebrates and invertebrates, harm from BPA occurred at exposures below the safe dose level of 50 µg/kg/day established by the Environmental Protection Agency (EPA).[53,56]

BPA's effects can be multigenerational, as first demonstrated in female mice exposed during fetal life that later produced aneuploid eggs and embryos.[48] Although BPA usually is discussed as an ED, arguments are made for additional classification as a human carcinogen based on the increased susceptibility to mammary and prostate cancers after early-life exposure of rodents at levels below the EPA's oral reference dose.[44]

The National Toxicology Program's 2008 assessment (NTP-CERHR Monograph on the Potential Human Reproductive and Developmental Effects of Bisphenol A, Sept. 2008, NIH Publication No. 08-5994, p. vii) of BPA safety concluded that there were "*some concerns* for effects on the brain, behavior, and prostate gland in fetuses, infants, and children"; only "*minimal concern* for effects on the mammary gland and an earlier age for puberty for females in fetuses, infants, and children"; and "*negligible concern* that exposure of pregnant women to bisphenol A will result in fetal or neonatal mortality, birth defects, or reduced birth weight and growth in their offspring." However, in testing for hazards posed by chemicals, regulatory agencies use intragastric gavage as the default approach, and less than 1% of BPA administered by this route is bioavailable in the blood. Much higher serum levels are reached when BPA exposure is dermal or sublingual, routes that bypass first-pass metabolism by the liver.[54]

The key findings of the hazardous health effects of BPA have been rejected by regulatory agencies; the claim is that the high levels of bioactive (unconjugated) serum BPA measured in human biomonitoring studies must be attributed to assay contamination because BPA is rapidly converted to inactive metabolites. In response, leading BPA researchers have provided convincing evidence that continuous exposure to BPA from multiple sources, not assay contamination, explains the alarmingly high levels measured in humans.[57]

There also is evidence that the fetus' immature BPA metabolic pathway effectively amplifies the impact of a given exposure level.[13] Regulatory agency assessments of BPA's toxicity are seriously out of date (see Chapter 12).

Under the U.S. Food and Drug Administration (FDA), BPA is regulated as a food additive because of the potential for migration into foodstuffs from packaging (see Chapter 11). The FDA's 2014 assessment (http://www.fda.gov/NewsEvents/PublicHealthFocus/ucm064437.htm) concluded that "BPA is safe at the current levels occurring in foods." However, the FDA disallowed polycarbonate baby bottles and sippy cups in 2012 and the use of BPA-based epoxy resins for lining infant formula containers in 2013, ostensibly because industry had already abandoned these uses in response to pressure from consumers—an example of what can be called *leading from behind*.

The European Union, Canada, and China are among the countries with similar restrictions placed on BPA, whereas in France, BPA is banned for use in food-contact materials. A new concern, however, is the industry's movement to replace BPA with the closely related compounds bisphenol S and bisphenol F, both of which are potent EDs with actions similar to BPA in vitro and in vivo.[38]

Vinyl Chloride. PVC is sometimes called the *poison plastic* because of toxicities associated with all stages of its life cycle, starting with synthesis. Its vinyl chloride monomer is made from chlorine and ethylene, and it is a highly flammable and explosive gas. By far, the number one use of vinyl chloride is in producing PVC polymer for plastics such as shower curtains, window frames, house sidings, household plumbing, garden hoses, medical tubing, carpeting, vinyl flooring, upholstery, school lunch boxes, and backpacks.

Many studies dating back as far as the 1930s demonstrated that even short-term exposure to vinyl chloride in laboratory animals and factory workers caused liver damage, and by the early 1970s, studies linking rare hepatic tumors (i.e., angiosarcomas) to chronic workplace exposure by inhalation or dermal contact had the attention of industry and governments.[22] Worldwide, air pollution in communities around factories using vinyl chloride also became an issue.

Recognition of vinyl chloride as an occupational carcinogen led to reductions but not elimination of residual monomer in PVC plastics as early as 1976. Because the FDA later reined in the use of PVC packaging and films in foodstuffs, there is a lower risk today of ingestion from foods. However, swallowing or inhalation of dust emitted from and direct dermal contact with the innumerable consumer products made of PVC remain routes of exposure.

The National Toxicology Program listed vinyl chloride as a known human carcinogen in 1980. In addition to the liver, other tissues in which cancers can appear after vinyl chloride exposure include the brain, lung, and lymphatic and hematopoietic systems.

Styrene. The styrene monomer is the building block of polystyrene plastics. The International Agency for Research on Cancer (IARC) has determined that styrene is a possible carcinogen, and the National Toxicology Program classifies styrene as "reasonably anticipated to be a human carcinogen." The State of California regulates styrene as a carcinogen under the Proposition 65 law. The major metabolite of styrene, styrene-7,8-oxide, is similarly listed and is thought to be responsible for the genotoxic effects of styrene.

Studies in mice exposed to styrene by inhalation or ingestion indicate that it causes cancers of the lung. Evidence of carcinogenicity in humans is more limited and is based primarily on increased lymphohematopoietic system cancers (e.g., leukemia, lymphoma) and DNA damage in circulating white blood cells in occupationally exposed workers. However, the central nervous system is deemed the most sensitive target of styrene toxicity in humans, with chronic occupational exposure causing tiredness, feeling drunk, slowed reaction time, and impaired concentration, balance, and color vision.[3]

Inhalation is the major route of occupational exposure, although styrene is readily absorbed and distributed throughout the body and concentrated especially in adipose tissue, whether encountered by inhalation, ingestion, or dermal contact. For the general public, breathing indoor air and ingestion of styrene migrants in foods and beverages packaged or served in polystyrene are the primary routes of exposure. Several studies have documented styrene contamination of hot beverages (e.g., tea, milk, coffee) served in crystal or foamed polystyrene cups and in water bottled in polystyrene, with increasing contamination as beverage temperature, fat content, and time in the container increase.[23]

ADDITIVES TO PLASTIC POLYMERS

The categorical list of allowed additives is alarming and includes catalyzers, hardeners, strengtheners, softeners, flame retardants, lubricants, antioxidants, colorants, texturizers, stabilizers, UV protectors, and blowing or foaming agents. There are multiple options within each category. Additives can account for more than one half of the mass of a product, and the number of additives in a finished product can easily be in the double digits. All of these are unknown to the consumer because the ingredients are deemed proprietary (see Chapter 12).

Some products, such as baby bottles with a nipple, ring, bottle, and cap, have many plastic parts, multiplying the number of additives present. Unlike a plastic's monomers, the additives are not chemically bonded to the polymer; they are simply mixed in and therefore are free to migrate out, depending on conditions the product encounters. Heating, freezing, acidity, microwaving, dishwashing, UV radiation, storage duration, and impact stress are conditions that can promote leaching of additives.

The following discussion focuses on two high-production-volume additives associated with health hazards: phthalate plasticizers and polybrominated diphenyl ether (PBDE) flame retardants.

Phthalates. Phthalates are a family of esters of phthalic acid used as softeners primarily in PVC plastics. They allow the polymer molecules to slide along one another. By weight, they can comprise one half or more of the final product. Common consumer items containing phthalates include food containers and wrappers, shower curtains, raincoats, floor tiles, rubbery or squishy toys (e.g., rubber ducky), vinyl upholstery, and car interior or dash components (e.g., "new car smell"). Plastic medical devices such as infusion bags and tubing often derive their flexibility from phthalates, a concern for adults undergoing hemodialysis and in neonatal intensive care units where exposure can be continuous for extended periods.[59] Phthalates are also used as plastic stabilizers, as in PVC machinery used in food processing, another dietary exposure route. Innumerable nonplastic items also contain phthalates, including nail polish, perfume, body lotions, adhesives, and enteric coatings of pills.

Phthalates are not thought to persist long in the environment after they are released from plastic waste, but because they are ubiquitous in manufactured products (i.e., billions of pounds per year), people are exposed continuously through ingestion, inhalation of contaminated dust or air, and dermal contact. Dermal uptake directly from volatilized phthalates also has been documented, illustrating that the skin is no guaranteed barrier to airborne pollutants.

At least eight common phthalates are thought to have antiandrogenic effects. They are rapidly metabolized to more stable monoester metabolites, and the latter are measured to assess tissue exposure levels. The monoesters have a half-life in humans of roughly 12 hours, and some are thought to be more toxic than their parent phthalates.

Phthalates are antiandrogenic EDs that act by disruption of androgen biosynthesis rather than blocking the androgen receptor.[18] To do this, they interfere with messenger RNA (mRNA) expression of key enzymes in androgen synthesis and the peptide hormone insulin-like peptide 3 (INSL3) from fetal Leydig cells. Any tissues targeted by androgen and INLS3 can be affected, but especially testicular Leydig cells. Early-life exposure of male rodents has identified a *phthalate syndrome,* with many features of andro-gen deficiency and feminization of male reproductive development; these include reduced testosterone production; decreased sperm counts; mal-formations of the epididymis, seminal vesicles, vas deferens, and prostate; and hypospadias, cryptorchidism, nipple or areola retention, and a reduced anogenital distance indicative of demasculinization of the perineum. Individuals are most vulnerable to phthalate syndrome in the fetal period, followed in decreasing order by the neonatal period, puberty, and adult-hood, in which testicular toxicity occurs only after exposure to much higher levels than those that cause permanent reproductive tract abnormalities after in utero exposure.[51]

Phthalates are also known obesogens in animal models. Exposure in utero, in the newborn period, or in adulthood causes weight gain with an increased number and size of adipocytes.[16]

Because of the clear-cut antivirilizing effect of early-life exposure in rodents and an emerging literature documenting similar effects in humans, the U.S. Congress, in 2008, placed permanent bans on three phthalates—di-2-ethylhexyl phthalate (DEHP), dibutyl phthalate (DBP), and benzyl butyl phthalate (BBP)—and an interim ban on three others—di-isononyl phthalate (DINP), di-isodecyl phthalate (DIDP), and di-n-octyl phthalate (DnOP)—in child care items designed for children 3 years of age or younger that can be placed in a child's mouth, including toys, baby bottles, sippy cups, sucking aids, and teethers. The permanent ban is most restrictive because it applies to children's toys. Similar bans on the same phthalates were enacted 3 years earlier in the European Union. Manufacturers of child care items are free to use any other phthalates or substitute plasticizers they deem safe, based on industry's internal assessment of safety.

Polybrominated Diphenyl Ethers. PBDEs arose as a replacement for the legacy pollutants PCBs. They are a family of flame retardants widely used in products such as upholstery, textiles, bedding, televisions, and electronic appliances for which flammability is an issue. There are more than 200 individual congeners, and those with fewer bromines off the phenyl ring (i.e., mono through penta forms) are considered more hazardous to humans.

PBDEs have been marketed as three commercial mixtures: penta-BDE, octa-BDE, and deca-BDE, although production of the penta and octa forms was halted in the United States and the European Union after they were shown to be lipophilic, persistent, bioaccumulative, toxic to humans and the environment, and capable of long-range atmospheric transport. Commercial deca-BDE production continues, and the chemical is prevalent in many con-sumer products, along with many congeners of PBDEs.[20]

Because they are not chemically bonded in plastics, PBDEs migrate into air and dust and are a worldwide environmental contaminant. PBDE levels are especially high in offices because of computers and other electronic devices. Whereas indoor air and diet are thought to be main routes of exposure for most adults, dust may be more important for toddlers because of greater hand-to-mouth activity (see Chapter 4).

Like PCBs, PBDEs are structurally similar to the thyroid hormone thyroxine (T_4), and laboratory studies have found thyroid-disrupting effects attributable to PBDEs. For example, the hydroxylated metabolites of PBDEs are potent competitors for T_4 binding to two human thyroid hormone–binding transport proteins in plasma; they thereby accelerate T_4 clearance and lower serum T_4 levels.[26,28] Prenatal or postnatal exposure in rodents to levels similar to those seen in more highly exposed human infants causes lasting changes in locomotor activity and performance on tests of learning and memory. It remains uncertain the extent to which these developmental neurotoxic effects on the brain are mediated indirectly by the reduction in circulating T_4 or directly by effects on the developing brain. The latter mechanism was suggested by in vitro and in vivo findings of oxidative stress (i.e., DNA damage and apoptotic cell death) in several brain cell types exposed to PBDEs.[7,8]

A PANDORA'S BOX OF OTHER ADDITIVES

The list of *intentional* plastic additives for which there is evidence of negative health effects is not limited to phthalates and PBDEs. Even BPA is sometimes used as a plasticizer or polymerization inhibitor in nonpolycarbonate plastics. Organotins and nonylphenols are additional examples.

Organotins. A family of substances previously used for antifouling paints on marine vessels, organotins were banned for this purpose worldwide because of proven toxicity to marine life, such as imposex (i.e., imposition of male sex characteristics in females) in mollusks and bioaccumulation throughout the marine food web, including marine mammals. In mammals, organotins interfere with aromatase and other steroidogenic enzymes, resulting in either androgen deficiency or a hyperandrogenized state, depending on the dose and developmental stage of exposure. Exposed rodents of both sexes show signs of developmental and reproductive toxicity and disruption of metabolic homeostasis because of additional actions on nuclear receptors that promote adipogenesis and weight gain.[14,16] Some organotins are still allowed in food-contact plastics, including PVC, in which they act as heat and light stabilizers.

Possible risks to humans of chronic exposure include obesity, metabolic syndrome, and liver and kidney damage.

Nonylphenols. A family of estrogen mimics, nonylphenols, are used as antioxidants and stabilizers in some PVC and polystyrene plastics. They are also used in toilet paper as softeners. Adverse effects reported in laboratory animals include testicular abnormalities, inhibition of ovarian development, and reduced reproductive organ weights. Human research points to interference with both hormonal feedback during pregnancy and normal fetal growth.[6]

Other Additives. In addition to the intentional additives, there is no guarantee that any polymer plastic product is free of potentially hazardous chemicals implemented at various stages of manufacturing. Ethylbenzene, for example, is used to synthesize styrene and is listed by the IARC as a possible human carcinogen. A 2008 study documented leaching of ethylbenzene into water from polystyrene cups, with greater contamination as the water temperature rose.[42]

The heavy metal antimony, used as a catalyst in the polycondensation of PET plastics, is another example. Condiments, water, and other beverages are most commonly bottled in clear PET plastics, a polymer the plastics industry usually touts as free of ED activity. However, using multiple bioassay techniques for detecting estrogenic activity, researchers have obtained clear evidence that xenoestrogens leach from PET bottles into the water contents in several brands of bottled water, attributable to antimony and phthalates.[43] Antimony is rated as a possible human carcinogen by the IARC. Higher temperature and longer storage duration promote greater antimony contamination. Antimony migration from PET oven-proof trays (used for ready-to-eat foods) into the foods as a consequence of microwaving or conventional-oven cooking has also been reported.[15]

Another study reported that intermediate-reaction products contributed to 19 migrants measured from commercial amber-colored PET bottles such as those used in bottling pharmaceuticals.[24] These observations suggest a very disturbing likelihood that even plastic manufacturers cannot know all of the side products of the manufacturing process—polymerization, molding, blowing, added colors—that contaminate an end product.

Human Biomonitoring

Probably no revelations about the potential health hazards from plastics are more worrisome than the degrees to which umbilical cord blood and breast milk are contaminated by industrial chemicals, including several attributable to the plastics industry. A benchmark study released by the Environmental Working Group in 2005 demonstrated that the placenta is not the barrier to chemical pollutants it was once thought to be. Cord blood from 10 babies born in U.S. hospitals was found to contain on average 200 industrial chemicals and pollutants falling into nine chemical categories. Among them were PBDEs and byproducts of the production and incineration of PVC and other plastics.

Breast milk draws on fatty tissues for nutrients, transferring fat-soluble pollutants stored in a mother's body directly to her infant. PBDEs have been particularly singled out for the study of breast milk contamination because, like other lipophilic persistent organic pollutants, they bioaccumulate in fatty tissues for days to years. A Swedish study revealed a doubling of PBDEs in breast milk every 5 years from 1972 to 1997.[29] BPA is also commonly detected in breast milk and possibly universally in cord blood.[13,30] Along with vital nutrients needed for normal fetal and postnatal development, cord blood and breast milk can deliver brews of toxic chemicals to fetuses and babies when they are most vulnerable to derailed development (Fig. 2.3).

Ongoing biomonitoring programs assaying human tissues for contamination with hazardous industrial chemicals include the Human Toxome Project (a collaborative effort of the Environmental Working Group and Commonweal) and the National Biomonitoring Program (NBP), which is

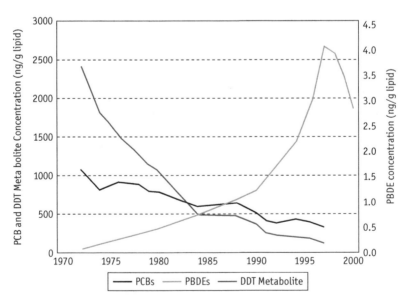

FIGURE 2.3. Trends in chemicals in breast milk in Sweden.
From the Natural Resources Defense Council (NRDC). IEM Book.

conducted through the Centers for Disease Control and Prevention (CDC). In the following sections, pertinent observations about human exposure to certain chemicals associated with plastics have been extracted primarily from summaries provided by the NBP.

The biomonitoring results available online impart only what the general population is exposed to and say nothing about the risks of such exposures. However, reference values for the general population should be useful to clinicians in assessing whether an individual has been exposed to unusually high levels of a chemical.

Antimony. Primary exposure is through food and, to a lesser extent, air and water. Dermal uptake also occurs. Urinary levels reflect recent exposure. Based on occupational exposure, the elimination half-life is about 95 hours.

Bisphenol A. BPA has a half-life in humans of about 6 hours. Most of 2517 people whose ages ranged from 6 years through adulthood who were tested exhibited BPA in their urine, indicating very recent universal exposure. Eating food and drinking water in plastic containers are important routes of exposure. Children, females, and lower-income people tend to exhibit higher urinary levels. In addition to breast milk and cord blood, BPA is detected in follicular and amniotic fluid, placental tissue, and fetal livers.

Ethylbenzene. Inhalation is a main route of exposure because ethylbenzene is ubiquitous in air due to its use in the synthesis of styrene and as a gasoline additive. It is also well absorbed through oral and dermal contact, which is relevant to its presence in polystyrene drink containers. Ethylbenzene is rapidly metabolized and is not known to bioaccumulate.

Polybrominated Diphenyl Ethers. PBDEs get into air, water, and soil during manufacture and persist in the environment. Because they bioaccumulate in fatty tissues, the dietary intake of fish, other fatty foods, and breast milk is a prime exposure route, as is intake of contaminated air and dust. U.S. residents have higher exposures than European residents by a factor of 3 to 10, with more than 60% of the U.S. population testing positive for at least one half of the 10 PBDEs measured by the NBP. In humans, the elimination half-life is several days to months, and blood levels reflect exposure over months to years. Blood levels in toddlers and children are typically several times those measured in adults.

Phthalates. Of the 13 phthalates measured in urine, many are widespread in the general population. Food and drink contamination from contact with phthalate-containing packaging is a prime exposure route, along with inhalation of phthalate vapors or contaminated dust and dermal contact. Women typically show greater exposure than men, and children likely have the greatest exposure because of more hand-to-mouth behaviors. Contaminated breast milk is an additional exposure route for infants. Phthalates do not accumulate in the body because they are rapidly converted to their monoester metabolites, some of which are thought to be responsible for the adverse outcomes attributable to phthalates.

In a nationally representative sample of the U.S. population (i.e., National Health and Nutrition Examination Survey [NHANES] 2003– 2004), all of the pregnant women sampled tested positive for at least one PBDE and four phthalates. The median number of PBDEs and phthalates detected were 6 and 9, respectively.[45] The levels of PBDEs and phthalates were similar to those reported in epidemiologic studies that found associations between prenatal exposure and adverse neurodevelopmental or reproductive outcomes.

Styrene. Because styrene is volatile, inhalation is a prime exposure route. Indoor air usually is more polluted than outdoor air because of the presence of photocopiers and other consumer products. Workplace exposure can produce blood levels 25 times greater than those in the general population. The highest levels are typically found in adipose tissues.[3] Styrene is rapidly metabolized by the liver (within hours).

Human biomonitoring is critical to gaining insight into how environmental chemicals affect health outcomes. However, our ability to track the environmental chemicals in our bodies is still far ahead of understanding the real risks they pose, singly or en masse, to humans at all life stages.

Human Health Studies

A survey of research findings of human health problems that correlate with exposure to chemicals associated with plastics reads like a catalog of modern Western diseases. However, epidemiologic studies are limited in their ability to assign causation to outcomes, and the fact that humans can be exposed to dozens, if not hundreds, of industrial chemicals every day adds to the challenge of deciphering the risks of exposure to any one chemical. This challenge is compounded when there are many chemically distinct members of a chemical family (e.g., phthalates) that do not have uniform physiologic effects.

Despite their limitations, epidemiologic study findings that are consistent with the research findings in laboratory animals can point to likely relationships between human exposures to chemicals and health outcomes. The largest bodies of human research have focused on BPA and phthalates, although human studies are still limited, with most conducted since the year 2000 and lag far behind the literature on laboratory animals. The more robust findings are listed in the following sections. They are largely based on cross-sectional studies in mostly nonoccupationally exposed populations and on spot sampling, which reveals only recent exposure to BPA or phthalates. However, there is evidence that spot sampling for these two chemicals can predict long-term exposure.

BISPHENOL A

Female Infertility. In women undergoing in vitro fertilization for infertility, higher urinary BPA levels have been associated with lower oocyte yield, fewer fertilized oocytes, and higher implantation failure.[37]

Male Sexual Function. Men exposed to BPA occupationally have lower self-reported sexual function (e.g., erectile function, orgasmic function, sexual desire) than controls in a dose-dependent manner, and the same may be true of men with normal environmental exposure.

Sperm Quality. Lower sperm quality (e.g., count, motility) is seen in men with higher urinary BPA levels from occupational or normal environmental exposure.

Sex Hormone Concentrations. Changes in endogenous concentrations of sex hormones (i.e., estrogens, androgens, and gonadotropins) and sex hormone–binding globulin in adults have been correlated with BPA exposure.

Polycystic Ovary Syndrome. Studies have consistently found higher BPA exposure in women with polycystic ovary syndrome, although it is not known whether adult or fetal exposure is more important.

Anogenital Distance. Boys of mothers occupationally exposed to BPA during pregnancy exhibit shorter anogenital distances in a dose-response relationship, suggesting antiandrogenic effects during embryonic development.

Altered Behavior and Neurodevelopment. Several longitudinal studies have found strong associations between in utero or early childhood BPA exposure and childhood behavior problems.

Type 2 Diabetes. Urinary BPA was positively correlated with insulin resistance and incidence of type 2 diabetes in both overweight or obese and normal-weight individuals in the large NHANES studies, which controlled for many demographic and other factors.

Cardiovascular Disease. Strong associations have been found in the NHANES studies between urinary BPA levels and both hypertension and cardiovascular disease (e.g., myocardial infarction, angina, coronary heart disease).

Obesity. Several studies, including multiple NHANES studies, have found a higher body mass index and waist circumference in children and adults with greater urinary BPA levels.

Other Effects. Human studies also link BPA to miscarriage, aneuploidy in the miscarried fetus, altered birth weight, childhood wheezing and asthma, altered liver and thyroid function, albuminuria, oxidative stress, inflammation, and altered epigenetic markers and gene expression, although the literature supporting these associations is limited and sometimes inconsistent.

PHTHALATES

Allergies, Wheezing, and Asthma. Rates of asthma and allergies have increased in recent decades. In developed parts of the world, people can spend 90% of their day indoors. Phthalates are suspected to act as allergens and adjuvants. PVC flooring and wall coverings, especially in the bedrooms of children and parents, have been associated with respiratory symptoms in younger children in many countries. Airway symptoms also correlated with certain phthalates (e.g., DEHP) in the child's bedroom dust (see Chapter 4).[21,36]

Androgen Levels. Phthalate exposure from breast milk has shown a positive correlation in newborn boys for sex hormone–binding globulin and luteinizing hormone (LH) levels as well as the ratio of LH to testosterone. A negative correlation with free testosterone levels was found.

Genital Development. Multiple studies in many cities have found reduced anogenital distance in boys (i.e., a measure of in utero androgen exposure) that was associated with prenatal exposure to several phthalates. Some studies also reported reduced penile dimension.

Semen Quality. An inverse relationship between phthalate exposure and sperm concentration and mobility has been reported in multiple studies of men visiting infertility clinics. Increasing exposure to phthalates has also been associated with sperm DNA damage as assessed by the neutral comet assay, which is used to measure double-strand breaks.

Gestational Age. A few studies have reported correlations between gestational age at birth and phthalate exposure, although the direction of correlation varies among phthalates.

Pubertal Gynecomastia and Premature Thelarche. Earlier onset of puberty in girls over the past few decades is a worldwide phenomenon. Elevated phthalate exposure has been reported in boys with pubertal gynecomastia and in girls with premature thelarche and other signs of precocious puberty, although the results are not consistent across all studies.

Children's Neurodevelopment. In several studies of children of various ages, phthalate exposure was associated with impairments in neurodevelopment, as reflected in poorer scores for conduct problems, attention or attention deficit hyperactivity disorder (ADHD), vocabulary, alertness in girls, and masculinity in boys. In neonates, alertness and orientation scores were inversely related to maternal urinary phthalate levels.

Thyroid Function in Children. Urinary phthalate levels were negatively correlated with serum levels of free and total triiodothyronine (T_3) and with height and weight in boys and girls. There also is evidence of interference with thyroid function in men and in pregnant women.

MEDICAL COMMUNITY AWAKENS TO RISKS OF ENVIRONMENTAL CHEMICALS

Obstetricians and pediatricians are uniquely positioned to inform parents about the potential risks to children of early-life exposure to environmental chemicals. Although pregnant women are routinely advised to avoid tobacco and alcohol, a nationwide survey of obstetricians found that fewer than 1 in 5 asked pregnant patients about exposure to environmental chemicals, and only 1 in 15 said they had received any training on taking an environmental health history.[47] Fewer than 1 in 10 obstetricians discussed their patients' exposure to BPA or phthalates, citing their own lack of knowledge among their reasons.

However, there are signs that health care professionals are beginning to view environmental factors as integral to preventive medicine.

The Federation of Gynecology and Obstetrics, whose members hail from 125 countries, released an opinion paper in 2015 stating that there was a threat to reproductive health from exposure to environmental chemicals during pregnancy and breastfeeding. They called on health professionals to advocate for policies to minimize these exposures. The Endocrine Society published its second scientific statement on EDs in 2015, which concluded there was strong scientific evidence linking EDs to obesity, diabetes, reproduction abnormalities, certain cancers, and disruptions in thyroid function and neurodevelopment. BPA, phthalates, and PBDEs were among the identified culprits. In 2015, the American Academy of Pediatrics signed a petition to the Consumer Products Safety Commission asking for a ban on PBDEs and related flame retardants in children's products, furniture, mattresses, and electronics casings.

REFERENCES

1. American Chemical Society. 2016. Polymer chemistry. https://www.acs.org/content/acs/en/careers/college-to-career/chemistry-careers/polymers.html.
2. Andrady, A.L. 2003. *Plastics and the Environment.* Hoboken, NJ: John Wiley & Sons.
3. Agency for Toxic Substances and Disease Registry, U.S. Department of Health and Human Services. 2010. Toxicological profile for styrene. http://www.atsdr.cdc.gov/toxprofiles/tp53.pdf.
4. Browne, M.A., Crump, P., Niven, S.J., Teuten, E., Galloway, T.S., & Thompson, R.C. 2011. Accumulation of microplastic on shorelines worldwide: Sources and sinks. *Environ Sci Technol* 45:9175–9179.
5. Cauwenberghe, L. & Janssen, C. 2014. Microplastics in bivalves cultured for human consumption. *Environ Pollut* 193:65–70.
6. Chang, C.H., Tsai, M.S., Lin, C.L., et al. 2014. The association between nonylphenols and sexual hormones levels among pregnant women: A cohort study in Taiwan. *PLoS One* 9:e104245.
7. Costa, L., & Giordano, G. 2007. Developmental neurotoxicity of polybrominated diphenyl ether (PBDE) flame retardants. *Neurotoxicology* 28:1047–1067.
8. Costa, L.G., de Laat, R., Tagliaferri, S., & Pellacani, C. 2014. A mechanistic view of polybrominated diphenyl ether (PBDE) developmental neurotoxicity. *Toxicol Lett* 230:282–294.
9. Ebbesmeyer, C., & Scigliano E. 2009. *Floatsametrics and the Floating World.* New York, NY: Harper Collins.

10. Ellen MacArthur Foundation. 2016. *The New Plastics Economy: Rethinking the Future of Plastics.* https://www.ellenmacarthurfoundation.org/publications/the-new-plastics-economy-rethinking-the-future-of-plastics.

11. Eriksen, M., Lebreton, L.C., Carson, H.S., et al. 2014. Plastic pollution in the world's oceans: More than 5 trillion plastic pieces weighing over 250,000 tons afloat at sea. *PLoS One* 9:e111913.

12. Gall, S.C., & Thompson, R.C. 2015. The impact of debris on marine life. *Mar Pollut Bull* 92:170–179.

13. Gerona, R.R., Woodruff, T.J., Dickenson, C.A., et al. 2013. BPA, BPA glucuronide, and BPA sulfate in mid-gestation umbilical cord serum in a northern California cohort. *Environ Sci Technol* 47:12477–12485.

14. Graceli, J.B., Sena, G.C., Lopes, P.F., et al. 2013. Organotins: a review of their reproductive toxicity, biochemistry, and environmental fate. *Reprod Toxicol* 36:40–52.

15. Haldimann, M., Blanc, A., & Dudler, V. 2007. Exposure to antimony from polyethylene terephthalate (PET) trays used in ready-to-eat meals. *Food Addit Contam* 24:860–868.

16. Heindel, J.J., Blumberg, B., Cave, M., et al. 2016. Metabolism disrupting chemicals and metabolic disorders. *Reprod Toxicol* xx:xxx–xxx. (Reprod Toxicol. 2016 Oct 16. pii: S0890-6238(16)30363-X. doi: 10.1016/j.reprotox.2016.10.001. [Epub ahead of print])

17. Hormann, A.M., vom Saal, F.S., Nagel, S.C., et al. 2014. Holding thermal receipt paper and eating food after using hand sanitizer results in high serum bioactive and urine total levels of bisphenol A (BPA). *PLoS One* 9:e110509.

18. Hu, G.X., Lian, Q.Q., Ge, R.S., Hardy, D.O., & Li, X.K. 2009. Phthalate-induced testicular dysgenesis syndrome: Leydig cell influence. *Trends Endocrinol Metab* 20:139–145.

19. Jambeck, J.R., Geyer, R., Wilcox, C., et al. 2015. Marine pollution: Plastic waste inputs from land into the ocean. *Science* 347:768–771.

20. Jinhui, L., Yuan, C., & Wenjing, X. 2015. Polybrominated diphenyl ethers in articles: A review of its applications and legislation. *Environ Sci Pollut Res Int.* Epub ahead of print.

21. Jurewicz, J., & Hanke, W. 2011. Exposure to phthalates: reproductive outcome and children health: A review of epidemiological studies. *Int J Occup Med Environ Health* 24:115–141.

22. Karstadt, M. 1976. PVC: Health implications and production trends. *Eniron Health Perspect* 17:107–115.

23. Khaksar, M.R., & Ghazi-Khansari, M. 2009. Determination of migration monomer styrene from GPPS (general purpose polystyrene) and HIPS (high impact polystyrene) cups to hot drinks. *Toxicol Mech Methods* 19:257–261.

24. Kim, H., Gilbert, S., & Johnson, J. 1990. Determination of potential migrants from commercial amber polyethylene terephthalate bottle wall. *Pharmaceutical Res* 7:176–180.

25. Lattin, G.L., Moore, C.J., Zellers, A.F., Moore, S.L., & Weisberg, S.B. 2004. A comparison of neustonic plastic and zooplankton at different depths near the southern California shore. *Mar Pollut Bull* 49:291–294.

26. Marchesini, G.R., Meimaridou, A., Haasnoot, W., et al. 2008. Biosensor discovery of thyroxine transport disrupting chemicals. *Toxicol Appl Pharmacol* 232:150–160.

27. Mato, Y., Isobe, T., Takada, H., Kanehiro, H., Ohtake, C., & Kaminuma, T. 2001. Plastic resin pellets as a transport medium for toxic chemicals in the marine environment. *Environ Sci Technol* 35:318–324.

28. Meerts, I.A., van Zanden, J.J., Luijks, E.A., et al. 2000. Potent competitive interactions of some brominated flame retardants and related compounds with human transthyretin in vitro. *Toxicol Sci* 56:95–104.

29. Meironyté, D., Norén, K., & Bergman, A. 1999. Analysis of polybrominated diphenyl ethers in Swedish human milk: A time-related trend study, 1972–1997. *J Toxicol Environ Health A* 58:329–341.

30. Mendonca, K., Hauser, R., Calafat, A.M., Arbuckle, T.E., & Duty, S.M. 2014. Bisphenol A concentrations in maternal breast milk and infant urine. *Int Arch Occup Environ Health* 87:13–20.

31. Moore, C. 2008. Synthetic polymers in the marine environment: A rapidly increasing, long term threat. *Environ Res* 108:131–139.

32. Moore, C. 2011. *Plastic Ocean*. New York, NY: Penguin Group.

33. Moore, C.J., Moore, S.L., Leecaster, M.K., & Weisberg, S.B. 2001. A comparison of plastic and plankton in the North Pacific central gyre. *Mar Pollut Bull* 42:1297–1300.

34. Moore, C.J., Moore, S.L., Weisberg, S.B., Lattin, G., & Zellers, A. 2002. A comparison of neustonic plastic and zooplankton abundance in southern California's coastal waters. *Mar Pollut Bull* 44:1035–1038.

35. Nagel, S.C., vom Saal, F.S., Thayer, K.A., Dhar, M.G., Boechler, M., & Welshons, W.V. 1997. Relative binding affinity-serum modified access (RBA-SMA) assay predicts the relative in vivo bioactivity of the xenoestrogens bisphenol A and octylphenol. *Environ Health Perspect* 105:70–76.

36. Robinson, L., & Miller, R. 2015. The impact of bisphenol A and phthalates on allergy, asthma, and immune function: A review of latest findings. *Curr Environ Health Rep* 2:379–387.

37. Rochester, J.R. 2013. Bisphenol A and human health: A review of the literature. *Reprod Toxicol* 42:132–155.

38. Rochester, J.R., & Bolden, A.L. 2015. Bisphenol S and F: A systematic review and comparison of the hormonal activity of bisphenol A substitutes. *Environ Health Perspect* 123:643–650.

39. Rochman, C.M., Hoh, E., Kurobe, T., & Teh, S.J. 2013. Ingested plastic transfers hazardous chemicals to fish and induces hepatic stress. *Sci Rep* 3:3263.

40. Rochman, C.M., Tahir, A., Williams, S.L., et al. 2015. Anthropogenic debris in seafood: Plastic debris and fibers from textiles in fish and bivalves sold for human consumption. *Sci Rep* 5:14340.

41. Sajiki, J., & Yonekubo, J. 2003. Leaching of bisphenol A (BPA) to seawater from polycarbonate plastic and its degradation by reactive oxygen species. *Chemosphere* 51:55–62.
42. Sanagi, M., Lu Ling, S., Nasir, Z., Ibrahim, W., & Naim, A. 2008. Determination of residual volatile organic compounds migrated from polystyrene food packaging into food simulant by headspace solid phase microextraction-gas chromatography. *Malay J Anal Sci* 12:542–551.
43. Sax, L. 2010. Polyethylene terephthalate may yield endocrine disruptors. *Environ Health Perspect* 118:445–448.
44. Seachrist, D.D., Bonk, K.W., Ho, S.M., Prins, G.S., Soto, A.M., & Keri, R.A. 2016. A review of the carcinogenic potential of bisphenol A. *Reprod Toxicol.* 59:167–182.
45. Shin, H.M., McKone, T.E., & Bennett, D.H. 2014. Attributing population-scale human exposure to various source categories: merging exposure models and biomonitoring data. *Environ Int* 70:183–191.
46. Staniszewska, M., Graca, B., & Nehring, I. 2016. The fate of bisphenolA, 4-tert-octylphenol and 4-nonylphenol leached from plastic debris inot marine water: Eexperimental studies on biodegradation and sorption on suspended particulate matter and nano-TiO2. *Chemosphere* 145:535–542.
47. Stotland, N.E., Sutton, P., Trowbridge, J., et al. 2014. Counseling patients on preventing prenatal environmental exposures: A mixed-methods study of obstetricians. *PLoS One* 9:e98771.
48. Susiarjo, M., Hassold, T.J., Freeman, E., & Hunt, P.A. 2007. Bisphenol A exposure in utero disrupts early oogenesis in the mouse. *PLoS Genet* 3:63–70.
49. Swift, G. 2003. Biodegradable water-soluble polymers. In: Andrady AL, ed. *Plastics and the Environment.* Vol 1. 2nd ed, p. 499. Hoboken, NJ: John Wiley & Sons.
50. United Nations Environment Program. 2001. Marine litter: trash that kills. Global Programme of Action Coordination Office, The Hague, Netherlands. http://www.unep.org/regionalseas/marinelitter/publications/docs/trash_that_kills.pdf.
51. U.S. Product Safety Commission. 2014. Chronic Hazard Advisory Panel on Phthalates and Phthalate Alternatives. https://www.cpsc.gov/PageFiles/169902/CHAP-REPORT-With-Appendices.pdf.
52. Vandenberg, L.N., Colborn, T., Hayes, T.B., et al. 2012. Hormones and endocrine-disrupting chemicals: Low-dose effects and nonmonotonic dose responses. *Endocr Rev* 33:378–455.
53. Vandenberg, L.N., Ehrlich, S., Belcher, S.M., et al. 2013. Low dose effects of bisphenol A: an integrated review of in vitro, laboratory animal and epidemiology studies. *Endocr Disrupt* 1:e25078.
54. Vandenberg, L.N., Welshons, W.V., vom Saal, F.S., Toutain, P.L., & Myers, J.P. 2014. Should oral gavage be abandoned in toxicity testing of endocrine disruptors? *Environ Health* 13:46.
55. vom Saal, F.S., Cooke, P.S., Buchanan, D.L., et al. 1998. A physiologically based approach to the study of bisphenol A and other estrogenic chemicals on the size

of reproductive organs, daily sperm production, and behavior. *Toxicol Ind Health* 14:239–260.

56. vom Saal, F.S., & Hughes, C. 2005. An extensive new literature concerning low-dose effects of bisphenol A shows the need for a new risk assessment. *Environ Health Perspect* 113:926–933.

57. vom Saal, F.S., & Welshons, W.V. 2014. Evidence that bisphenol A (BPA) can be accurately measured without contamination in human serum and urine, and that BPA causes numerous hazards from multiple routes of exposure. *Mol Cell Endocrinol* 398:101–113.

58. Wallace, N. 1984. Debris entanglement in the environment. In: Shomura RS, Yoshida HO, eds. *Proceedings on the Fate and Impact of Marine Debris*. NOAA Technical Memo NMFS,NOAA-TM-NMFS-SWFC-54. Washington, DC: U.S. Department of Commerce; 259–277.

59. Weuve, J., Sanchez, B.N., Calafat, A.M., et al. 2006. Exposure to phthalates in neonatal intensive care unit infants: urinary concentrations of monoesters and oxidative metabolites. *Environ Health Perspect* 114:1424–1431.

60. Zoeller, R.T., Brown, T.R., Doan, L.L., et al. 2012. Endocrine-disrupting chemicals and public health protection: A statement of principles from the endocrine society. *Endocrinology* 153:4097–4110.

3

Environmental Chemicals and their Effects on Human Physiology

JOEL A. MARUNIAK

Key Concepts

- The human body depends on complex, layered sets of homeostatic control systems to maintain internal conditions within the narrow range of parameters compatible with life.
- The activities of cells, tissues, and organs are regulated by myriad messenger molecules that are crucial for maintaining homeostasis in the face of a wide range of external conditions.
- Messenger molecules are transported in the blood and extracellular fluid, often in association with binding proteins. Plasma-binding proteins frequently interact with chemicals from the environment, which alters bioactive levels of hormones.
- Messenger molecules cause effects by binding to receptors on or in a cell. The binding event can lead to changes in gene expression and initiate one of many possible cascades of biochemical reactions that change the activity of the cell. At each step along the pathways, there is the potential for disruption by environmental chemicals.
- The expression of our genes can be permanently altered by life experiences or environmental chemicals through a process called *epigenetic modification*. Some epigenetic changes in DNA are heritable and passed on to successive generations.
- Fetuses, neonates, children, and adolescents are particularly vulnerable to environmental chemicals because of the ability of exogenous chemicals to influence genetic imprinting and organizational events that occur during critical stages in development.

This chapter examines some of the biologic portals through which environmental chemicals impact homeostatic, communication, and epigenetic systems.

Homeostasis

Homeostasis is the property of one or more physiologic control systems that ensures the maintenance of a more or less constant and optimal set of internal conditions despite broad variations in external conditions. Humans can survive in a large range of external environments but only when their internal environment is maintained within a surprisingly narrow range of conditions. Homeostatic maintenance within narrow ranges of variance involves layered sets of control systems.

At the most basic level of homeostasis, each cell performs autonomous activities to maintain optimal functioning. Such a basic system is sufficient for single-celled organisms but not for large, complex organisms. There are many situations in which the health of the individual cells is good but the health of the organism is not. For example, a person can be in a vegetative state for years, during which time most individual cells continue to thrive. Because it is not sufficient for individual cells to maintain their own homeostasis in a large organism, hierarchical regional and global control systems evolved to maintain whole-body homeostasis. Higher-level control systems include the autonomic nervous system, hormonal feedback loops, thermoregulatory systems, osmoregulatory systems, acid-base balance, and buffer systems.

To understand the maintenance of homeostasis and the ways in which environmental chemicals can perturb it, we begin with the individual cell. A basic tenet of physiology is that all cells are ignorant and have to be instructed by messenger molecules when it is necessary to make local changes for the good of the body. Each of the approximately 37 trillion cells in the human body must be continuously informed of the state of the organism of which it is part. Although processing systems such as the brain often know what is going on, even their individual cells do not. Orchestration of changes in the activities of individual cells, which are the components of tissues and organs ultimately maintains optimal functioning of the body.

Whole-body homeostasis is accomplished through the control of a large number of physiologic parameters whose levels are monitored by sensing cells that detect when a variance occurs from a set point. Set points include a variety of values such as a blood pH of 7.4, body temperature of 37°C, blood osmolarity of 300 mOsm, and blood glucose levels of about 90 mg/dL. Set points vary between individuals due to a variety of factors, and they can be adjusted up and down according to the body's developmental, life cycle, health, stress, metabolic, and traumatic states and in response to drug or chemical exposures. Homeostatic control systems monitor variance from set points and respond with corrective messages that are sent to target tissues, instructing them to upregulate or downregulate activity. In this way, the levels of physiologic parameters are maintained within a narrow optimal range on either side of a set point.

Most homeostatic control systems operate automatically and without conscious control. They perform their jobs subliminally to keep the body performing optimally in response to changing internal and external conditions. To monitor changing conditions, technologies were designed to sense and analyze physiologic parameters. Modern medicine is based on the ability to gather and respond to data acquired by these technologies.

Messenger Molecules and the Information Systems of the Body

Many types of messenger molecules, including hormones, growth factors, neurotransmitters, and cytokines, are used to convey information in the body. The messenger molecules typically connect with antenna-like receptors arrayed on the outer membranes of cells. Most messages are chemicals that reach a cell through the extracellular fluid, often after traveling in the bloodstream.

Messenger systems are a remnant of the type of communication used by the first cells that evolved about 3.8 billion years ago. For about the first 2 billion years that life existed on earth, it consisted only of unicellular prokaryotes living in brackish seawater. The earliest life forms communicated by releasing a chemical from their surface that diffused into the surrounding water. If the chemical reached a fellow prokaryote that had a receptor for it, communication transpired. Billions of years later, cells mostly communicate in the same way. Even in advanced organisms such as humans, individual cells know only what is brought to their attention by messenger molecules arriving at the receptors on their plasma membrane by way of the extracellular fluid that surrounds them.

BINDING PROTEINS

Some of the endogenous messenger molecules employed by cells are stored in vesicles inside the cells and are exported by exocytosis into the extracellular fluid. Others are manufactured on demand and diffuse across the cell's outer membrane into the extracellular fluid. The chemistry and transport systems of the body take place in a water-based matrix, and most of the body's messenger molecules are water soluble. However, many, such as the steroid and thyroid hormones and endocannabinoid neurotransmitters, are not. The body solves the problem of transporting water-insoluble messenger molecules by attaching them to water-soluble carriers called hormone-binding proteins (HBPs) (Fig. 3.1). HBPs perform other important functions, and some of the water-soluble hormones also circulate in the blood attached to HBPs.[32]

HBPs have several roles in homeostasis. Only messenger molecules that are not bound to binding proteins are active, and HBPs help to regulate the effective concentrations of the messenger molecules they bind. When messenger molecules are bound to HBPs, they cannot be filtered into the urine or broken down by the liver, which extends their half-lives.

The binding proteins in blood include albumin, globulins, lipoproteins, and glycoproteins. They can be further subdivided into binding proteins that have a high affinity and high specificity for one or a few messenger molecules or low-affinity, low-specificity binding proteins such as albumin, which can associate more loosely with a variety of compounds.

An example of how hormones interact with binding proteins can be seen with the water-insoluble hormone testosterone, which associates with both low- and high-affinity binding proteins in blood. Testosterone moves through the circulation in three main states.[7] About one half of the testosterone in the bloodstream is bound to sex hormone–binding protein (SHBG), which is a special carrier for two of the sex steroids, testosterone and estradiol. Somewhat less than one half of the testosterone is bound to albumins, and

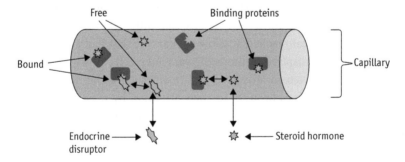

FIGURE 3.1. A few of the actions of plasma-binding proteins in the blood are shown. Some hormone-binding proteins and globulins are very specific for certain endogenous messenger molecules such as steroid or thyroid hormones. Others are less specific and can bind many different compounds, including exogenous chemicals from the environment such as endocrine disruptors.

only about 2% is free or unbound, which is the active form. Anything that affects the amount of SHBG or albumin in the bloodstream can have a significant effect on the amount of free testosterone and its activity. For example, as men age, the levels of SHBG increase, and because of the higher affinity of SHBG for testosterone relative to estradiol, a greater proportion of circulating testosterone is bound to SHBG compared with estradiol, reducing the ratio of free (active) testosterone to estradiol.[24]

Many environmental chemicals and drugs function as endogenous messengers; like testosterone, they circulate in the bloodstream free, bound to HBPs, or bound to albumins (Fig. 3.1). This affects the activity levels, catabolism, and half-lives of the exogenous chemicals. Because they compete with endogenous messengers for access to HBPs, these chemicals can also affect the activity and clearance of the endogenous messengers.[5,19] One example is the flame retardant tetrabromobisphenol A (TBBPA), which has about a 50-fold greater affinity for transthyretin (i.e., HBP for thyroxine) than thyroxine (T_4) does and therefore alters the normal regulation of active T_4 in blood.[22]

MESSENGER MOLECULE RECEPTORS AND THEIR EFFECTS

When a messenger molecule binds to a receptor on the surface of a cell, its effects are communicated to the cell through a limited number of second messengers, including cyclic adenosine monophosphate (cAMP), cyclic guanosine monophosphate (cGMP), inositol triphosphate, calcium ions (Ca^{2+}), diacylglycerol, phosphatidylinositols, and the gases nitric oxide (NO) and carbon monoxide (CO). Second messengers can influence the cell through a dizzying array of pathways and cascades of biochemical steps (>60) along each pathway (Fig. 3.2). In individual pathways, specific cellular responses occur as a result of activation of a receptor by an endogenous messenger or, in some cases, an exogenous chemical.

In each of these pathway and at each step along the pathway, there is the potential for influence by environmental chemicals. Some chemicals can enhance the action in one pathway but inhibit it in others. Others have more complex actions. For example, bisphenol A (BPA) stimulates insulin production and release from pancreatic beta cells through separate receptors and cell-signaling pathways,[2] but in other tissues, BPA inhibits the action of thyroid hormone by recruiting a co-repressor protein to the thyroid receptor that blocks thyroid hormone from activating the receptor.[23] Because homeostatic mechanisms attempt to maintain set-point values within narrow ranges, the excitatory and inhibitory influences of environmental chemicals at any point in the cascades can produce negative consequences.

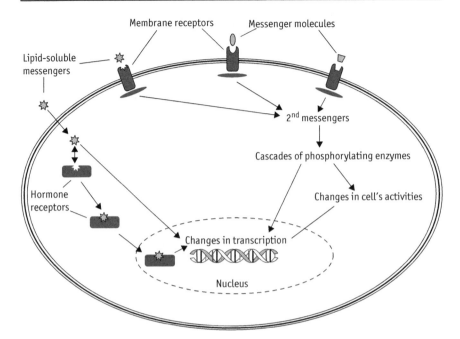

FIGURE 3.2. The cell has different cell membrane receptors for three messenger molecules. When the receptors bind a messenger molecule, they activate second messenger pathways. The second messengers activate a cascade of phosphorylating enzymes that ultimately change an activity in the cell. Messenger molecules that are lipid soluble can diffuse through the outer membrane into the cell and bind to receptor proteins that escort them to the nucleus, where they can affect DNA transcription, ultimately causing a change in cellular activity.

Exogenous environmental chemicals can affect almost any cellular activity.[37] For example, in addition to affecting beta cell and thyroid hormone function, the endocrine-disrupting chemical BPA can influence all of the cell communication pathways shown in Figure 3.2.[1] Although the consequences of environmental chemicals begin with their effects on individual cells, it is the cumulative impact on higher organizational units of the body that is most dramatic. The effects of BPA and other environmental chemicals on the reproductive, metabolic, and immune systems and on brain development and behavior can adversely affect human health.[31,6,18]

In most steps in the biochemical cascades shown in Figure 3.2, macromolecules that are involved in controlling a cell's operations are activated or inactivated or have their function altered by undergoing a chemical interaction that causes a morphologic change. Under normal conditions, this is accomplished by phosphorylation of the macromolecule or by binding of the macromolecule with a ligand or divalent cation. The powerful effects that an exogenous environmental chemical can have on the body may be seen in the mechanism by which selective serotonin reuptake inhibitors (SSRIs) change human affect. Many antidepressants act by binding to the macromolecular reuptake transporter for serotonin located in the synapses of neurons in mood networks of the brain. Reuptake transporters normally retrieve serotonin after it is released by neurons. When an SSRI binds to a reuptake pump, it changes the stereochemistry of the pump, reducing the pump's ability to retrieve serotonin after it is released.[4] The levels of serotonin in the synapses rise, causing increased stimulation of the target neurons, which at a conscious level ameliorates the symptoms of depression. As in this example, any exogenous chemical that binds to a macromolecule that is part of a messenger or metabolic pathway can have a pronounced influence on the entire system,

Epigenetic Effects

The field of epigenetics studies the changes in gene expression caused by developmental differentiation, life experiences and exposures, whereas classic genetics studies genes and how the information encoded in them changes as a result of mutations and natural selection. Environmental chemicals and drugs can cause permanent, and sometimes heritable, epigenetic changes. The epigenetic and genetic changes are transferred from one cell to its daughter cells during mitosis and from stem cells of the ovaries and testes to their daughter cells during meiosis.

Humans begin as a fertilized egg that divides into two identical new cells, which divide into four identical new cells and so on until some of these pluripotent cells, which can become any type of cell in the adult body, begin to undergo changes that render them nonidentical to their progenitors. At that point, their fates separate from those of their progenitors and sister cells that enter other differentiation pathways. The mechanisms that allow divisions of the fertilized egg and its daughter cells to produce the diverse tissues and organs of the body (even though all of the cells have the same genome) involve epigenetic changes.

In the coding parts of genes, each successive block of three nucleotides (i.e., codon) specifies an amino acid that can become part of a polypeptide manufactured from the genetic information. If each codon in the human genome were equivalent to a word in a book, the total information in the 46 human chromosomes would be about the same as in 4000 books that are each 1000 pages long. Offspring inherit this large set of instructions (i.e., genome) on how to build a human body from their parents.

Until the discovery of epigenetic effects, it was thought that the inherited set of instructions encoded in genes was fixed and immutable. However, epigenetics provides a fine-tuning system that can adjust the inherited instructions in response to life experiences and exposures.

Two major epigenetic mechanisms can permanently change the way in which genes are read. First, the inherited instructions can be altered by chemical modification of the histone proteins that package and wind DNA into compact structural units called nucleosomes (Fig. 3.3). Modification of histones by the addition of chemical groups makes the genes wound around the histones easier to read by providing better access to them. In contrast, in stretches of DNA with reduced addition of those chemical groups to histones, the genetic information is much less accessible and the genes are said to be *silenced*. The second way that genetic instructions are rendered more or less readable is by methylation or demethylation of nucleotides in DNA. Histone modifications and methylation or demethylation occur in a coordinated manner to determine whether the genes are expressed or silenced.

Epigenetic changes during fetal development are generally more profound than those occuring after birth.The making of a big toe is an example. Every cell in the body has the entire library of genetic information (i.e., 46 chromosomes) in it, except for sperm and eggs, which contain only one half of the library (i.e., 23 chromosomes). However, because big toes do not need to know how to make stomach acid and many other things, only those genes that are needed for the formation and function of a big toe are read in its cells. Most unnecessary instructions in big toe cells remain unread. The regulatory mechanism by which they are made unreadable is the epigenetic changes that occur during development. A line of cells that becomes part of the big toe could have become any kind of cell in the body during embryonic life, but at some point, progressive epigenetic changes cause the cells to differentiate, and they irreversibly become big toe cells.

The epigenetic adjustments to gene expression that direct cells early during development also occur throughout life. Epigenetically active environmental chemicals are a concern because of their potential to affect development of the body, especially the endocrine, reproductive, and nervous systems, and because of their etiologic role in a variety of diseases, including cancer. Many of these chemicals can cross from the mother's circulation into the fetal circulation. There is ample evidence for the negative consequences of exposure to these chemicals during fetal development and for delayed effects on the body and brain later in life.[15]

Other factors can cause epigenetic effects, including the nutritional status of the mother and father,[8,34] illnesses,[30] smoking,[16] medical drugs,[20] stress,[38] physical and mental abuse,[35] and other traumas. A striking example comes

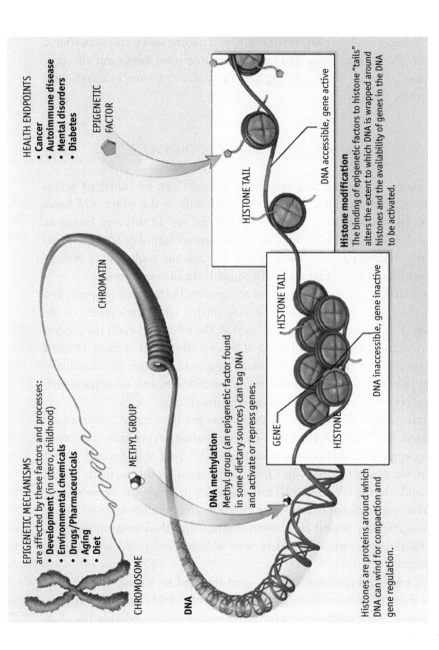

EPIGENETIC MECHANISMS
are affected by these factors and processes:
- **Development** (in utero, childhood)
- **Environmental chemicals**
- **Drugs/Pharmaceuticals**
- **Aging**
- **Diet**

CHROMOSOME

CHROMATIN

METHYL GROUP

DNA

DNA methylation
Methyl group (an epigenetic factor found in some dietary sources) can tag DNA and activate or repress genes.

Histones are proteins around which DNA can wind for compaction and gene regulation.

GENE

HISTONE TAIL

HISTONE

DNA inaccessible, gene inactive

HEALTH ENDPOINTS
- **Cancer**
- **Autoimmune disease**
- **Mental disorders**
- **Diabetes**

EPIGENETIC FACTOR

HISTONE TAIL

DNA accessible, gene active

Histone modification
The binding of epigenetic factors to histone "tails" alters the extent to which DNA is wrapped around histones and the availability of genes in the DNA to be activated.

FIGURE 3.3. Methylation and histone modifications can change gene expression. The enzyme DNA dimethyl transferase adds methyl groups to the cytosines of DNA, which can enhance or inhibit gene expression. Histone modification occurs when certain chemical groups are added to the histone tails by methylation, acetylation, phosphorylation, or ubiquitination, rendering the affected stretches of DNA more or less tightly wound around histones and therefore more or less easily accessed.

from research on the effects of heroin on mouse brains and on the postmortem brains of heroin abusers.[14,17,27] Prominent changes have been reported in the brains of heroin addicts in the genes and neuronal networks related to areas commonly linked to drug abuse. These differences resulted from epigenetic changes in those parts of the brain, and the changes were proportional to length of drug use. These findings suggest that some long-term effects of drug abuse and addiction (including high rates of relapse) may be attributable to epigenetic changes.

INHERITANCE OF EPIGENETIC CHANGES

Accumulated data show that epigenetic changes can be inherited across generations, and epigenetic changes in stem cells in the ovary and testes are retained across meiotic divisions throughout life. In this way, chemical, emotional, dietary, and other exposures can impact future generations. This surprising finding has sent shock waves through the evolutionary biology community and the broader medical and public health community.[33]

Most of the epigenetic changes that accumulate in the genes of sperm and eggs in the course of a lifetime are erased during fetal development of the offspring of those sperm and eggs. After that, the offspring repeat the process of differentiation, and the fine-tuning of genes begins anew in them. In some cases, however, not all of the accumulated epigenetic changes are erased, and they are instead passed on to children, grandchildren, and subsequent generations[33] (i.e., transgenerational epigenetic inheritance).

Several notable examples of heritable changes have been demonstrated or inferred. For example, if parents or grandparents experience starvation, resulting epigenetic changes can be inherited by their children and grandchildren. Studies of famines—in China in the 1950s, in the northern part of Netherlands during World War II, and in Sweden in the 1800s—revealed profound transgenerational effects.[21] The children and grandchildren of people who were starving tended to be born smaller, and their rates of diabetes, heart disease, and mental disorders were elevated compared with control populations.

Other profound epigenetic effects were revealed in a study that showed that the abuse of a mother during pregnancy or of a child could cause epigenetic changes in the cortisol receptor genes of the child, rendering the child more susceptible to stress.[3] In addition, high stress levels in the mother during a child's first year of life was shown to cause 139 epigenetic changes in the child.[9] Although it is not known through how many generations these epigenetic changes can persist in humans, transgenerational studies show that transmission of epigenetic imprints can remain stable for several generations in plants.[12] An alarming aspect of the accumulation of epigenetic changes during one's life, whether they are passed on to one's children or not, is the discovery that many environmental chemicals can induce epigenetic changes.

Fetal, Infant, Childhood, and Adolescent Vulnerability

Fetuses, neonates, children, and adolescents are uniquely vulnerable to environmental chemicals. These groups show more widespread and exaggerated effects of chemical exposures than adults do, in large part because of the ability of exogenous chemicals to influence critical imprinting and organizational events that occur during developmental stages. Such effects are exacerbated by the sensitivity of differentiating stem or progenitor cells, immaturity of the immune system and the blood-brain barrier, and limited ability of the immature liver to detoxify chemicals.

The homeostatic and protective systems that operate in fetuses, infants, and children are not capable of responding to environmental insults in a manner similar to that of adults. The maxim in pediatric medicine is that "babies are not little adults." Research has revealed associations between many long-latency diseases (e.g., obesity, type 2 diabetes, cardiovascular disease, reduced fertility, reproductive organ cancers, neurobehavioral abnormalities) and early-life exposure to endocrine-disrupting chemicals.[10,39]

A particularly onerous example of in utero exposure to endocrine-disrupting and epigenetically active chemicals is the estrogenic drug diethylstilbestrol (DES). DES was prescribed to millions of pregnant women from the 1940s through 1960s in the mistaken belief that it could reduce the incidence of miscarriage.[25] Because of the delayed onset of exposure effects on the reproductive system, the disastrous effects on fetuses of DES did not become obvious until decades later.[26] Some female offspring (i.e., DES daughters) developed clear cell adenocarcinoma of the vagina and cervix in adolescence or young adulthood, and virtually all male and female offspring showed some type of adverse consequence of exposure to DES.[25,26] Follow-up studies revealed that by the age of 50 years, DES daughters had a threefold increase in breast cancer incidence.[29] DES and other estrogenic compounds caused delayed-onset and transgenerational effects by altering the epigenetic imprints underlying normal reproductive system differentiation.[26]

Study of delayed-onset effects led to the formulation of a hypothesis called developmental origins of health and disease (DOHaD).[13] This proposition holds that many diseases that are not expressed until adulthood originate during earlier periods when organs are differentiating. The concept that some long-term adverse effects result from exposure to environmental chemicals or stressors during critical periods in organogenesis is now understood to extend beyond cancers of reproductive organs to metabolic diseases (i.e., those affecting cardiovascular, liver, adipocyte, and pancreatic function and pathobiology) including heart attack, fatty liver, obesity, insulin resistance, and diabetes.[13]

There is extensive evidence for long-term effects of chemicals and other stressors on the brain, learning, and behavior.[11] An interesting aspect of the effects of fetal exposure to endocrine-disrupting chemicals on neurobehavioral development is that very different and sometimes opposite outcomes are observed for males and females, although this phenomenon remains unexplained.[28]

Conclusions

The modern environment is a chemical soup generated by the industries and technologies that allow many people to survive in comfortable and pleasing conditions. However, the side effects and byproducts of these conveniences are often not good for human health. Many manufactured chemicals are functionally indistinguishable from the naturally occurring messenger molecules that are used by cells to communicate with each other. Therefore, biochemical cascades and gene expression can be altered by the many environmental chemicals that disrupt normal cellular, physiologic, developmental, and hereditary processes and adversely affect human health.

REFERENCES

1. Acconcia, F., Pallottini, V., & Marino, M. 2015. Molecular mechanisms of action of BPA. *Dose Response.* 13:1559325815610582.
2. Alonso-Magdalena, P., Ropero, A.B., Soriano, S., et al. 2012. Bisphenol-A acts as a potent estrogen via non-classical estrogen triggered pathways. *Mol Cell Endocrinol.* 355:201–207.
3. Babenko, O., Kovalchuk, I., & Metz, G.A. 2015. Stress-induced perinatal and transgenerational epigenetic programming of brain development and mental health. *Neurosci Biobehav Rev.* 48:70–91.
4. Davis, B.A., Nagarajan, A., Forrest, L.R., & Singh, S.K. 2016. Mechanism of Paroxetine (Paxil) inhibition of the serotonin transporter. *Sci Rep.* 6:23789.
5. Déchaud, H., Ravard, C., Claustrat, F., Perrière, A.B., & Pugeat, M. 1999. Xenoestrogen interaction with human sex hormone-binding globulin (hSHBG). *Steroids.* 64:328–334.

6. Desai, M., Jellyman, J.K., & Ross, M.G. 2015. Epigenomics, gestational programming and risk of metabolic syndrome. *Int J Obes.* 39:633–641.

7. Diver, M.J. 2006. Analytical and physiological factors affecting the interpretation of serum testosterone concentration in men. *Ann Clin Biochem.* 43:3–12.

8. Dominguez-Salas, P., Moore, S.E., Baker, M.S., et al. 2014. Maternal nutrition at conception modulates DNA methylation of human metastable epialleles. *Nat Commun.* 5:3746.

9. Essex, M.J., Boyce, W.T., Hertzman, C., et al. 2013. Epigenetic vestiges of early developmental adversity: Childhood stress exposure and DNA methylation in adolescence. *Child Dev.* 84:58–75.

10. Gore, A.C., Chappell, V.A., Fenton, S.E., et al. 2015. EDC-2: The Endocrine Society's second scientific statement on endocrine-disrupting chemicals. *Endocr Rev.* 36:E1–E150.

11. Grandjean, P., & Landrigan, P.J. 2014. Neurobehavioural effects of developmental toxicity. *Lancet Neurol.* 13:330–338.

12. Heard, E., & Martienssen, R.A. 2014. Transgenerational epigenetic inheritance: Myths and mechanisms. *Cell.* 157:95–109.

13. Heindel, J.J., & vom Saal, F.S. 2009. Role of nutrition and environmental endocrine disrupting chemicals during the perinatal period on the aetiology of obesity. *Mol Cell Endocrinol.* 304:90–96.

14. Hurd, Y.L. Quoted in Akst, J. 2013, November 11. The epigenetics of drug abuse. *The Scientist.*

15. Kaita, M., & Woitowicz A.K. 2013. Impact of endocrine-disrupting chemicals on neural development and the onset of neurological disorders. *Pharmacol Rep.* 65:1632–1639.

16. Klebaner, D., Huang, Y., Hui, Q., et al. 2016. X chromosome-wide analysis identifies DNA methylation sites influenced by cigarette smoking. *Clin Epigenet.* 8:20.

17. Koo, J.W., Mazei-Robison, M.S., LaPlant, Q., et al. 2015. Epigenetic basis of opiate suppression of *Bdnf* gene expression in the ventral tegmental area. *Nat Neurosci.* 18:415–422.

18. Kreitinger, J.M., Beamer, C.A., & Shepherd, D.M. 2016. Environmental immunology: Lessons learned from exposure to a select panel of immunotoxicants. *J Immunol.* 196:3217–3225.

19. Liu, X., Miao, M., Zhou, Z., et al. 2015. Exposure to bisphenol-A and reproductive hormones among male adults. *Environ Toxicol Pharmacol.* 39:934–941.

20. Lötsch, J., Schneider, G., Reker, D., et al. 2013. Common non-epigenetic drugs as epigenetic modulators. *Trends Mol Med.* 19:742–753.

21. Lumey, L.H., Stein, A.D., & Susser, E. 2011. Prenatal famine and adult health. *Annu Rev Public Health.* 32:237–262.

22. Meerts, I.A., van Zanden, J.J., Luijks, E.A., et al. 2000. Potent competitive interactions of some brominated flame retardants and related compounds with human transthyretin in vitro. *Toxicol Sci.* 56:95–104.

23. Moriyama, K., Tagami, T., Akamizu, T., et al. 2002. Thyroid hormone action is disrupted by bisphenol A as an antagonist. *J Clin Endocrinol Metab.* 87:5185–5190.

24. Nagel, S.C., & vom Saal, F.S. 2003. Endocrine control of sexual differentiation: Effects of the maternal-fetal environment and endocrine disrupting chemicals. In: Miller V, Hay M, eds. *Principles of Sex-Based Physiology,* pp 15–37. New York, NY: Elsevier.

25. Newbold, R. 1995. Cellular and molecular effects of developmental exposure to diethylstilbestrol: Implications for other environmental estrogens. *Environ Health Perspect.* 103:83–87.

26. Newbold, R.R., Padilla-Banks, E., & Jefferson, W.N. 2006. Adverse effects of the model environmental estrogen diethylstilbestrol are transmitted to subsequent generations. *Endocrinology.* 147:S11–S17.

27. Ökvist, A., Fagergren, P., Whittard, J., et al. 2011. Dysregulated post-synaptic density and endocytic zone in the amygdala of human heroin and cocaine abusers. *Biol Psychiatry.* 69:245–252.

28. Palanza, P., Nagel, S.C., Parmigiani, S., & vom Saal, F.S. 2016. Perinatal exposure to endocrine disruptors: Sex, timing and behavioral endpoints. *Curr Opin Behav Sci.* 7:69–75.

29. Palmer, J.R., Wise, L.A., Hatch, E.E., et al. 2006. Prenatal diethylstilbestrol exposure and risk of breast cancer. *Cancer Epidemiol Biomarkers Prev.* 15:1509–1514.

30. Reddy, M.A., Zhang, E., & Natarajan, R. 2014. Epigenetic mechanisms in diabetic complications and metabolic memory. *Diabetologica.* 58:443–455.

31. Rogers, J.A., Metz, L., & Yong, V.W. 2013. Review. Endocrine disrupting chemicals and immune responses: A focus on bisphenol-A and its potential mechanisms. *Mol Immunol.* 53:421–430.

32. Seasholtz, A.F., Valverde, R.A., & Denver, R.J. 2002. Corticotropin-releasing hormone-binding protein: Biochemistry and function from fishes to mammals. *J Endocrinol.* 175:89–97.

33. Skinner, M.K. 2014. A new kind of inheritance. *Sci Am.* 311:44–51.

34. Soubry, A., Guo, L., Huang, Z., et al. Obesity-related DNA methylation at imprinted genes in human sperm: Results from the TIEGER study. *Clin Epigenet.* 8:51.

35. Suderman, M., Borghoi, N., Pappas, J.J., et al. 2014. Childhood abuse is associated with methylation of multiple loci in adult DNA. *BMC Med Genomics.* 7:13.

36. Toppari, J., Virtanen, H.E., Main, K.M., Skakkebaek, N.E. 2010. Cryptorchidism and hypospadias as a sign of testicular dysgenesis syndrome (TDS): Environmental connection. *Birth Defects Res A Clin Mol Teratol.* 88:910–919.

37. Yang, O., Kim, H.L., Weon, J., Seo, Y.R. 2015. Endocrine-disrupting chemicals: Review of toxicological mechanisms using molecular pathway analysis. *J Cancer Prev.* 20:12–24.

38. Zannas, A.S., & West, A.E. 2014. Epigenetics and the regulation of stress vulnerability and resilience. *Neuroscience.* 264:157–170.

39. Zoeller, R.T., Brown, T.R., Doan, L.L., et al. 2012. Endocrine-disrupting chemicals and public health protection: A statement of principles from the endocrine society. *Endocrinology.* 153:4097–4110.

SECTION 2

Sources and Clinical Aspects of Environmental Exposures

4

Sources of Contaminants in the Home: Indoor Air Quality and Human Health

JAMES S. DENNINGHOFF AND FREDERICK S. VOM SAAL

Key Concepts

- Many sick people in compromised environments could be well; indoor air is essential for good health.
- Inflammation is central to the pathogenesis of asthma, allergy, and sinusitis.
- Inflammation can be triggered by exposure to dust, mold, and environmental chemicals.
- Identifying the sources and health consequences of dust is critical.
- Understanding the hazards of exposure to toxic man-made chemicals is part of the solution.
- The health costs of preventable diseases are huge.

Introduction

The incidence of asthma, allergy, and sinusitis has been increasing for decades. The number of people diagnosed with asthma increased by 4.3 million from 2001 to 2009. The Centers for Disease Control and Prevention (CDC) reported that in 2014, 17.7 million adults (7.4% of adults) and 6.3 million children (8.6%) in the United States had asthma, with 3651 deaths annually attributed to this disease. Patients with asthma as their primary diagnosis made 10.5 million visits to physician offices annually. The estimated annual cost to the health care system (based on 2007 data) was $56 billion.[9]

A relationship between asthma and environmental and lifestyle factors is indicated by the fact that the childhood asthma prevalence more than doubled from 1980 to the mid-1990s.[1] Because the occurrence of respiratory diseases is related to pollutant exposures, outdoor and indoor air quality is a concern. People do not have good control over the quality of outdoor air, but there are practical ways to reduce daily exposure to pollutants at home, in the workplace, and in other indoor spaces or environments.

It is commonly assumed that the products we buy and put in our homes are safe. Although we assume that public water supplies are safe, the 2016 lead contamination crisis in Flint, Michigan, and subsequent findings about high lead levels in drinking water in many other communities showed this to not necessarily be true. The assumption of safety is also clearly invalid for common household products[13] and for indoor air quality.[23] Health risks associated with indoor air quality exist in both old and new houses, although the types of problems encountered can differ based on the age of the house.[7] Many modern building materials, as well as the chemicals used in the manufacture of common household items, are assumed by most people to be safe, but, as discussed in a number of other chapters, this is not always the case. It is up to clinicians, who are frequently asked for health advice, and the public to become knowledgeable about these issues; our health is in the balance.

Respiratory Diseases

SINUS INFLAMMATION

A "sinus problem" is a symptom of upper respiratory inflammation. Illnesses that are treated as an allergy or sinus problem are usually symptoms of other issues, including environmental air contamination and chemical and food intolerances. Most people think that they know the causes of sinus and allergy problems, based on TV advertisements, but what most people don't realize is that there is always a reason for tissue irritation and inflammation in sinus infections, and recognizing this is key to seeking a specialist for diagnosis and treatment.

It is essential to determine whether upper respiratory inflammation is a chronic condition or a recurring acute condition. Upper respiratory epithelium is self-cleaning and functions normally until it becomes irritated. On examination, a common finding is objective evidence of tissue breakdown, nasal crusting, pharyngeal lymphoid tissue studding, voice changes, postnasal drainage, and eye irritation. Most of these findings can be diagnosed on visual examination, looking for tenderness, swelling, redness, labored breathing, and cough. Other diagnostic tools include spirometry and nasal endoscopy. The point is to compare the physical findings with the patient's history; in most patients there is a history of repetitive sinus-nasal-lung problems. Questions to ask include: would this patient benefit from antibiotics, inhalers, allergy medications or nasal decongestants for these symptoms?

ALLERGY

Allergy is a commonly used word, but what does it mean to have an allergy? Airborne allergies are caused by the reaction of the immune system to inhaled dust, pollen, mold spores, animal dander, and other allergens. These are everyday occurrences, but some of us are predisposed to react strongly enough to trigger an immune response, often involving the lungs, nose, sinuses, ears, throat, and skin. As with most diseases, allergies result from an interaction between genetic predisposition (i.e., nature) and environmental factors (i.e., nurture). There is no longer a dispute that only one or the other is the sole factor.[32]

Airborne allergies can occur at any age. Factors that play major roles include heredity, a family history of allergy, and environmental exposures. An allergic predisposition and repetitive exposure (e.g., dust mites, mold, cat dander) result in an allergic load, which triggers an immune response. Inflammation of delicate upper and lower respiratory tissues results from exposure to allergens. After these tissues are inflamed, they cannot function normally or heal themselves, and disease, including bacterial infection, can result. Controlling exposures is critical to good health.

Common symptoms of allergy include fatigue, cough, ear blockage, snoring, congestion, wheezing, sneezing, postnasal drainage, gastric reflux, halitosis, headache, itching, skin inflammation, and recurring sinus infection. Obtaining a comprehensive patient history is an important part of the diagnosis, and symptoms may vary among individuals. Repetitive exposures contribute greatly to physical complaints.

Symptoms are often worse seasonally (i.e., spring and fall) and depend on a patient's geographical location. Perennial allergens as a cause of allergy can be deceptive due to extended periods without relief, which complicates evaluation of exposure patterns. Cross-reactivity between food and pollen allergies also occurs. For example, ragweed cross-reacts with watermelon, cantaloupe, and chamomile. Cross-reactivity occurs between latex and a wide variety of foods, including fruits, vegetables, and nuts.[12]

The goal of all allergy treatment is to obtain healed, uninflamed, normally functioning respiratory epithelium. An accurate diagnosis is essential to avoid prescribing medications that treat symptoms rather than the underlying cause.

ASTHMA

Asthma is a chronic inflammatory disease that is triggered by exposure to allergens or other irritants. The airway becomes hyperreactive, with bronchial muscle spasm, mucus hypersecretion, and edema. These factors combine to produce cough, wheezing, chest pain, and general respiratory distress. Asthma differs from chronic obstructive pulmonary disease (COPD), which is typically associated with smoking, and onset is later in life relative to asthma, although it can be a concomitant illness of a reactive airway. Acute asthmatic reactions occur in response to airborne allergens, chemicals used in fragrances, and gastric reflux.

DIET AS A CONTRIBUTING FACTOR IN RESPIRATORY DISEASES

True food allergies are rare, but food intolerances are prevalent. True food allergies result in an immunoglobulin E (IgE) reaction, which can cause an anaphylactic reaction and in extreme cases can result in death. Food intolerances correlate with indigestibility, which occurs with casein (i.e., dairy), egg whites, and gluten (i.e., bread products). Gluten intolerance or sensitivity results in an immune response to gluten; information can be obtained online from the Celiac Disease Foundation. It is possible that most patients prescribed reflux medications (e.g., omeprazole) are unknowingly intolerant of common foods, and this is a significant issue given the prevalence of this class of medications in clinical practice.

In contrast to true food allergies, food sensitivities can be determined by testing for an immunoglobulin (IgG) reaction caused by repetitive exposures to specific foods. Food intolerances are common in the standard Western diet, which has now spread to the rest of the world. Food intolerances are particularly difficult to treat because patient resistance is high; patients are often unwilling to believe a possible food-symptom relationship or unable to make a sustained change in diet. People are rarely without favorite foods for which they have cravings and which likely are the culprits for their food intolerance. One solution is to keep a food journal, listing any associated symptoms that arise from various foods and specific ingredients. Clinicians can teach patients how to read food labels, which is easier since changes were incorporated into the U.S. 2016 Nutrition Facts Label requirements.

Indoor Air Quality

DUST

Dust is a commonly used term that encompasses a large amount of heterogeneous material. It consists of pulverized airborne particulates from biologic and inorganic sources. Organic materials in dust include insect feces, skin fragments, packaging, paper products, pet dander, dust mites, mold spores, and volatile organic pollutants. Inorganic materials in dust include volatile cleaning agents, carpet fragments, and limestone. Dust is so common as to be taken for granted, but this should not be the case, given the enormous impact dust can have on the health of the inhabitants who share the same space.

Because most people work, live, sleep, eat, and breathe in dusty environments, understanding the health consequences of dust is important, and identifying the sources of exposure is necessary to make improvements. As part of a comprehensive history and physical examination, clinicians should ask patients where they spend time. They should be questioned about how much time they spend at home or work; in school, church, other public buildings, or an automobile; and outdoors. All indoor and outdoor spaces have the likelihood of exposure to environmental toxins, although the specific toxins that impact allergy and asthma in outdoor air are different from those that create problems indoors.[10,37] For example, there are health effects of living near a freeway with high traffic volumes and exhaust levels from vehicles[39] or near construction sites with high levels of airborne particulates that can produce respiratory diseases such as silicosis and other inflammatory diseases such as obesity and diabetes.[40]

Opening windows in the home for fresh air ventilation seems like a reasonable idea, but it can have negative effects depending on the home's location. For example, in an area without paved roads, the amount of dust that is generated by passing cars and comes into the home through open windows can be significant. Living near a factory that releases polluting chemicals into the air and surrounding streams can also be dangerous.[18]

CONTROLLING DUST IN THE HOME

How do you assess the risk of living in your house? Do you consider your house dusty? Because controlling house dust is a critical factor, the question should be considered again after reading the information in this chapter. Modern houses provide a climate-controlled environment with recirculating air, which affects air quality in many ways. Minimizing illness and reducing medication use is the primary health goal, but most people do not realize that the amount of dust in their homes is related to the risk of airway inflammation resulting in asthma, allergy, and infection.

Methods used to identify and reduce dust exposure in everyday life focus primarily on the home, although they also apply to workplaces, schools, and indoor environments of all other buildings in which people spend time. Some well-known solutions include eliminating mold, removing carpets, and giving away pets to which members of the family have become allergic. Other concerns include the chemicals used in furniture, carpets, and construction materials (see Chapter 2); pesticides (see Chapter 8); fragrances (air fresheners); toxic antiseptic and disinfecting agents (see Chapter 9); and the interaction of chemicals with commonly used medications (see Chapter 7). Such sources are likely not as commonly recognized as being carried by dust or causing disease.

Endocrine-Disrupting Chemicals Associated with Dust in Homes. Dust is a transport vehicle for toxic chemicals and biologic debris, and it can greatly increase the concentrations of toxins that are inhaled. Chemicals stick to airborne particles and can cause respiratory inflammation and other systemic effects. For numerous chemicals, the airborne concentration is positively associated with the amount of dust. These are chemicals that off-gas or leach out of construction materials, carpets, adhesives, furniture, and other common household items (Fig. 4.1). Many of these chemicals are classified as endocrine disruptors (see Chapter 12), which can disrupt the hormonal control systems that regulate the functioning of cells, tissues, organs, and organ systems.[13,42]

In a house that has good air flow with limited insulation and few sealed windows, off-gassing of indoor toxic materials is not as critical an issue because particles are unable to concentrate. However, modern homes, which are designed to be energy efficient with limited indoor-outdoor airflow to improve costs, may increase chemical concentrations to levels that can be harmful to inhabitants.

One example of a toxic or carcinogenic group of chemicals that off-gasses from numerous household items is flame retardants.[3] The polybrominated diphenyl ethers (PBDEs) used as flame retardants are being phased out due to their neurobehavioral[17] and reproductive[15] toxicities. Unfortunately, the flame retardants used in beds, furniture, and carpets have been shown to be ineffective at the concentrations used in these products.

Flame retardant chemicals were widely introduced in 1975 under the California TB-117 law to reduce fires most commonly caused by unextinguished cigarettes. The law, however, was based on fraudulent data linked

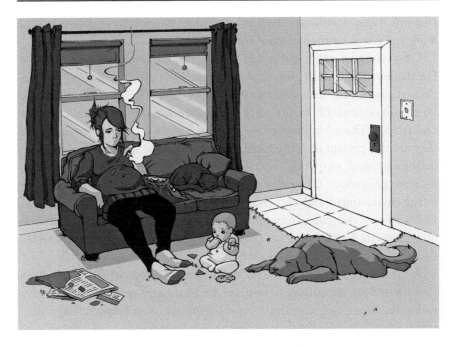

FIGURE 4.1. Sources of dust and toxic pollutants associated with dust levels in homes. The pregnant woman who is smoking is exposing her fetus and herself to nicotine and other components of cigarettes that are developmentally and metabolically disruptive chemicals and are also associated with asthma and cancer. The baby is sitting and eating food on a carpet that contains neurotoxic flame retardants. The fabric, sofa, and drapes also contain flame retardants. The carpet and sofa are sources of dust. The baby is holding a plastic doll that contains phthalates and BPA, both of which are developmental toxicants whose concentration in indoor air is related to levels of dust, to which the chemicals stick. Cat and dog dander on the couch and carpet is associated with asthma and allergy. Vinyl chloride flooring in front of the door and vinyl chloride window shades release the endocrine-disrupting chemical di-2-ethylhexyl phthalate (DEHP), the most toxic of the phthalates. Newspapers left on the floor are a source of mold and dust.

to the tobacco industry, which went on to orchestrate years of lobbying to prevent lawmakers from revising the law to no longer require toxic flame-retardant chemicals in couches, home furnishings, and baby products such as crib mattresses, baby car seats, and nursing pillows. More information is available in the California Technical Bulletin 117-2013 (Flammability Standard Requirements for Upholstered Furniture) and a series of articles documenting the role of the tobacco industry in orchestrating the fraud (http://articles. chicagotribune.com/keyword/flame-retardants). Despite turnover of TB-117, many products used for babies and children are still made with foam that contains flame retardants. The flame-retardant chemicals migrate out of the foam and are a common component in house dust.[43]

Off-gassing of other chemicals (e.g., formaldehyde) is also a concern. Formaldehyde is used in pressed-wood products. Highly fluorinated (perfluorinated) chemicals, such as perfluorooctanoic acid (PFOA) and perfluorooctane sulfonic acid (PFOS) are compounds found in stain-resistant carpeting and fabrics. These highly persistent compounds are being phased out, but they are still present in many products. They are used in cookware, clothing, outdoor apparel, carpeting, and food packaging to provide oil- and water-resistant properties. Like many other modern chemicals, they are persistent in the environment and have been detected in humans, other animals, and plants all over the globe. In humans, some highly fluorinated chemicals have been associated with cancers of the liver, pancreas, prostate, bladder, and testis and with metabolic diseases.[16,19,28]

Air fresheners are often used in homes to mask odors, which may indicate that the indoor air quality is suspect. Air fresheners may contain harmful endocrine-disrupting chemicals, especially those often found in fragrances, which are a class called phthalates that are not included on product packaging labels. Most cleaning products are scented, including facial and toilet tissue (see Chapter 9).

U.S. government regulatory agencies routinely classify these chemicals as "generally regarded as safe (GRAS)" without testing to determine whether they are actually safe (see Chapter 11). How did this happen? When data questioning the safety of a commercially used chemical appear, the tobacco industry tactic of manufacturing doubt is employed by paying for studies that support the safety of the chemical.[24,27,30]

Bisphenol A (BPA) is an estrogenic endocrine-disrupting chemical used to make polycarbonate plastic, and it is an additive in a wide range of other products as well. BPA sticks to dust and is inhaled.[35,36] BPA exposure in fetuses, infants, and children has been shown in a prospective study of children to be associated with a wide range of diseases, including impaired immune function, inflammation, asthma, and allergy.[11,33]

More than 1000 experiments with laboratory animals (i.e., fish, amphibians, reptiles, birds, and mammals, including monkeys) and 100 other epidemiologic studies, both prospective and cross-sectional, have shown that exposure to BPA during development or in adulthood is linked to an remarkable list of diseases that have been increasing in the United States and worldwide since the advent of the post–World War II chemical revolution (see Chapter 1). These diseases include obesity, type 2 diabetes, hypertension, coronary heart disease, impaired liver and kidney function, and reproductive effects in women, including endometrial disorders, polycystic ovary syndrome, reduced fertility, implantation failure, reduced embryo quality, miscarriage, premature delivery, breast cancer, and neural deficits. In human females and animals, fetal exposure to BPA increases aggressiveness and hyperactivity and impairs learning. Reproductive effects in men and male animals due to BPA exposure include reduced libido, reduced sperm quality, reduced embryo quality, altered thyroid hormone concentrations, and prostate cancer.[31,38,41]

Phthalates are a class of chemicals that are used as plasticizers in polyvinyl chloride (PVC) plastic found in building materials (e.g., flooring, shower curtains), cosmetics, dyes, artificial leather, adhesives, and a host of other common household products including fragrances (see Fig. 4.1). This class of chemicals off-gas and are associated with indoor dust levels and asthma (i.e., di-2-ethylhexyl phthalate [DEHP]), rhinitis, and eczema (i.e., butylbenzyl phthalate [BBzP]).[6] The levels of phthalates in homes correlate with the use of building materials, such as PVC flooring, shower curtains, and plastic window shades, and with many other characteristics of homes.[7] Other chemicals of concern for respiratory diseases that are found at elevated levels in indoor air are the aromatic hydrocarbons benzene, toluene, ethylbenzene, and xylene isomers (BTEX).[5]

Regulation

In the United States, there are no regulations regarding the selection of chemicals to replace known toxic chemicals such as DEHP and BPA after they are found to pose a human health hazard. DEHP is gradually being replaced with di-isononyl phthalate (DINP), which has been associated with atopic dermatitis and a variety of adverse neurobehavioral and reproductive effects similar to those of DEHP.[4,20] BPA is being replaced with other bisphenols, such as bisphenol S (BPS) and bisphenol F (BPF), and these replacements are now being found to pose human health risks similar to those of BPA,[34] although the public is being misled by advertising suggesting that a product is safe because it is BPA or DEHP free. This is a serious deficiency in the U.S. chemical regulation system (see Chapter 11).

The chemical industry sponsored a revision to the outdated Toxic Substance Control Act originally passed in 1976. The new legislation, called the Frank R. Lautenberg Chemical Safety for the 21st Century Act, prohibits states from passing legislation to regulate chemicals if federal regulators have placed them on a list of chemicals that they are examining. If a similar prohibition of local control had been placed on tobacco products, the reduction in smoking in the United States over the past 2 decades from 25% to 15% of the population, which was entirely driven by local ordinances restricting smoking in public places without any federal action, would never have occurred.

In 2007, the European Union (EU) mandated much stronger chemical regulation by passing the Regulation on Registration, Evaluation, Authorization, and Restriction of Chemicals (REACH) law, but EU chemical corporations have successfully managed to interfere with implementation of this law. Similarly, although in 1996 the U.S. Congress passed, almost unanimously, the Safe Drinking Water Act and Food Quality Protection Act, which mandated that the Environmental Protection Agency (EPA) (which is currently in sole control of chemical safety in the United States) address the issue of identifying the health effects of endocrine-disrupting chemicals, chemical corporations have successfully blocked all attempts by the EPA to implement the requirements of the law. This has led to harsh criticism by medical societies, including The Endocrine Society, which consists of clinicians and scientists with expertise in drugs and chemicals (e.g., BPA, DEHP) that disrupt normal endocrine function.[42]

Keeping a Clean House

Keeping a clean, dust-free house requires a plan. The amount of dust existing in modern homes is impressive but is not apparent to the average person. In Japan, it is customary to remove one's shoes before entering a house. Shoes track in a large amount of organic and inorganic material. This is just one of many practical approaches to reduce dust in the home.

HEATING, VENTILATION, AND AIR CONDITIONING SYSTEM

A critical detail is whether there is continuous air movement through the air-handling system or whether it turns on only when heat or cool air is needed. It is optimal to have air constantly circulating in the house rather than on-demand circulation. Adequate ventilation and an outside air source are important, with the air feeding through the air-handling system to filter dust.

Filters. The heating, ventilation, and air conditioning (HVAC) system requires a high-quality filter that is checked regularly and changed as needed. Air filters for HVAC systems have a minimum efficiency reporting value (MERV rating) to assess their effectiveness. The MERV rating (i.e., 1 to 16) identifies the size of particles trapped. Typical filters used in a home trap particles in the range of 0.3 to 10 μm). The higher the MERV rating, the greater the percentage of particles captured on each pass.

A MERV rating of 9 is sufficient to remove indoor air particles larger than 0.3 μm, including pollen, dust mites, cockroach debris, sanding dust, spray paint dust, textile fibers, carpet fibers, mold, spores, and cat and dog dander. Higher MERV ratings can also remove odors, smoke, and finer particles. Filters that meet high-efficiency particulate arrestance (HEPA) filter standards trap 99.7% of particles greater than 0.3 μm, which are dust particles that commonly carry toxic chemicals.

HUMIDITY CONTROL: MOLD AND MITES

Assessment of humidity in the home is critical to minimize mold and the infiltration of dust mites and other insects. Maintaining an airtight home at a humidity of less than 45% is important because a high humidity level is an indication of water infiltration. Keeping a dry house is more difficult in homes in tropical climates where the outside air is hot with a high relative humidity, compared with homes in nontropical climates.

If the relative humidity in a home is greater than 70%, dust mites can thrive in the absence of moisture from humans, such as in a bed with moisture from human sweat. Dust mite feces are the major source of mite allergens. High humidity levels in the home can lead to a vicious cycle. The mites feed on mold that grows in high-humidity conditions, and the mite feces contain mold spores that can germinate in a humid environment, producing more food for mites.[25]

A small, portable hygrometer is used to measure humidity. Humidity control is essential to discourage mold and dust mites that thrive in a moist environment but cannot thrive in a dry environment. Mold prefers moisture and cellulose from any carbon-containing product, such as boxes, newspapers, mail, or paper bags (see Fig. 4.1), which are common sources of dust in homes. There are many types of mold, and some species are particularly dangerous. Infants are most affected by the mycotoxins, and in rare cases, exposure can be fatal.[26]

Other places where mold is found in the home are windows and door sills, chimneys, leaking roofs, ducts with air-conditioning condensation, laundry rooms with damp items, storage areas under sinks, damp sponges or cleaning cloths, and carpeting with pet or vermin (mouse) urine. The most important issue regarding mold infestation after flooding or other events is its safe removal. Improper mold remediation can spread mold spores instead of eliminating them. High humidity levels after catastrophic water events can also increase exposure to mold spores, which can be ameliorated with the use of a dehumidifier. Knowing the home's humidity level can also reveal whether a humidifier may be needed in the winter, when a very low humidity level can lead to nose and lung irritation.

ITEMS TO FACILITATE KEEPING A HOUSE CLEAN

Free-Standing Air Purifiers. An air purifier should meet HEPA filter standards (i.e., clearing 99.7% of particles >0.3 µm) to adsorb dust particles that commonly carry chemicals. These filters adsorb chemical odors along with dust, and many are equipped with ultraviolet (UV) light that kills microorganisms and with ozone generation, although ozone has both positive and negative effects.[23] Ozone can be helpful in water-damaged buildings, but care should be taken because ozone is a common lung irritant associated with asthma and other respiratory diseases.[22]

Chemicals Off-Gassing from Carpets. Carpets contain toxic chemicals and are a significant source of dust. After purchase of a new carpet, it is important to provide an opportunity for off-gassing of toxic chemicals by opening windows and avoiding breathing the air for a few days or longer, depending on the product. One of the most striking examples of the impact of toxic carpets on health occurred at the EPA headquarters in the late 1980s.[29] In response to severe illnesses associated with the installation of carpets, the employees sued the EPA and prevailed.

Carpet padding, a major source of flame retardant chemicals, should be vetted for brands that do not use these harmful chemicals. Shoppers should look for labels on home furnishings (e.g., couch, pillows) that refer to the TB-117-2013 law, indicating that flame-retardant chemicals are not present. This California labeling requirement became mandatory on January 1, 2015.

Vacuums. It is important to minimize dust production and dispersal in air during cleaning. This requires use of a vacuum cleaner that is designed to contain the dust; information is available from Consumerreports.org. The vacuum cleaner should be designed so that the air blows through the filter and does not stir up more dust than it picks up. The device can be tested on dust found in locations not usually vacuumed, such as around the edges of carpeting, inside closets, under sinks, underneath furniture, behind bookshelves, and under beds.

If a good vacuum is not available, having the carpets and fabric coverings of chairs and sofas professionally cleaned is a good idea. This can be done without the use of cleaning chemicals (i.e., using only water), although professional cleaners may prefer chemicals that are, unknown to them, quite toxic (see Chapter 9). This deep cleaning can reveal how much dust is not being removed by vacuuming.

Dusting Products. Dusting products can rapidly pick up dust, but brands that contain fragrances, which consist of toxic chemicals, should be avoided. Because these products are easy to use, they can provide a solution for increasing the frequency of cleaning if there are substantial areas that are not carpeted.

Home Furnishings. Items brought into homes often remain in the home for many years, especially flooring (i.e., vinyl, synthetic wood, or pressboard), carpeting and carpet backing, and large or expensive objects such as couches, dressers, and bookshelves. It is wise to make informed choices before deciding on these purchases to avoid chronic exposure to toxins for many years.

Insecticides. Indoor use of insecticides is a particular concern if it leads to exposure of fetuses during pregnancy or exposure of infants, children, or adolescents[14] (see Chapter 8). Insecticides can lead to neurobehavioral and reproductive abnormalities. For example, the organophosphate insecticides chlorpyrifos (Dursban) and diazinon have been linked to abnormal neurobehavioral development, including small head circumference at birth, and to significantly reduced scores on tests of working memory, processing speed, verbal comprehension, perceptual reasoning, and full-scale intelligence quotient (IQ). Children exposed as fetuses in the highest quartile had a 7-point IQ deficit compared with children who as fetuses were in the lowest quartile for exposure.[8,14] The same concerns about these types of adverse effects are true for fungicides used to kill mold and rodenticides used to kill rodents.

Care needs to be taken regarding the use of herbicides on lawns and plants around the home. These pesticides pose a danger to infants, children, and pets. Infants and children are more likely than adults to be in direct contact with the ground, and they engage in more frequent hand-to-mouth behaviors.

Cleaning Materials. Cleaning materials are a source of dust. Most cleaning materials are scented and can directly irritate the upper airway (see Chapter 9). Sensitization to fragrances in cleaning materials, which contain phthalates that are associated with myriad adverse health effects, is also a health concern.[2]

Cookware. Teflon and high heat do not go well together. The manufacture of Teflon involves use of the carcinogenic chemical PFOA, also known as C8, which off-gasses from Teflon at high temperatures. This chemical is acutely toxic (deadly) to birds and can cause cancers and other diseases in humans. A troubling characteristic of PFOA is that it is highly persistent (i.e., resistant to breakdown), and its widespread use as a water and oil repellant in fabrics has resulted in measurable levels of PFOA in the bodies of almost everyone who is tested.[21]

Lead Paint. Houses built during or before 1978 should be checked for the presence of lead-containing paint. There are still thousands of U.S. homes that contain lead paint. Even very low levels of exposure to lead during early life, when the brain is developing, can permanently impair brain function and reduce IQ.[14,24]

Pets. Like humans, all animals shed. Birds and cats shed feathers, fur, and other dander even more than dogs do. Warm-blooded animals also carry many microorganisms and macroorganisms on their bodies.

For pet owners, symptoms can be deceptively minor and difficult to identify because the exposures are chronic. Subclinical symptoms, such as tissue swelling and chronic sinus or nasal inflammation, can result from chronic exposure to pet dander and reduce quality of life. This is a difficult issue for clinicians because suggesting that a family pet is the source of illness is often met with strong resistance to taking action (Fig. 4.2).

Reducing Allergic Symptoms Due to Indoor Air

- Determine the tightness of construction of the house and whether there is adequate air movement through the home (i.e., air exchange rate).
- Determine the insulation material used in the walls.
- Determine what type of HVAC system is installed and what type of filter is used.
- Check air ducts associated with the HVAC.
- How often is the house dusted? The accumulation of dust can be rapid.
- Drapes are a common source of dust, and they are difficult to clean.
- Get a glass cover for the chimney.
- In wood-burning stoves and fireplaces, firewood is a food source for various forms of life and creates dust.

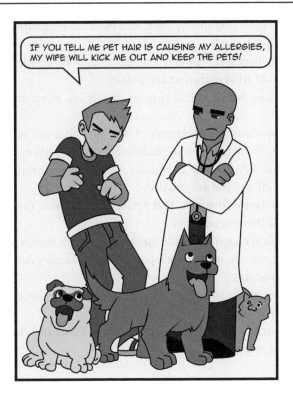

FIGURE 4.2. Pets are sources of allergies.

- Cooking is a source of dust; grilling inside is a bad idea because it generates smoke.
- Is there an exhaust fan to reduce dust or soot from cooking?
- Clean ceiling fans.
- Air purifiers reduce airborne dust but require maintenance of the filters to function properly.
- Keep the humidity of the home at about 45%. Check for mold.
- Do not keep paper products in areas with elevated moisture levels.
- Boxes are continually coming into peoples' houses. If stored, they can be a source of mold.
- Remove shoes when entering the home to reduce the level of outdoor contaminants.
- Mattresses, mattress covers, comforters, and pillows require protection against dust mites.
- If the house was built during or before 1978, check for lead paint.
- In older homes, lead in water pipes can result in lead-contaminated water.

- Inventory food containers, cups, and plates to determine how much plastic is being used.
- Food and beverages should not be heated in plastic containers, regardless of what manufacturers claim.
- Avoid having babies spend time on, crawl on, or eat food off vinyl floors.
- Reduce or eliminate children's plastic toys that are manufactured from PVC (which contains phthalates) or polycarbonate (which is made from BPA). These chemicals are absorbed through the skin; they also off-gas and are inhaled.
- Minimize fabric furniture and petrochemical foam that likely contains toxic flame retardants.
- Use chemical cleaning agents that have not been shown to be toxic.
- Limit the use of cosmetics, carpet powders, laundry detergents, and similar products.
- Do not ignore the impact of good nutrition and its benefit for resisting airborne allergens.
- Keep a journal tracking the health of inhabitants and changes in the home that might be associated with illness.

REFERENCES

1. Akinbami, L.J. 2006. The State of Childhood Asthma, United States, 1980–2005. Advance data from vital and health statistics, no. 381. Hyattsville, MD: National Center for Health Statistics.
2. Barrett, E.S., Parlett, L.E., Wang, C., Drobnis, E.Z., Redmon, J.B., & Swan, S.H. 2014. Environmental exposure to di-2-ethylhexyl phthalate is associated with low interest in sexual activity in premenopausal women. *Horm Behav.* 66:787–792.
3. Betts, K.S. 2008. Unwelcome guest: PBDEs in indoor dust. *Environ Health Perspect.* 116:A202–A208.
4. Boberg, J., Christiansen, S., Axelstad, M., et al. 2011. Reproductive and behavioral effects of diisononyl phthalate (DINP) in perinatally exposed rats. *Reprod Toxicol.* 31:200–209.
5. Bolden, A.L., Kwiatkowski, C.F., & Colborn, T. 2015. New look at BTEX: Are ambient levels a problem? *Environ Sci Technol.* 49:5261–5276.
6. Bornehag, C.G., Sundell, J., Weschler, C.J., et al. 2004. The association between asthma and allergic symptoms in children and phthalates in house dust: A nested case-control study. *Environ Health Perspect.* 112:1393–1397.
7. Bornehag, C.G., Lundgren, B., Weschler, C.J., Sigsgaard, T., Hagerhed-Engman, L., & Sundell, J. 2005. Phthalates in indoor dust and their association with building characteristics. *Environ Health Perspect.* 113:1399–1404.

8. Bouchard, M.F., Chevrier, J., Harley, K.G., et al. 2011. Prenatal exposure to organophosphate pesticides and IQ in 7-year-old children. *Environ Health Perspect.* 119:1189–1195.

9. Centers for Disease Control and Prevention, National Center for Health Statistics. 2016. Asthma. http://www.cdc.gov/nchs/fastats/asthma.htm.

10. den Dekker, H.T., Sonnenschein-van der Voort, A.M., de Jongste, J.C., et al. 2016. Early growth characteristics and the risk of reduced lung function and asthma: A meta-analysis of 25,000 children. *J Allergy Clin Immunol.* 137:1026–1035.

11. Donohue, K.M., Miller, R.L., Perzanowski, M.S., et al. 2013. Prenatal and postnatal bisphenol A exposure and asthma development among inner-city children. *J Allergy Clin Immunol.* 131:736–742.

12. Ferreira, F., Hawranek, T., Gruber, P., Wopfner, N., & Mari, A. 2004. Allergic cross-reactivity: From gene to the clinic. *Allergy.* 59:243–267.

13. Gore, A.C., Chappell, V.A., Fenton, S.E., et al. 2015. EDC-2: The Endocrine Society's Second Scientific Statement on Endocrine-Disrupting Chemicals. *Endocrine Rev.* 36:E1–E150.

14. Grandjean, P., & Landrigan, P.J. 2014. Neurobehavioural effects of developmental toxicity. *Lancet Neurol.* 13:330–338.

15. Harley, K.G., Marks, A.R., Chevrier, J., Bradman, A., Sjodin, A., & Eskenazi, B. 2010. PBDE concentrations in women's serum and fecundability. *Environ Health Perspect.* 118:699–704.

16. Heindel, J.J., Blumberg, B., Cave, M., et al. 2016. Metabolism disrupting chemicals and metabolic disorders. *Reprod Toxicol.* Online October 2016.

17. Herbstman, J.B., Sjodin, A., Kurzon, M., et al. 2010. Prenatal exposure to PBDEs and neurodevelopment. *Environ Health Perspect.* 118:712–719.

18. Kassotis, C.D., Alvarez, D.A., Taylor, J.A., Vom Saal, F.S., Nagel, S.C., & Tillitt, D.E. 2015. Characterization of Missouri surface waters near point sources of pollution reveals potential novel atmospheric route of exposure for bisphenol A and wastewater hormonal activity pattern. *Sci Total Env.* 524–525:384–393.

19. Klaunig, J.E., Hocevar, B.A., & Kamendulis, L.M. 2012. Mode of action analysis of perfluorooctanoic acid (PFOA) tumorigenicity and human relevance. *Reprod Toxicol.* 33:410–418.

20. Koike, E., Yanagisawa, R., Sadakane, K., Inoue, K., Ichinose, T., & Takano, H. 2010. Effects of diisononyl phthalate on atopic dermatitis in vivo and immunologic responses in vitro. *Environ Health Perspect.* 118:472–478.

21. Lam, J., Koustas, E., Sutton, P., et al. 2014. The Navigation Guide. Evidence-based medicine meets environmental health: Integration of animal and human evidence for PFOA effects on fetal growth. *Environ Health Perspect.* 122:1040–1051.

22. Malig, B.J., Pearson, D.L., Chang, Y.B., et al. 2016. A time-stratified case-crossover study of ambient ozone exposure and emergency department visits for specific respiratory diagnoses in California (2005–2008). *Environ Health Perspect.* 124:745–753.

23. Manuel, J. 1999. A healthy home environment? *Environ Health Perspect.* 107:A352–A357.

24. Markowitz, G., & Rosner, D. 2000. "Cater to the children": The role of the lead industry in a public health tragedy, 1900–1955. *Am J Public Health.* 90:36–46.

25. May, J. C. 2001. *My House Is Killing Me: The Home Guide for Families with Allergies and Asthma.* Baltimore: Johns Hopkins University Press.

26. May, J.C., & May, C.L. 2004. *The Mold Survival Guide: For Your Home and for Your Health.* Baltimore: Johns Hopkins University Press.

27. Michaels, D. 2005. Doubt is their product. *Sci Amer.* 292:96–101.

28. Nakayama, S., Harada, K., Inoue, K., et al. 2005. Distributions of perfluorooctanoic acid (PFOA) and perfluorooctane sulfonate (PFOS) in Japan and their toxicities. *Environ Sci.* 12:293–313.

29. National Federation of Federal Employees. 1989. Indoor air quality and work environment study: EPA headquarters buildings. https://nepis.epa.gov/Exe/ ZyNET.exe/91014F8Z.TXT?ZyActionD=ZyDocument&Client=EPA&Index=1986 +Thru+1990&Docs=&Query=&Time=&EndTime=&SearchMethod=1&TocRest rict=n&Toc=&TocEntry=&QField=&QFieldYear=&QFieldMonth=&QFieldDay =&IntQFieldOp=0&ExtQFieldOp=0&XmlQuery=&File=D%3A%5Czyfiles%5C Index%20Data%5C86thru90%5CTxt%5C00000027%5C91014F8Z.txt&User=AN ONYMOUS&Password=anonymous&SortMethod=h%7C-&MaximumDocume nts=1&FuzzyDegree=0&ImageQuality=r75g8/r75g8/x150y150g16/i425&Display= hpfr&DefSeekPage=x&SearchBack=ZyActionL&Back=ZyActionS&BackDesc=R esults%20page&MaximumPages=1&ZyEntry=1&SeekPage=x&ZyPURL.

30. Oreskes, N., & Conway, E.M. 2010. *Merchants of Doubt: How a Handful of Scientists Obscured the Truth on Issues from Tobacco Smoke to Global Warming.* New York, NY: Bloomsbury Press.

31. Peretz, J., Vrooman, L., Ricke, W.A., et al. 2014. Bisphenol A and reproductive health: Update of experimental and human evidence, 2007–2013. *Environ Health Perspect.* 122:775–786.

32. Polderman, T.J., Benyamin, B., de Leeuw, C.A., et al. 2015. Meta-analysis of the heritability of human traits based on fifty years of twin studies. *Nat Genet.* 47:702–709.

33. Robinson, L., & Miller, R. 2015. The impact of bisphenol A and phthalates on allergy, asthma, and immune function: A review of latest findings. *Curr Environ Health Rep.* 2:379–387.

34. Rochester, J.R., & Bolden, A.L. 2015. Bisphenol S and F: A systematic review and comparison of the hormonal activity of bisphenol A substitutes. *Environ Health Perspect.* 123:643–650.

35. Rudel, R.A., Brody, J.G., Spengler, J.D., et al. 2001. Identification of selected hormonally active agents and animal mammary carcinogens in commercial and residential air and dust samples. *J Air Waste Manag Assoc.* 51:499–513.

36. Rudel, R.A., Camann, D.E., Spengler, J.D., Korn, L.R., & Brody, J.G. 2003. Phthalates, alkylphenols, pesticides, polybrominated diphenyl ethers, and other endocrine-disrupting compounds in indoor air and dust. *Environ Sci Technol.* 37:4543–4553.

37. Schultz, E.S., Hallberg, J., Bellander, T., et al. 2016. Early-life exposure to traffic-related air pollution and lung function in adolescence. *Am J Respir Crit Care Med.* 193:171–177.
38. Seachrist, D.D., Bonk, K.W., Ho, S.M., Prins, G.S., Soto, A.M., & Keri, R.A. 2016. A review of the carcinogenic potential of bisphenol A. *Reprod Toxicol.* 59:167–182.
39. Shirinde, J., Wichmann, J., & Voyi, K. 2015. Allergic rhinitis, rhinoconjunctivitis and hayfever symptoms among children are associated with frequency of truck traffic near residences: A cross sectional study. *Environ Health.* 14:84.
40. Sun, Q., Yue, P., Deiuliis, J.A., et al. 2009. Ambient air pollution exaggerates adipose inflammation and insulin resistance in a mouse model of diet-induced obesity. *Circulation.* 119:538–546.
41. Vandenberg, L.N., Ehrlich, S., Belcher, S.M., et al. 2013. Low dose effects of bisphenol A: An integrated review of in vitro, laboratory animal and epidemiology studies. *Endocr Disrupt.* 1:e25078.
42. Zoeller, R.T., Brown, T.R., Doan, L.L., et al. 2012. Endocrine-disrupting chemicals and public health protection: A statement of principles from the endocrine society. *Endocrinology.* 153:4097–4110.
43. Zota, A.R., Rudel, R.A., Morello-Frosch, R.A., & Brody, J.G. 2008. Elevated house dust and serum concentrations of PBDEs in California: Unintended consequences of furniture flammability standards? *Environ Sci Technol.* 42:8158–8164.

5

Chemical Water Pollution and Human Health

CHRISTOPHER P. WEIS AND DONALD E. TILLITT

Key Concepts

- The overall quality of water in the United States surpasses that in most developed and developing countries of the world, but is threatened by increased demand for recycling, poorly controlled use and disposal of pharmaceuticals, as well as urban and agricultural runoff.
- The largest challenges for the future of water in the United States are aging infrastructure and increasing reliance on water recycling. If uncontrolled, leaching of lead and other metals from aging pipes poses a serious threat to children, pregnant women, and fetuses. Low levels of anthropogenic chemicals pose a poorly characterized threat to human health.
- Overuse and uncontrolled disposal of pharmaceuticals in agriculture and human medicine threaten water quality nationwide.
- Exposure to endocrine-disrupting chemicals can result in long-latency adverse effects, which have surpassed acute toxicity as a greater focus of regulatory reviews and re-registration of pesticides in recent years.
- Use of pesticides and fertilizers poses acute challenges to maintaining a healthy water supply because of direct exposures (e.g., atrazine in the Corn Belt, nitrates from ammonia application).
- Chronic threats to water quality from pharmaceuticals, antibiotics, household products, and pesticides require enhanced monitoring efforts and screening approaches.
- Increased vigilance for water security is needed to avoid catastrophic health occurrences.

Water Quality in the United States

Ample quantities of high-quality water are required for human health and the health of the environment. Threats to water quality and water security have increased globally in recent years, paralleling population growth and economic development. Many factors influence water quality and security. The greatest threats globally and in the United States are pollution and water diversion or management. These two drivers of water quality correlate with reductions in biodiversity in North America and across the world. Causal linkages between water pollution, water diversion, and poor water security or water quality have not been established, but correlations among these drivers are consistently observed across countries.[37]

In the United States, the threat index is reduced compared with similarly populated countries due to investments in water and wastewater treatment facilities and regulations such as the Clean Water Act, the Federal Water Pollution Control Act, the Safe Drinking Water Act, the National Environmental Policy Act, and the Federal Insecticide, Fungicide, and Rodenticide Act. These laws and others have helped guide the use of water, discharge of wastewater, and reduction of environmental pollution from chemicals and nutrients. The quality of surface water and drinking water in the United States is better because of such legislation and the resulting changes to water and waste handling systems.

The regulations in the Clean Water Act of 1972 gave the U.S. Environmental Protection Agency (EPA) authority to regulate the discharge of chemical pollutants into public waters and to set water quality standards "to restore and maintain the chemical, physical, and biological integrity of the nation's waters." These regulations fundamentally changed how water pollution regulation occurred in the United States. The authority for these regulations is delegated to the states, with the stipulation that each state must maintain standards that are at or above those of the EPA national standards.

The Clean Water Act defines water quality as the "suitability for a particular use." The Act requires states to adopt water quality standards that "provide, wherever attainable, water quality for the protection and propagation of fish, shellfish, and wildlife and recreation in and on the water" and that "consider the use and value of state waters for public water supplies, propagation of fish and wildlife, recreation, agricultural and industrial purposes, and navigation."[4] Physical characteristics (e.g., temperature, dissolved solids, pH), chemical characteristics (e.g., dissolved minerals, dissolved chemicals, dissolved oxygen), and biologic characteristics (e.g., bacteria, viruses, algae) of water quality are defined and regulated in receiving waters of the state based on the intended use (i.e., designated use) of those receiving waters.

Water quality criteria are established for chemical pollutants, based on scientific information of the known or potential effects of that chemical pollutant on the intended uses of the receiving waters, to achieve, maintain, or protect the water quality. Currently, EPA attempts to attain water quality standards by regulating the release of individual chemical pollutants through discharge permits at point sources and setting cumulative or total maximum daily loading (TMDL) of a pollutant for a watershed. The TMDL is the maximum amount of an individual chemical pollutant that may be in the water without adversely affecting water quality, as defined by the intended uses. A TMDL is calculated based on a safe concentration and allocation of loadings of the chemical into the waters from point and nonpoint sources within the drainage basin—essentially a pollutant budget for that water body.[4]

Even though the Clean Water Act and its enforcement have helped maintain and in some cases improve water quality in the United States, this type of regulatory system has challenges. An immense amount of information is required for understanding and predicting the fate of the chemical in the environment and its potential toxicity to fish, wildlife, humans, and the environment. Additionally, each chemical is regulated individually under the assumption of independent, noninteractive action on exposed organisms.

The intense data requirements for adequate regulation of chemical pollutants is magnified by the ever-increasing number of chemicals used in commerce, personal care products, agriculture, and industry. It is estimated that more than 2500 new chemicals enter the market each year and are added to the Toxic Substance Control Inventory.[6] The current Tox21 program is an intensive effort by the EPA, National Institutes of Health (NIH), and U.S. Food and Drug Administration (FDA) to develop toxicity data based on in silico predictions, in vitro screening assays, and high-throughput toxicologic assays.[7] Through this program, scientists are testing 10,000 chemicals and developing a battery of rapid, high-throughput testing protocols.

Drinking Water

METROPOLITAN WATER SUPPLIES

Approximately 86% of the U.S. population rely on water for domestic use from approximately 156,000 public water supplies. The EPA defines a public water supply as one having at least 15 connections or serving an average of at least 25 people. Most of this water is from surface sources, with less than 20% derived from publicly maintained groundwater wells. In 2010, there were about 51,000 U.S. community water delivery systems (i.e., systems serving water to the same population year round). However, only 8% of these systems supply water for 82% of the population.[2]

Overall, fresh water use in the United States is estimated at 355 billion gallons per day, almost one half of which is devoted to the generation of thermoelectric power through coal-fired or other secondary steam-generating systems. Another one third is for irrigation of crops, with most irrigation occurring in the drier, western regions of the country.

Although community water treatment systems vary in their approach to ensuring the purification and delivery of clean water, the process usually includes the following steps:

- *Coagulation and flocculation:* This step neutralizes the negative charge of dissolved particles, causing them to precipitate and settle from the water column.
- *Sedimentation:* Precipitated floc settles to the bottom of the water supply.
- *Filtration:* After floc has settled out of the water column, clean water can be mechanically filtered using a variety of substances and techniques to remove contaminants. This step may involve filtration through sand, gravel, or charcoal to remove dusts, organic chemicals, parasites, bacteria, or viruses.
- *Disinfection:* After filtration is complete, disinfectants such as chlorine or chloramine may be added to kill remaining pathogens and suppress further contamination in the distribution system.

As many as 40% of U.S. households also employ point-of-entry or point-of-use treatment systems to further ensure purification of their household water. These systems include filters, water softeners, distillation systems, and disinfection systems. The Centers for Disease Control and Prevention (CDC), the EPA, and the National Sanitation Foundation recommend these systems for people with compromised immune systems.

More than 97% of the 156,000 U.S. public water systems serve fewer than 10,000 people. These small water producers face complex challenges to ensure the delivery of clean water to customers connected to the system. Finding the financial, technical, and operational resources to sustainably manage these systems is difficult and requires knowledge and investment from the entire community. Compliance with federal and state drinking water regulations is required but not always monitored as effectively as necessary.

Federal drinking water regulations are promulgated by the EPA and include the National Primary Drinking Water Regulations (NPDWRs) and limits for microorganisms, disinfectants, disinfection byproducts, inorganic chemicals, organic chemicals, and radionuclides.[8] The cost and availability of treatment and laboratory analysis may be difficult, if not cost-prohibitive. Often, administrators of these drinking water systems find it more cost-effective and practical to use nontreatment options employing multiple barriers rather than install expensive treatment systems requiring maintenance and skilled operators. Nontreatment options include careful protection of the source of water and well-maintained storage and distribution systems, along with clear communication to the public.

INDIVIDUAL WELLS

More than 15 million U.S. households rely on private wells for delivery of drinking water. The wells are not covered by regulatory requirements of the NPDWRs. The siting and initial construction of wells is critical to protect them from contamination. State and county regulations and supportive information on well depth and placement offer individuals some protection against foul water and potential threats.

Inappropriate siting of domestic wells near sources of bacteriologic contamination, dysfunctional wastewater treatment systems, industrial wastes, or areas of chemical groundwater contamination can make well water unsafe or unusable. Nearby use of fertilizers and pesticides and disposal of other household or automobile chemicals can easily contaminate a shallow well. In some areas of the United States, naturally occurring minerals can contaminate wells with substances such as arsenic, lead, and radon. The CDC recommends testing domestic wells at least once each year for pathogens and possible contamination from natural or man-made contaminants.

AGRICULTURAL USE OF WASTEWATER AND BIOSOLIDS

Approximately 127 billion gallons of water per day are used for agricultural purposes in the United States. Approximately 30% of this water is devoted to irrigation, with the balance attributed to livestock and aquaculture. U.S. irrigation practices are varied and include flood or furrow irrigation, drip irrigation, and spraying techniques, which are the most wasteful because much of the water sprayed or misted into the air evaporates before reaching the ground.

Application, irrigation, overland flow, and percolation through the soil are common wastewater disposal practices in the United States. These processes strain suspended solids by filtration through the soil. Organic matter and colloids are adsorbed to soil particles, and nutrients are used by vegetation.

Ground and surface water quality for overland disposal of wastewater is protected by the National Pollutant Discharge Elimination System (NPDES) permitting program, which is designed to ensure that receiving waters (i.e., surface or ground waters) meet applicable water quality standards. The sewage sludge (i.e., solids) generated during the disposal process is managed by approved practices and operational standards, and it is treated by aerobic or anaerobic digestion until contaminant and pathogen reduction standards are met. Treated sludge is often referred to as *biosolid* and is available for recycling, for use as fertilizer, or for soil improvement. Sludge that is applied on land or disposed of in unlined surface sites is monitored for inorganic contaminants, pathogen indicators (e.g., *Escherichia coli*), and odors that may attract disease vectors such as rodents.

Unfortunately, recalcitrant man-made organic chemicals such as the perfluoroalkyls (PFAs) are highly resistant to degradation in the environment and are not efficiently removed during commonly employed wastewater treatment processes. These and other recalcitrant chemicals and pesticides are not regulated by federal biosolid rules. They can find their way through the system and into foods, livestock, and water supplies. A nationwide study[36] found PFA concentrations in biosolids collected from 32 states as high as 990 ng/g.

ACUTE AND CHRONIC THREATS TO THE WATER SUPPLY

Acute Threats. Unauthorized discharges into public wastewater pose a threat to human and ecologic health downstream. Examples include accidental spills, terrorist activities, disposal of persistent toxic compounds into the system. Treatment plant operators work to reduce or eliminate the impact of sudden upsets to their biologic treatment operations by establishing early warnings of anomalies in the system through sophisticated algorithms that rely on a clear understanding of the system's history and past performance. Despite efforts to predict anomalies, upsets and threats to waste treatment and water delivery systems remain a significant problem.

Chemical Accidents. On April 17, 2013, a wooden warehouse in the city of West, Texas, exploded, killing 15 total casualties as described by the United States Chemical Safety Board report (http://www.csb.gov/assets/1/7/West_Fertilizer_FINAL_Report_for_website_021216.pdf). The explosion flattened more than 500 homes and displaced 2800 residents in the small farming community. The crater created by the blast destroyed the main water line, eliminating access to water and causing the city to issue a multiweek boil order after service was restored.

The explosion was caused by the inappropriate storage of a strong oxidizer, the common fertilizer ammonium nitrate. The nitrate was stored in wooden barrels near an organic fuel source—seeds stored overhead that were being staged for spring planting. A fire attributed to arson by the Bureau of Alcohol, Tobacco, Firearms, and Explosives provided a source of ignition for the deadly chemical mixture. The massive explosion, equivalent to a 2.1 magnitude earthquake, left a crater 93 feet wide.

In the wake of the chemical explosion disaster in West, Texas, President Barack Obama issued an executive order[28] forming an interagency working group to improve chemical safety at storage facilities nationwide. Despite significant efforts by this new interagency working group, between 2013 and 2015, there were more than 165 major chemical spills, fires, and oil pipeline leaks that damaged or threatened drinking water systems for thousands of Americans. Fortunately, not all chemical accidents are as spectacular or as deadly as the incident in West, Texas. However, over the years, these large and small events have demonstrated that populations use and live near chemical storage facilities that can pose significant threats if their physicochemical characteristics are misunderstood or if they are mishandled. These avoidable accidents, malicious spills, and uncontrolled chemical leaks can cause acute and sometimes disastrous threats to water supplies.

On January 9, 2014, the residents of Charleston, West Virginia, awoke to the acrid odor of licorice in their drinking water supply. The smell was caused by 4-methylcyclohexanemethanol (MCHM), a chemical used in industry to separate usable coal from mining debris and coal dust. Ten thousand gallons of MCHM had leaked from a storage tank into the Elk River one-half mile upstream from the Charleston municipal surface water intake.

So little information was available about this unusual chemical that the National Library of Medicine in Bethesda, MD, had no records of its use or potential toxicity. Because of the regulatory structure in the United States, this proprietary information about MCHM was held confidentially by the chemical manufacturer and released only after urgent requests by the NIH, which initiated studies of the chemical by the National Toxicology Program (Fig. 5.1).

In response to the Charleston spill and coupled with the lack of toxicologic data on MCHM, the CDC and the state of West Virginia issued a *Do Not Use* recommendation, preventing more than 300,000 West Virginians from accessing water for any household use. The Do Not Use order caused residents to search desperately for water for drinking and for clothes washing, bathing,

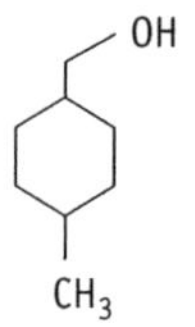

National Toxicology Program Studies on MCHM:

- High throughput screening.
- Structure-activity relationship analysis
- Bacterial mutagenicity assays
- Zebrafish developmental toxicity tests
- 5-Day rat toxicogenomic analysis
- Mouse dermal irritation and hypersensitivity
- Prenatal developmental toxicity
- Nematode toxicity

FIGURE 5.1. Studies concerning 4-methylcyclohexanemethanol (MCHM), a chemical that contaminated the Elk River near Charleston West Virginia, in January 2014. Only afterward was MCHM subjected to research by the U.S. National Toxicology Program.

and cooking. The National Guard of West Virginia instituted a massive effort to provide water to the population.

Such incidents provide an urgent reminder that safe water is critical for good health and essential to the social structure in urban communities. Fortunately for the citizens of Charleston, the National Toxicology Program determined MCHM to have low toxicity at the exposure levels recorded there, with little possibility of chronic health effects.

A similar tragedy occurred in Flint, Michigan, when in the spring of 2014, city officials switched the primary water supply from Lake Huron to the Flint River in an apparent[39] attempt to economize on the cost of drinking water. The water in the Flint River, with a history of significant pollution, is considerably more corrosive[40] than the water in Lake Huron. The corrosive water of the Flint River caused iron to leach from the distribution lines and lead to leach from proximity water supply lines to an estimated 45,000 homes.

On January 16, 2016, President Obama signed an emergency declaration ordering federal assistance to support state and local responses to the crisis. By April of 2016, more than 1700 of the samples collected by the state of Michigan had returned analytic results at concentrations greater than the EPA-recommended limit for lead in drinking water (i.e., 15 ppb).[26] Some of the highest-level samples collected exceeded the EPA limit by more than 1000 times.

The U.S. Department of Health and Human Services (HHS) led an effort supported by emergency response teams from the EPA. According to the National Toxicology Program, even at blood concentrations of 10 µg/dL or lower, lead is known to cause a variety of health effects, including delayed puberty, decreased IQ, and increased incidence of neurobehavioral problems including attention deficit hyperactivity disorder (ADHD).[41]

Acute threats to the water supply remind us of the importance of this precious resource. Lack of access to community water due to a chemical incident is terrifying and potentially dangerous. Understanding the vulnerabilities of access to water is a shared responsibility among members of the community. That responsibility starts with learning how and from where this precious resource comes, who is caring for it, and what the options are if it suddenly disappears.

Plating Operations. A large fraction of hazardous waste cleanup projects are initiated in response to failure of waste control at metal finishing (plating) operations. Metals associated with plating systems include cadmium, chromium, copper, cyanide, nickel, silver, and zinc. Zinc and copper in these wastes are particularly toxic to aquatic organisms that are essential for efficient biologic degradation of wastes. In the absence of sophisticated treatment systems to remove metals and acid-contaminated waters from the plating process waste, these facilities pose a destructive threat to the aerobic biologic systems of wastewater treatment plants (WWTPs).

Terrorist Threats. The potential vulnerabilities of systems that supply safe drinking water have not escaped the authorities responsible for protecting them. There is a long history of such attacks, including physical threats and incidents of biologic and chemical contamination of public systems.[16] Although the use of chemical or biologic substances to cause mass casualties in a large urban drinking water supply would be technically difficult, localized contamination is entirely possible, as was illustrated by a thwarted 2002 attack on the U.S. Embassy in Rome. In that case, fortunately, the chemical agent was poorly selected. Potassium ferricyanide, which the Salifist terror group was planning to use in the attack, is not particularly poisonous and would not have been likely to harm the residents or workers in the embassy.[23] The likelihood of purposeful contamination of a municipal supply with a biologic pathogen or toxin, although not impossible, is greatly reduced by the overall volume of water in most systems coupled with existing treatment and filtration systems designed to remove such contaminants.

In the wake of the terror events of September 2001, most systems have improved surveillance and security measures, further diminishing the possibility of a terror event of any significance. The Bioterrorism Act of 2002[11] requires drinking water utilities that serve more than 3300 people to conduct vulnerability assessments and develop plans to respond to emergencies affecting drinking water supplies. Nonetheless, the Federal Bureau of

Investigation, in cooperation with the Department of Homeland Security and EPA's Criminal Investigations Division, has established a well-exercised program for the identification and assessment of threats against the water supply.

Chronic Threats

Persistent Organic Pollutants. An ongoing threat is presented by low-level contamination from man-made organic chemicals that make their way into the potable water supply through complex environmental pathways, including the decay of aging distribution infrastructure. These low-level toxicants include agricultural and human medicines, pesticide residues, and household and industrial organic or metallic wastes. Engineering approaches to remove low-level organic and metallic contaminants are costly to install and maintain.

A study conducted by the U.S. Geological Survey in 2002 identified the presence of organic chemicals derived from wastewater in more than 80% of 139 streams across 30 states.[21] Many of these compounds include chemicals that are known to have androgenic and estrogenic activity at very low concentrations. Pharmaceutical chemicals that are disposed down the drain or deposited in agricultural and domestic waste streams eventually make their way into drinking water sources. As pressures to recycle water for industrial and domestic use increase, the importance of treatment technologies that can effectively remove these contaminants at biologically significant concentrations grows (see Chapter 13).

As concerns grow about the scarcity of water in regions susceptible to drought and water shortages, the need to effectively recycle water is increasing. Florida currently leads the nation in the amount of water recycled and reused. In 2013, the state reclaimed more than 700 million gallons of water each day for beneficial purposes.[21]

To save on costs associated with the purchase of water, many industrial facilities and utilities that supply water to drought-prone communities are researching treatment methods for indirect potable use of recycled water. *Indirect potable use* refers to the addition of purified recycled water to domestic water drinking water. This practice is common in larger utilities and is expected to increase as demands on the drinking water supply increase. Some utilities are exploring feasibility and methods for 100% reuse of water resources.

Unfortunately, the infrastructure necessary to produce and distribute clean water is aging rapidly at the same time that water resources are being threatened by population growth, climate change, and increasing contamination.

New methods for filtering and purifying drinking water at the level of the utility suppliers are negated by deterioration of distribution systems and the questionable quality of pipes near the drinking water tap. As highlighted by the 2014 tragedy in Flint, subtle changes in water chemistry can have drastic consequences for users who rely on this aging distribution system.

As the population of the United States grows, so does the demand for clean, safe water, but we continue to use this precious drinking water resource for industrial processes, disposal of domestic and industrial wastes, avenues for urban storm water runoff, and the unconventional extraction of fossil fuels by hydraulic fracturing. The burden of cleaning and recycling these wastewaters increasingly relies on effective engineering solutions and treatment systems that can recycle wastewaters into a resource fit for reuse, including drinking water.[24]

ENDOCRINE-DISRUPTING CHEMICALS AND THREATS TO ECOLOGIC AND HUMAN HEALTH

Chemical pollutants that interact with endocrine signaling pathways and subsequently alter normal homeostasis of organs and their function are referred to as *endocrine-disrupting chemicals* (EDCs). Evidence for the ability of environmental pollutants to alter hormone control and function has been found in wildlife populations, laboratory animals, and humans. Hormones exert regulatory actions and signaling functions at low blood serum concentrations (i.e., nanomole to picomole range). EDCs, particularly those that mimic hormone structure and function, can disrupt endocrine-controlled systems at very low exposure concentrations.[35] Small concentrations of EDCs can bring about complete reproductive failure in wildlife and cause population collapse.[20]

Evidence for disruption of endocrine systems in wildlife was first documented in the mid-20th century. However, recognition of the widespread nature of EDC impacts did not occur until the 1990s with the publication in 1996 of the book, *Our Stolen Future*.[3] Since then, regulatory screening and toxicologic testing protocols for chemicals have been completely changed based on the chronic, low-dose effects of EDC exposure.

Over the past 2 decades, an extensive amount of research into the effects and mechanisms of EDCs on humans and wildlife has clarified the threats these chemicals pose to water quality and environmental health. In addition to the low-dose effects of EDCs, chemicals that act through disruption of normal endocrine function often elicit nonmonotonic dose-response relationships. Classic toxicologic paradigms are based on linear dose-response relationships, with increasing chemical doses leading to linear increases in symptoms of toxicity. All regulatory actions, including determination of safe concentrations of chemicals in consumer products, foods, drugs, and releases to the environment, are based on the concept of linear dose-response relationships.

In this context, EDCs pose an uncertain risk that may or may not be quantified correctly because their graded dose-response relationships do not follow a linear form. EDCs can have U-shaped or inverted U–shaped dose-response curves, meaning that there can be greater effects at low doses. This has posed an extreme challenge to regulatory agencies in making certain the threshold concentrations of chemicals they define are safe.

EDCs can have effects on development, with adverse health outcomes occurring at a later time in adults, which also has troublesome implications for defining public safety and protecting human and environmental health. Development is sensitive to endocrine signaling, particularly during certain critical windows such as organogenesis. An example of the delayed consequences of EDC exposure during development was the exposure of pregnant women to diethylstilbestrol (DES), a drug that was widely prescribed in the mistaken belief that it would help maintain pregnancy and reduce complications. Daughters born to women who took this drug had high rates of vaginal clear cell carcinoma beginning at age 16 after exposure in utero. The latency of effects is an additional challenge to understanding the risk posed by EDC contamination of surface and drinking waters.

The chemical structures and physical properties of chemicals that can disrupt normal endocrine function do not fall into a single class or category. The structures of EDCs vary greatly due to the wide variety of biochemical mechanisms and molecular targets along the endocrine signaling pathways (Fig. 5.2). Disruption of endocrine communication systems occurs through multiple mechanisms. Among the possible mechanisms through which EDCs can exert their effects are activation of hormone receptors (i.e., agonist or mimetic chemicals), blockade of receptor signaling (i.e., antagonist), inhibition of hormone synthesis and degradation pathways, and displacement of hormones from serum carrier proteins. This wide array of biochemical and molecular targets for disruption of endocrine function by EDCs is a result of a multitude of chemical structures capable of interactions with the various receptors, carrier proteins, and enzymes. This becomes important because the structure of the chemical dictates where it will go in the environment (e.g., stay in water, accumulate in fish).

EDCs fall into two broad categories: those that are persistent and bioaccumulate and those with chemical structures that are more water soluble and do not bioaccumulate or persist. Both types of EDCs can be problematic as water

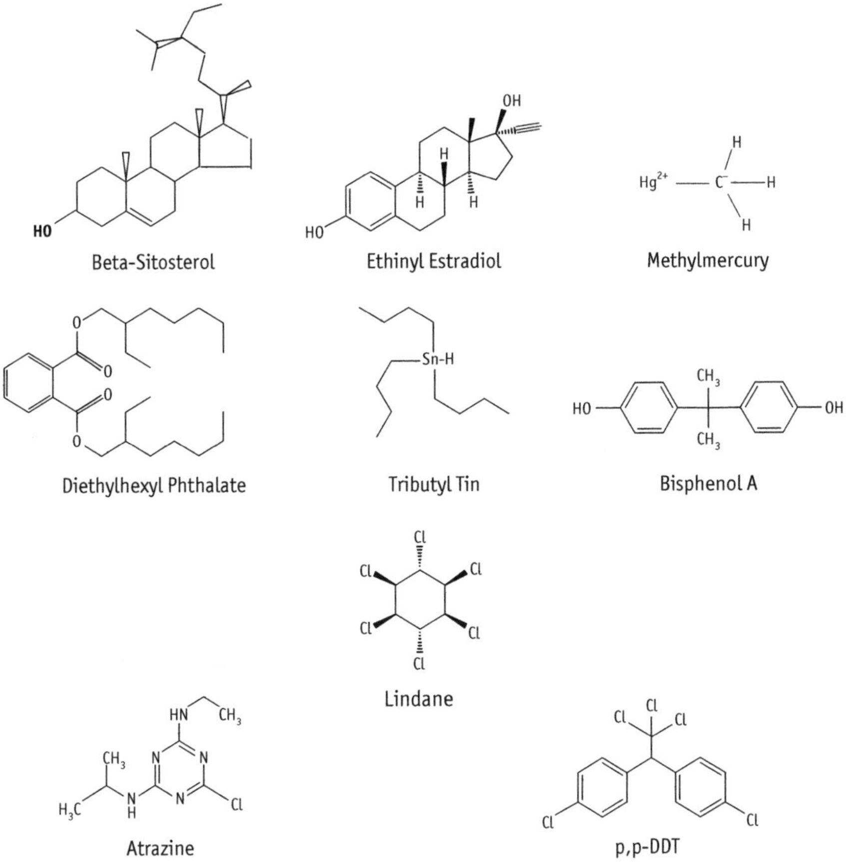

FIGURE 5.2. Structural diversity of endocrine-disrupting chemicals, which are common surface and ground water pollutants.

pollutants. The persistent EDCs are often *legacy contaminants,* most of which have been banned because they are persistent, effective at low concentrations, and bioaccumulate in the environment. Examples of these EDCs are the poly-chlorinated biphenyls (PCBs), which were formerly used in industry, and the agricultural pesticides dichlorodiphenyltrichloroethane (DDT) and lindane. Chronic exposure of wildlife to legacy chemicals occurs through water pollution and bioaccumulation, but human exposures are largely from dietary intake, such as consumption of fish from a contaminated area. In the United States, fish consumption advisories occur in all 50 states[10] and are usually based on legacy contaminants. State fish advisories offer guidance on reducing exposure and identifying risks posed through consumption of contaminated fish.

The less persistent EDCs can still pose an exposure concern based on the fact that they are continually used and released into surface or ground waters. Chronic exposure to these less-persistent EDCs can be more insidious to predict and their risk more difficult to evaluate due to ever-changing concentrations and minimal monitoring.

An example of a less-persistent EDC with continuous environmental release is the birth control agent ethinyl estradiol (EE2), which is found in most birth control pills. Humans excrete EE2 as a sugar conjugate (i.e., glucuronide), a portion of which is passed through wastewater treatment facilities. The original chemical (EE2) can be regenerated (i.e., deconjugated) in the effluent or sediments through bacterial enzymes and released into the environment.[5] This was first discovered based on effects observed in fish downstream from wastewater treatment facilities in certain streams in the United Kingdom.[17] Small concentrations (i.e., low nanogram per liter amounts) of potent estrogens such as EE2 can have dramatic effects on wildlife populations, including intersex, reproductive failure, and population crashes.[20]

Small amounts of potent pharmaceuticals can elicit adverse effects on wildlife populations. The same molecular targets (i.e., receptors) that the pharmaceuticals were designed to affect in humans are often conserved phylogenetically, and it is therefore not surprising that wildlife continuously exposed to EDCs under environmental conditions can have altered endocrine function and adverse health outcomes.

Exposure Pathways

Chemical pollutants are released into surface and ground waters from a diverse array of sources. Millions of tons of pesticides are intentionally applied to agricultural lands or used in urban household settings each year. Fertilizers with nitrogen and phosphorous are applied to farmlands and run off into streams, rivers, and lakes, producing harmful algal blooms, oxygen depletion, and nitrates in ground water at toxic levels.

Municipal use of water, even after treatment in WWTPs, releases a wide variety of pharmaceuticals, macronutrients, personal care products, household cleaners, and pesticides into surface waters, often with uncharacterized degrees of risk. Industrial use of freshwater is approximately 5% of total use in the United States[19]; another 37% is used for power generation, and ever-increasing amounts are used in oil and gas operations for hydraulic fracturing and extraction techniques.

Mining operations mobilize millions of tons of mineral and earth elements and often are associated with moderate to extensive environmental contamination of surface and ground waters.[42] Hazardous waste sites and chemical or oil spills are another source of pollutant release into water resources. Each source of chemical contamination to water and drinking water supplies adds risk to our water security.

Enhanced industrialization of countries such as in China, India, and Brazil puts more stress on waterways and threatens water security and quality because the regulatory framework for water protection is not in place in these countries. Although the United States has greater water consumption per capita, regulations such as the Clean Water Act and other statutes have provided much greater protection for water quality and water security.

The following sections address some common sources of pollution to ground and surface waters that threaten water quality and water security.

PHARMACEUTICAL USE AND DISPOSAL AND OCCURRENCE IN MAJOR DRINKING WATER SUPPLIES

A growing number of pharmaceuticals are being consumed annually for human health care and intensive agriculture production. More affluent societies have increased life spans, with greater use of medications and drugs. The use of pharmaceuticals, particularly antibiotics, in intensive livestock operations for growth promotion and disease prevention is the greatest use of antibiotics in the United States.[25,34] Waste from the animals contains up to 80% of the administered amount of the antibiotic and is applied to crop land as fertilizer.[12] As a result of these greater uses, more pharmaceuticals are being found in water, soil, sediments, and biologic compartments of the environment. Most observed concentrations are small or minimal, usually in the range of nanograms per liter and sometimes reaching low micrograms per liter concentrations.

Pharmaceuticals are designed specifically to be active at a specific target or mode of action. In some cases, pharmaceuticals in the environment affect fish and wildlife populations. Examples include EE2 from WWTPs causing intersex in fish[17] and diclofenac-induced crashes of vulture populations in Eurasia.[27] The estimated human risks from exposure to pharmaceutical chemicals in water are expected to be low.[1] No systematic monitoring for pharmaceuticals in drinking water exists in any country, which exaggerates the uncertainty of estimates of risk. Continued vigilance is required to ensure these threats to water quality remain low for humans. The greatest threat of pharmaceuticals in water for human health is the potential for antibiotic resistance to develop in microbes near intensive animal feeding operations.

AGRICULTURAL CHEMICAL USE AND THE CONTAMINATION OF STREAMS, RIVERS, AND RURAL WELLS OR DISTRIBUTION FACILITIES

Intensive agricultural practices around the world have led to increased use of pesticides over the past 4 decades to enhance productivity and crop yield. Annually in the United States alone, more than 230 million kg of fungicides, herbicides, and insecticides are used and released into the environment.[33]

The benefits of pesticide use have been observed in a number of crops, but the unintentional and unpredicted consequences of pesticides on water quality are the subject of routine monitoring and investigation in the United States. The U.S. Geological Survey (USGS) National Water-Quality Assessment (NAWQA) Program was instituted as a national program to monitor pesticides and other aspects of water quality in rivers and streams across the United States.[15] Over the period during which the NAWQA Program has been monitored (1992 to present), pesticide concentrations in surface waters have paralleled trends in usage. There have been declines in concentrations of several pesticides (e.g., cyanazine, alachlor, metalochlor, chlorpyrifos, malathion, diazinon, carbaryl, carbofuran) nationally, but concentrations of the high-use herbicides simazine and atrazine have remained constant over this period.[31]

In these cases, the human health concerns related to exposure to pesticides in water come from contamination of ground water. Chemicals that might be expected to degrade in surface waters can be more persistent in ground water.[15] For example, the drinking water standard for atrazine and its metabolites is predicted to be exceeded in large areas of the Corn Belt, as well as in portions of the mid-Atlantic region in the Chesapeake Bay watershed and in sections of the San Joaquin Valley of California.[32]

Contamination of ground water occurs over long periods and offers a significant challenge for state and federal regulatory agencies and affected communities. Communities affected by atrazine contamination of their drinking water supplies have had to sue the manufacturer (Syngenta Corporation) in efforts to have the company pay for technologies to adapt treatment facilities for removal of these contaminants from their water supply systems.[13] The adverse health outcomes of atrazine in drinking water at or above the standard (3 μg/L) are yet to be fully resolved. This example demonstrates the need for continued and in some cases enhanced protection of water supplies from unsuspected contamination resulting from agricultural practices. The benefits of agricultural pesticides need to be balanced against the threats they may pose to water quality and security.

INDUSTRIAL AND MUNICIPAL EFFLUENTS, WASTE DISPOSAL, AND URBAN RUNOFF

Surface water discharges of effluents from municipal and industrial facilities have historically been major concerns as sources for chemical water pollution. In the United States, regulations controlling the release of toxic substances from point sources come from the Clean Water Act of 1972, under provisions of the NPDES. According to the legislation, "it is national policy that the discharge of toxic pollutants in toxic amounts be prohibited."[22] The NPDES is a program that develops standards for industrial and municipal effluent discharges. Although imperfect in many respects, the NPDES program has been largely successful in reducing and in some cases identifying pollutant discharges into surface waters of the country.

Municipal WWTPs were largely designed to remove nutrient pollution but not toxic chemicals. It has been challenging for water treatment managers to meet the intent of the Clean Water Act. However, changes in WWTP facility design to include treatment processes, technologies, and operations that can reduce certain chemical pollutants have greatly improved their function over the past 3 decades. Through these regulations and investments in physical infrastructure, the United States has maintained certain aspects of water quality and water security in the face of ever-expanding populations and water use. With greater water use and greater numbers of chemicals entering municipal wastewater systems in developed and undeveloped countries, investment and re-investment in water treatment technologies and systems is more important than ever.

Urban runoff containing pesticides, nutrients, and road-related chemicals such as oil, salts, and coal-tar sealants has long been recognized as an important source of pollution of streams and rivers.[38] Only recently has the extent and quantification of nonpoint source runoff from urban landscapes been appreciated for its contributions to declining water quality.[14] Examination of threats to water quality from urban sources of chemicals, like much of the past assessments of water quality related to chemical contamination, has focused on acute toxicity. However, chronic effects such as those caused by EDCs have been the greater focus of regulatory reviews and re-registration of pesticides in recent years.

FRACKING CHEMICALS AND THE THREAT TO SURFACE AND GROUND WATER

The combination of oil and gas technologies of hydraulic fracturing (hydrofracturing or fracking) and horizontal drilling has revolutionized this

industry around the world. Oil and gas are extracted from geologic forma-
tions after high-pressure hydraulic fracturing. The practice has opened up
areas to oil and gas extraction that had never previously been economically
feasible to exploit, such as the Marcellus Shale formation in Pennsylvania and
the Williston Basin in North Dakota.

Threats to water quality from fracking are manifold. The practice of hydrofracturing oil and gas requires the use of millions of gallons of fresh water
and creates millions of gallons of wastewater. Large amounts of chemicals
are used at different stages of the process and contaminate the water used. In
the United States, these chemicals are considered proprietary and often are
undisclosed. Because U.S. industry was granted exemption from key statutes
of the Clean Water Act and Safe Drinking Water Act, many standard protec-
tions have been lost. Hydrofracturing in certain regions poses a high risk
of contamination by injection of hydrofracturing fluids directly into ground
water aquifers. Disposal of the wastewaters requires transport and handling
of millions of gallons, which are subject to spills and mishandling. Many
types of chemicals are used in hydrofracturing oil and gas operations.[18]

PATHWAYS FOR HUMAN EXPOSURE
TO CONTAMINANTS IN WATER

Effective maintenance of public health and prevention of environmental disease rely heavily on a detailed analysis of exposure. Without a clear understanding of each component of the exposure pathway, steps taken to minimize
or eliminate environmentally associated disease are necessarily limited and
may miss the mark altogether. Understanding the outcome of an exposure
requires a detailed analysis of the set and setting of the pathway along which
the exposure occurs. The *set* is the susceptibility of the individual (e.g., health
status, age), and the *setting* refers to the environmental factors (e.g., temperature, transformation, route of exposure) that may influence an individual's
reaction to the toxicant (Fig. 5.3).

Chemicals of concern may be altered as they move through the environment, and they can be metabolically activated or deactivated by the environmental microbiome or within the body (see Chapter 6). Ecologic and human
target receptors can vary widely in their response to chemical exposures in
different individuals and species. A classic example of differential interspe-
cies effects is the extreme toxicity of the compound theobromine to dogs.
Exposure to this ingredient in chocolate can cause muscle rigidity, increased
heart rate, seizures, or death in dogs, yet the substance is pleasurable to
most humans. Some chemicals may be transformed in the environment by

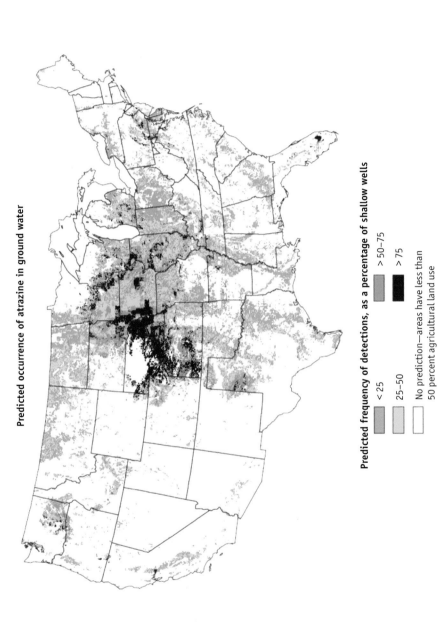

Predicted occurrence of atrazine in ground water

Predicted frequency of detections, as a percentage of shallow wells

< 25   > 50–75

25–50   > 75

No prediction—areas have less than
50 percent agricultural land use

FIGURE 5.3. Map shows where the herbicide atrazine has been detected in shallow drinking water wells in the United States. Adapted from Gilliom, R.J., Barbash, J.E., Crawford, C.G., et al. 2006. *The Quality of Our Nation's Waters—Pesticides in the Nation's Streams and Ground Water, 1992–2001.* U.S. Geological Survey Circular 1291. https://pubs.usgs.gov/circ/2005/1291/pdf/circ1291.pdf.

microbial degradation, oxidation processes, or sunlight, causing them to have increased or reduced toxicity. Other chemicals may be medically useful via one route of exposure and toxic via another. For example, dermal exposure to aloe can be medically useful, but certain components of the plant are potent carcinogens when ingested.

Understanding the inherent physicochemistry and toxicology of chemical exposures is critical to determining threats from drinking water. Unless clarifying information about the exposure pathway is available, the EPA assumes that only about 20% of the exposure to a drinking water contaminant comes from ingestion. The other 80% is considered to come from dermal contact and inhalation during showering, washing dishes, or washing clothes and ingestion of garden vegetables that have been irrigated with contaminated water. Such extraneous exposures are known to have contributed to the extreme exposures to perfluorooctanoic acid (PFOA) experienced by the residents of Parkersburg, West Virginia, living near the DuPont De Nemours Washington Works chemical facilities. This highly persistent chemical is man-made and does not occur in nature, yet it has been found in food, drinking water, and mammalian tissues worldwide.[43]

The concepts of exposure and dose are often confused in the exposure sciences. Although *dose* normally refers to a chemical concentration measured internally, *exposure* more accurately describes an external measure used as an index of the dose. Although measurements of internal dose are often more useful to the toxicologist, they are difficult to collect and usually involve ethical issues, invasive medical procedures, and discomfort for the subject. In contrast, external exposure measurements can often be collected with minimal disturbance to the individual, but they do not always provide the type of information desired by the toxicologist.

Monitoring of exposure to chemicals in the environment is commonly performed using techniques conducive to estimation of external concentrations. Although this process may seem simple, it can be quite complicated in practice, often requiring specialized tools and expertise. As an example, the National Institute for Occupational Safety and Health (NIOSH) has for decades recommended that exposure to airborne contaminants be monitored by collection of samples in the breathing zone using a filtration or capture device located on the shirt collar. Despite this recommendation, in practice a stationary monitor placed somewhere in the vicinity of the subject of study is often used. This practice of proximity sampling invariably underestimates inhalation exposures to dusts, mists, and aerosols, sometimes by an order of magnitude.

Monitoring of water quality at the source may provide useful information to the water utilities, but waterborne chemical exposures in the home are influenced by the age and condition of the proximity plumbing. Many older homes were plumbed with lead pipes that can release high concentrations of metal if the source water is corrosive and not carefully monitored or controlled.

With the advent of handheld smartphone devices such as the iPhone or Android, a new world of exposure monitoring is emerging. Many attachments on these devices and the device itself can report valuable information to the user or to a remotely located exposure scientist or physician. With available attachments, environmental contaminants can be associated with an accurate location determined by the global positioning system. This information presents opportunities to understand personal environmental exposure and appropriate medication on levels never previously imagined. Social media is adding value to environmental medicine by allowing exposure scientists to observe the migration of epidemics. By monitoring key words in the microblogging community of Twitter or by tracking Google search inquiries associated with symptoms such as fever or headache, epidemiologists have improved forecasting for exposure and epidemics.[29] Massive quantities of data can be collected from community exposures, highlighting geographic regions of concern and relationships between economic factors and environmental disease.

Collection and communication of environmental exposure data by citizens have the potential to greatly expand understanding of contaminant occurrence and community exposures. The application of citizen science has had major impacts in other natural sciences. For example, it has been used by the Audubon Society to track bird migrations and by the National Weather Service for real-time reporting of extreme weather by prequalified citizen-scientists. Similarly, we can expect a revolution in the collection of environmental data in the immediate future.

STEPS FOR REDUCTION OF PERSONAL EXPOSURE TO WATERBORNE CHEMICALS

Little can be done to mitigate the inherent toxicity of a chemical, but reductions in exposure can decrease the risks associated with chemical toxicity. After a chemical has made its way through an environmental pathway and been absorbed into the body, the response of the individual or organism is defined by the chemical's inherent toxicity. However, as demonstrated in Figure 5.4, there are often several points along the exposure pathway that provide opportunities to reduce or eliminate exposure to chemicals in water. The most effective and desirable strategy is to remove the chemical at the

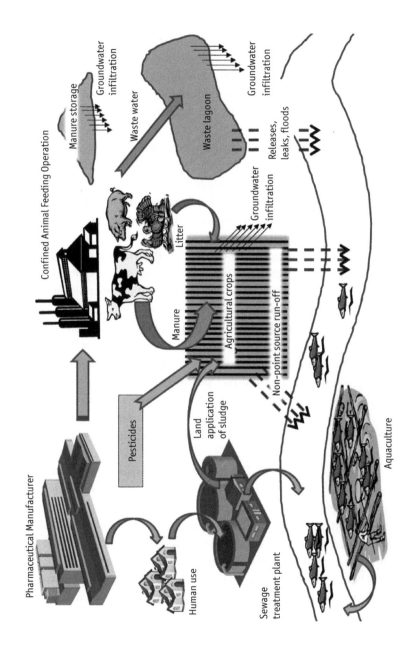

FIGURE 5.4. Agricultural sources and pathways of contaminants of emerging concern.

source (see Chapter 13) or, better, to prevent contamination from occurring in the first place.

Ecologic receptors depend more on our ability to prevent rather than remediate environmental contamination, but prevention is not always possible. Removal of contaminants from a large surface water source may be too costly or difficult to consider. Contaminants can bind to soils, resulting in persistent release of toxicants into wells. As the people of Flint, Michigan experienced, aging distribution systems can release contaminants as a result of changes in water chemistry. Replacement of distribution networks in towns and cities is a monumental task.

The complexity of exposure pathways depends on the set and setting and on the nature of the toxicant at the point of exposure. Chemicals that are less volatile may be of concern in drinking water, whereas volatile contaminants may result in significant exposure through dermal and inhalation pathways. In such cases, supplying bottled drinking water may eliminate only a fraction of the exposure.

Emerging filtering technologies are extremely effective at removing contaminants from domestic water for individual users and major utilities. Advances in reverse osmosis systems and nanofiltration membranes and improvements in the use of granular activated carbon (GAC) have provided highly effective physical and chemical mechanisms for purification of contaminated drinking water.[9] In cities where water resources are limited, these technologies provide a feasible option for sustainable management of water. Direct potable reuse (DPR) and indirect potable reuse (IPR) of wastewater are viable options for increasing water resources in areas of shortage while reducing exposure to uncontrolled contaminants. Combinations of these technologies are emerging to provide for the IPR of precious water resources in drought-stricken regions.[30]

Table 5.1 lists areas of the United States that are using or piloting IPR systems to improve availability of clean water. Although these tools can provide effective treatment, they are often expensive and are not widely available to all segments of the population. These filtering systems and technologies are aimed at reducing chemical contaminants or biologic materials that are present at *low concentrations*. They work effectively when the amount of the contaminants being removed is low to moderate. Most of these systems can be saturated when chemical concentrations become greater and cause breakthrough of the targeted agents. Although clean water remains extremely inexpensive in the United States, we can expect the costs for this precious resource to increase in the near future.

As water resources become stressed by climate change, overpopulation, and related contamination, it will be important for citizens to be actively

Table 5.1. **Indirect Potable Reuse of Water for Increasing Reserves in Areas of Water Shortage and Drought**

Location	Type of System	Operational Status	Population Served	Percent Blended
Orange County, CA	Multimedia filtration with lime clarification	Built in 1975 and decommissioned in 2004	<2 million	3.2% of total Orange County water
Denver, CO	High pH lime clarification, sedimentation, recarbonation, filtration, selective ion exchange, UV irradiation, activated carbons, others	Demonstration program concluded that potable reuse is a viable option	NA	NA
West Basin Municipal Water District, CA	Full-scale project that produces three types of tertiary treated, recycled water for industrial and irrigation uses and three types of RO water, groundwater recharge	Operational since 1995	950,000	10%–15%
Upper Occoquan Sewage Authority, Virginia	Lime clarification two-stage recarbonation, flow equalization, sand filtration, granular activated carbon, ion exchange, postfiltration chlorination	Full-scale project supplies about 50% of the population's water supply; during drought periods, recycled water provides up to 90% of reservoir inflow	1.2 million	10%–45%

(continued)

Table 5.1. Continued

Location	Type of System	Operational Status	Population Served	Percent Blended
Tampa Water Resource Recovery Project. Florida	Pre-aeration, lime clarification recarbonation, gravity filtration, and ozone disinfection; granular activated carbon, RO, and ultrafiltration were evaluated	Operational 1987–1989; discharged to reservoir, where water augmented the reservoir	NA	NA

NA = Not applicable; RO = reverse osmosis; UV = ultraviolet.
Modified from Rodriguez, C., Van Buynder, P., Lugg, R., et al. 2009. Indirect potable reuse: A sustainable water supply alternative. *Int J Environ Res Public Health.* 6:1174–1209.

involved in ensuring the availability of clean water. Clean water resources are beginning to disappear worldwide and have already done so in many geographic regions. More than a billion people have no access to clean water, and one of five childhood deaths occurs due to exposures to contaminated water.[44] It is no longer possible to take the availability of safe, clean water for granted. Everyone must become aware and involved in the steps necessary to protect the sources and pathways to clean water.

Conclusions

Threats to water quality in the United States and across the globe have increased with increasing human populations and associated activities. In the United States, these threats have been mitigated and higher water quality maintained based solely on regulatory programs and investments into clean water infrastructure such as WWTPs and drinking water treatment plants.

Replacement of clean water infrastructure systems is inevitable and will be a daunting task. New technologies can help, but there must be strong support by citizens. Because costs of these systems continue to rise, investments require long-term planning and commitments by local, state, and federal planners. Such commitment will occur only through the will of citizens and an outlook for future generations.

Acute and chronic threats to drinking water quality from chemical contamination are increasing in the United States and elsewhere in the world. Enhanced chemical monitoring and further development of forensic capabilities will be required to allow appropriate characterization and diagnosis of these threats. The complexity of chemical exposures has increased in recent years, but modern technologies are aiding health care professionals and epidemiologists in assessing and tracking chemical exposures and disease.

Reducing chemical exposures continues to be an important regulatory activity for state and federal agencies. The Clean Water Act, the Safe Drinking Water Act, and the Food Quality Protection Act are critical tools for keeping our food and water clean. Updates to the Toxic Substances Control Act (TSCA) now provide also for use of high-throughput screening of chemicals. This added information helps to prevent or limit the use of toxic chemicals in business and commerce. This is another piece of important legislation aimed at reducing chemical exposure.

Water filtration technologies for municipalities and for personal use at home have improved and continue to offer ways to reduce personal exposure to chemicals in drinking water.

REFERENCES

1. Bergman, A., Heindel, J.J., Jobling, S., Kidd, K.A., & Zoeller, R.T. 2013. State of the science of endocrine disrupting chemicals 2012: An assessment of the state of the science of endocrine disruptors prepared by a group of experts for the United Nations Environment Programme and World Health Organization. http://www.who.int/ceh/publications/endocrine/en/.
2. Center for Sustainable Systems, University of Michigan. 2016. U.S. Water Supply and Distribution Factsheet. Pub. No. CSS05-17. http://css.snre.umich.edu/factsheets/us-water-supply-and-distribution-factsheet.
3. Colborn, T., Dumanoski, D., & Myers, J.P. 1996. *Our Stolen Future: Are We Threatening Our Fertility, Intellgence, and Survival? A Scientific Detective Story.* New York, NY: Dutton/Penguin Books.
4. Czarnezki, J.J., Lam, S.T., & Ahmad, N.B. 2016. A primer: Air and water environmental quality standards in the United States. *William Mary Environ Law Policy Rev.* 40:115.
5. Desbrow, C., Routledge, E.J., Brighty, G.C., Sumpter, J.P., & Waldock, M. 1998. Identification of estrogenic chemicals in STW effluent. 1. Chemical fractionation and in vitro biological screening. *Environ Sci Technol.* 32:1549–1558.
6. Environmental Protection Agency. 2016. TSCA Chemical Substance Inventory. https://www.epa.gov/tsca-inventory.

7. Environmental Protection Agency. 2016. Toxicology Testing in the 21st Century (Tox21). https://www.epa.gov/chemical-research/toxicology-testing-21st-century-tox21.

8. Environmental Protection Agency. 2016. Table of regulated drinking water contaminants. https://www.epa.gov/ground-water-and-drinking-water/table-regulated-drinking-water-contaminants.

9. Environmental Protection Agency. 2016. Drinking Water Treatability Database: Granular Activated Carbon. https://iaspub.epa.gov/tdb/pages/treatment/treatmentOverview.do?treatmentProcessId=2074826383.

10. Environmental Protection Agency. 2016. Fish and shellfish advisories and safe eating guidelines. https://www.epa.gov/choose-fish-and-shellfish-wisely/fish-and-shellfish-advisories-and-safe-eating-guidelines.

11. Food and Drug Administration. 2009. Bioterrorism Act of 2002. http://www.fda.gov/RegulatoryInformation/Legislation/ucm148797.htm.

12. Food and Drug Administration. 2015. FDA Annual Summary Report on Antimicrobials Sold or Distributed in 2013 for Use in Food-Producing Animals. http://www.fda.gov/AnimalVeterinary/NewsEvents/CVMUpdates/ucm440585.htm.

13. FindLaw. Atrazine lawsuit overview. 2016. http://injury.findlaw.com/product-liability/atrazine-lawsuit-overview.html.

14. Fraga, I., Charters, F.J., O'Sullivan, A.D., & Cochrane, T.A. 2016. A novel modelling framework to prioritize estimation of non-point source pollution parameters for quantifying pollutant origin and discharge in urban catchments. *J Environ Manage.* 167:75–84.

15. Gilliom RJ, Barbash JE, Crawford CG, et al. 2006. *The Quality of Our Nation's Waters—Pesticides in the Nation's Streams and Ground Water, 1992–2001.* U.S. Geological Survey Circular 1291. https://pubs.usgs.gov/circ/2005/1291/pdf/circ1291.pdf.

16. Gleick, P.H. 2006. Water and terrorism. *Water Policy.* 8:481–503.

17. Jobling, S., Nolan, M., Tyler, C.R., Brighty, G., & Sumpter, J.P. 1998. Widespread sexual disruption in wild fish. *Environ Sci Technol.* 32:2498–2506.

18. Kassotis, C.D., Tillitt, D.E., Lin, C.H., McElroy, J.A., & Nagel, S.C. 2016. Endocrine-disrupting chemicals and oil and natural gas operations: Potential environmental contamination and recommendations to assess complex environmental mixtures. *Environ Health Perspect.* 124:256–264.

19. Kenny, J.F., Barber, N.L., Hutson, S.S., Linsey, K.S., Lovelace, J.K., & Maupin, M.A. 2009. *Estimated Use of Water in the United States in 2005.* U.S. Geological Survey Circular 1344. http://pubs.usgs.gov/circ/1344/.

20. Kidd, K.A., Blanchfield, P.J., Mills, K.H., et al. 2007. Collapse of a fish population after exposure to a synthetic estrogen. *Proc Natl Acad Sci U S A.* 104:8897–8901.

21. Kolpin, D.W., Furlong, E.T., Meyer, M.T., et al. 2002. Pharmaceuticals, hormones, and other organic wastewater contaminants in U.S. streams, 1999–2000: A national reconnaissance. *Environ Sci Technol.* 36:1202–1211.

22. Kovalic, J.M., & Hennelly, A. 1987. *The Clean Water Act of 1987.* 2nd ed. Alexandria, VA: Water Pollution Control Foundation.

23. Kroll, D. 2006. *A Reinterpretation of the 2002 Attempted Water Terror Attack on the U.S. Rome Embassy: Don't Underestimate the Enemy.* http://hachhst.com/wp-content/uploads/2010/07/White-Paper_-WATER-TERROR-ATTACK1.pdf

24. Liu, Z., Kanjo, Y., & Mizutani, S. 2009. Removal mechanisms for endocrine disrupting compounds (EDCs) in wastewater treatment—physical means, biodegradation, and chemical advanced oxidation: A review. *Sci Total Environ.* 407:731–748.

25. Mellon, M., Benbrook, C., & Benbrook, K.L. 2001. *Hogging It: Estimates of Antimicrobial Abuse in Livestock.*, Cambridge, MA: Union of Concerned Scientists Publications.

26. State of Michigan. 2016. Flintwater Test Results for lead and copper in water [database].   http://www.michigan.gov/documents/deq/Copy_of_deq-fw-Flint-Home-Owner-Data-Sept-3-thru_Nov-5-15_505529_7_505579_7.pdf

27. Oaks, J.L., Gilbert, M., Virani, M.Z., et al. 2004. Diclofenac residues as the cause of vulture population decline in Pakistan. *Nature.* 427:630–633.

28. Obama, B. 2013. Executive Order: Improving Chemical Facility Safety and Security. https://www.whitehouse.gov/the-press-office/2013/08/01/executive-order-improving-chemical-facility-safety-and-security.

29. Paul, M.J., Dredze, M., & Broniatowski, D. 2014, October 28. Twitter improves influenze forecasting. *PLOS Curr Outbreaks.*

30. Rodriguez, C., Van Buynder, P., Lugg, R., et al. 2009. Indirect potable reuse: A sustainable water supply alternative. *Int J Environ Res Public Health.* 6:1174–1209.

31. Ryberg, K.R., & Gilliom, R.J. 2015. Trends in pesticide concentrations and use for major rivers of the United States. *Sci Total Environ.* 538:431–444.

32. Stackelberg, P.E., Barbash, J.E., Gilliom, R.J., Stone, W.W., & Wolock, D.M. 2012. Regression models for estimating concentrations of atrazine plus deethylatrazine in shallow groundwater in agricultural areas of the United States. *J Environ Qual.* 41:479–494.

33. Stone, W.W., Gilliom, R.J., & Ryberg, K.R. 2014. Pesticides in U.S. streams and rivers: Occurrence and trends during 1992–2011. *Environ Sci Technol.* 48:11025–11030.

34. Swartz, M.N. 1989. *Committee on Human Risk Assessment of Using Subtherapeutic Antibiotics in Animal Feeds, Institute of Medicine, Division of Health Promotion and Disease Prevention. Human Health Risks with the Subtherapeutic Use of Penicillin or Tetracyclines in Animal Feed.*, Washington, DC: National Academy Press.

35. Vandenberg, L.N., Colborn, T., Hayes, T.B., et al. 2012. Hormones and endocrine-disrupting chemicals: Low-dose effects and nonmonotonic dose responses. *Endocr Rev.* 33:378–455.

36. Venkatesan, A.K., & Halden, R.U. 2013. National inventory of perfluoroalkyl substances in archived U.S. biosolids from the 2001 EPA National Sewage Sludge Survey. *J Hazard Mater.* 252–253:413–418.

37. Vorosmarty, C.J., McIntyre, P.B., Gessner, M.O., et al. 2010. Global threats to human water security and river biodiversity. *Nature.* 467:555–561.

38. Weibel, S.R., Anderson, R.J., & Woodward, R.L. 1964. Urban land runoff as a factor in stream pollution. *Journal of the Water Pollution Control Federation.* 36:914–924.

39. Kurtz, E.M. 2013. Declaration by the Emergency Manager. EM Submission No. 2013 EM140. June 21.

40. EPA. 2015. Memorandum from Miguel A. Del Toral to Thomas Poy. June 24, 2015. "High Lead Levels in Flint, Michigan—Interim Report." https://www.aclumich. org/sites/default/files/Original%20EPA%20memo.%20062514.pdf

41. Department of Health and Human Services (DHHS). 2012. National Toxicology Program. NTP Monograph: Health Effects of Low-Level Lead. June, 2012. https:// ntp.niehs.nih.gov/ntp/ohat/lead/final/monographhealtheffectslowlevellead_ newissn_508.pdf

42. Nuss, P., & Eckelman, M.J. 2014. Life cycle assessment of metals: a scientific synthesis. PLOS one, July 7. http://journals.plos.org/plosone/article?id=10.1371/journal.pone.0101298

43. EPA. 2016. Drinking Water Health Advisory for Perfluorooctanoic Acid (PFOA). U.S. EPA Office of Water. EPA 822-R-16-005. https://www.epa.gov/sites/production/files/2016-05/documents/pfoa_health_advisory_final-plain.pdf.

44. WHO. 2015. World Health Organization Fact Sheet No. 391. Drinking Water Key Facts. Published on line as: http://www.who.int/mediacentre/factsheets/fs391/en/.

6

Diet, Environmental Chemicals, and the Gut Microbiome

MARVIN M. SINGH AND GERARD E. MULLIN

Key Concepts

- The gut microbiome is a versatile organ that is affected by various factors, particularly diet and environmental exposures, and it can contribute to health or illness, depending on its composition.
- The root cause of many chronic conditions and symptoms stems from inflammation, which is modulated by the gut microbiome.
- Diet, food choices, and method of food preparation can affect the gut microbiome and influence disease.
- Environmental exposures and food chemicals can contribute to dysbiosis and have an adverse effect on health.

Introduction

The gut microbiome has taken center stage with regard to understanding disease and what causes chronic medical conditions and symptoms. More than 100 trillion microorganisms coexist within each of us. They can affect our health, and we can modulate their existence by our actions and the things we are exposed to. The gut microbiome, composed of various fungi, viruses, and bacteria, is a vital part of the human host. The gut flora provide vitamins and short-chain fatty acids and play a significant role in the intestinal immune system and inflammation.[46]

In normal, healthy intestinal mucosa, tight junctions seal the spaces between cells and form ion- and size-selective gateways. Various parts of the gastrointestinal tract allow different degrees of permeability through these junctions. A wide variety of triggers can cause increased intestinal permeability, which can lead to mucosal inflammation, chronic symptoms, and various medical conditions. The gut microbiome is one of the layers of defense in the intestinal tract that contributes to the intestinal barrier, and it helps determine what can cross the epithelium by usual and regulated means.[11]

A significant amount of research is being done to better understand how changes to the gut microbiome can modulate disease. Epigenetic changes are thought to occur in response to a wide variety of factors, including weight, physical activity, nutrition, and environmental and emotional exposures. The microbiome can affect these factors, and vice-versa. Low-molecular-weight substances produced by the gut microbiota can interact with the cellular environment, affecting the signaling pathways and gene expression that regulate cell death, inflammation, and differentiation.[54] It is nearly impossible to have a discussion on genetics and health and not include the gut microbiome. This is a rapidly growing area in medicine and research. Understanding the gut microbiome and its interaction with the epigenome and diseases will help physicians to improve disease prevention and treatment.

Chopra and Tanzi[18] eloquently described how high-fat, high-carbohydrate diets can contribute to intestinal permeability and allow endotoxin and other harmful substances to cross into the bloodstream and provoke an immune response that results in inflammation. This proinflammatory state is thought to contribute to insulin resistance and obesity, even in the face of normal caloric intake.[18]

Changing the diet to include more healthy foods, such as fiber, fruits, and vegetables, can intervene in the process by cultivating a more favorable gut microbiome. This has implications for management of a wide variety of conditions, including obesity, diabetes, heart disease, allergy, and autoimmune disorders. The gut microbiota can produce substances such as vitamins that are favorable to health, but they can also produce harmful substances such as toxic metabolites. The mucous barrier of the intestinal tract works together with a diverse microbiome to favor a strong proportion of beneficial bacteria and to keep the harmful bacteria from causing disease.[20] A healthy diet is an excellent way of maintaining a robust and diverse microbiome.

It is not just diet and nutrition that can modulate the gut microbiome and have an impact on health. Environmental toxins, exposures, and stressors can influence the gut microbiota, and it seems prudent to include the gut microbiome when assessing how environmental factors can affect human health.[22] For example, antibiotic use early in life can alter the gut microbiome and is associated with later obesity.[70] One study demonstrated how seasonal changes can contribute to shifts in the composition of the gut microbiome in a special population of communal-living people known as the Hutterites in North America. It was postulated that dietary changes due to the availability of fresh produce during a particular season contributed to changes in the gut microbiome. Other factors such as outdoor activity, sun exposure, and temperature should also be considered, although they were not directly measured.[57]

Although pesticide exposure was not considered or evaluated in the Hutterite study, there are data regarding the importance of considering this issue when evaluating changes in the gut microbiome. One experiment with female rats showed that maternal exposure to chlorpyrifos, an insecticide that can cross the placenta, resulted in several effects in newborn rats that lasted into adulthood, including microbial dysbiosis, alteration of nutrient absorption, changes in the intestinal barrier, and stimulation of the immune system.[19] Although many factors can influence the gut microbiome during a lifetime, exposure to pesticides is a particularly important one because the impact can have both short-term and longer-lasting effects.

This information highlights the significance of the gut microbiome and factors that can influence it. Eating an appropriate diet and avoiding certain types of environmental exposures can improve the composition of the gut microbiome, thereby modulating inflammation and the incidence of certain diseases and conditions. Understanding these influences on the gut microbiota is a key concept that can help guide clinicians when counseling patients about following a healthy diet and lifestyle.

Diet

The gut microbiome is versatile. Many factors can influence the composition of the gut microbiome on a daily basis. The diversity of bacterial species in the gut microbiome is affected by changes in diet through competition for substrates and tolerance of intestinal conditions.[28] Dysbiosis, an imbalance of the flora in the gut microbiome, has been associated with many different conditions (Box 6.1), including, but not limited to, diabetes, colon cancer, colon polyps, inflammatory bowel disease, and obesity.[72]

Data support the influence of the gut microbiome on mood and behavior,[53] neurologic conditions such as Parkinson disease,[49] and coronary artery disease.[8,30,75] Research has also demonstrated the influence of the microbiome on a wide array of other medical conditions. The American Heart Association has stated that the gut microbiome is a potential risk factor for diabetes, obesity,

Box 6.1 Medical Conditions Associated with Dysbiosis

- Allergies
- Alzheimer's dementia
- Anxiety
- Asthma
- Autism
- Autoimmune conditions
- Cancer (e.g., colorectal, breast, ovarian, endometrial)
- Celiac disease
- Chronic fatigue syndrome
- Colon polyps
- Coronary artery disease (CAD)
- Depression
- Diabetes mellitus
- Eczema
- Inflammatory bowel disease (e.g., ulcerative colitis, Crohn disease)
- Irritable bowel syndrome (IBS)
- Metabolic syndrome
- Multiple sclerosis
- Obesity
- Parkinson disease
- Small intestinal bacterial overgrowth (SIBO)
- Thyroid disease

and heart disease because microbial dysbiosis can alter intestinal permeability and induce systemic inflammation.[24] The statement also emphasized the significant impact of diet on the composition of the gut microbiome. For example, bacterial species from the phylum Tenericutes and the genus *Desulfovibrio* have been associated with the production of trimethylamine-*N*-oxide (TMAO), a metabolite implicated in cardiovascular risk that is produced as a result of metabolic reactions driven by the microbes when they encounter dietary components such as carnitine and phosphatidylcholine.[24] Although much research is still needed, the evidence on the importance of diet and nutrition in human health is compelling. Understanding how diet and proper nutrition influence this most important "organ" in the human body could have a substantial impact on the clinical course of patients with many different conditions.

Plant nutrients (i.e., phytonutrients) are effective in preventing infection by pathogenic organisms. They can be taken as supplements or integrated into a well-balanced diet. A recent study demonstrated how anethole, carvacrol, cinnamaldehyde, eugenol, capsicum oleoresin, and garlic extract lead to changes in gene expression in the colon. In particular, eugenol, which can be found in cloves, nutmeg, cinnamon, and basil, stimulates the inner mucus layer, a key barrier to microbes in the colon. The investigators thought that this occurred by means of "microbial stimulation" because there was an abundance of bacterial families in the order Clostridiales present. This change led to resistance of colonization by *Citrobacter rodentium*, which has pathogenic similarities to *Escherichia coli*.[73]

Lactobacillus supplementation has reduced inflammation and proteinuria associated with renal dysfunction in rats, suggesting that it can play a protective role against the progression of chronic kidney disease.[76] Another study showed that rats that had segmented, filamentous bacteria as part of their gut microbiomes had improved immunity and resistance to *Staphylococcus aureus* pneumonia. The presence of this type of bacteria also led to increased levels of interleukin-22 (IL-22), which was also protective against severe staphylococcal pulmonary infection.[29] The evidence supporting the effects of alterations in the gut microbiome in the setting of various diseases is growing.

One of the easiest ways to modulate the gut microbiome is through the diet. Including certain foods and nutrients in the diet to promote particular species of microbes can offer positive health effects. Prebiotics, which are nondigestible foods that provide nourishment for beneficial bacteria, and probiotics, which are supplements of beneficial microbes that can improve the microbial balance, can help to maintain good gut health. Nutritional supplements that combine prebiotics and probiotics are called *synbiotics*, and they are thought to work synergistically together to improve human health.[75] Chapter 14 provides a comprehensive list of prebiotics and probiotics.

When an infant is born, the sterile gut of the fetus is colonized by the maternal gut microbiome from the genital tract and colon in addition to the birth environment. Commonly identified bacteria include *Bifidobacterium*, *Ruminococcus, Enterococcus, Clostridium*, and *Enterobacter*.[54] There can be a substantial influence on the gut microbiome of the infant based on whether the delivery was vaginal or via cesarean section and whether the infant is breast fed or bottle fed. Maternal diet and infant nutrition play a role very early on in the establishment of a child's gut microbiome, which can influence the child's epigenome and predispose to conditions such as obesity and cardiovascular disease later in life.

The gut microbiome is dynamic. A diet that is high in fiber can produce more short-chain fatty acids in the colon. Butyrate, a short-chain fatty acid, can act as a chemotherapeutic agent.[54] Alternatively, a diet high in fat and red meat can increase the risk of colon cancer and cardiovascular disease by means of *N*-nitroso compounds and heterocyclic aromatic amines. Bacteria digest the L-carnitine in red meat and convert it to toxic substances that can promote heart disease and other problems.[54]

The importance of the gut microbiome can not be overstated; researchers and clinicians continue to explore ways to influence the course of many chronic health issues facing patients today. The following sections review special topics related to the dietary influences on the gut microbiome, as well as the importance of nutrition on the gut microbiome for overall health.

Water Safety

ARSENIC

Water is a vital part of the human diet and a critical route for chemical exposure. Millions of Americans drink water containing more than the recommended levels of arsenic (>10 µg/L). This problem largely reflects the lack of regulations regarding private wells. Diabetes, cardiovascular disease, and several malignancies have been associated with arsenic ingestion. In a study using mice, arsenic exposure contributed to a significant change in the gut microbiome which was strongly associated with changes in the flora-related metabolites that impact energy harvesting, short-chain fatty acid production, and adipogenesis.[40] The specific composition of the gut microbiome has also been associated with susceptibility to toxins such as arsenic.[39]

One study found that although the levels of arsenic in water may not be enough to directly cause hepatotoxicity, low levels could contribute to sensitization to nonalcoholic fatty liver disease and enhance damage to the liver caused by a diet high in fat. However, supplementation with the prebiotic oligofructose contributed to changes in the gut microbiome that had protective effects in the liver when there was arsenic exposure.[44] Oligofructose is part of a class of soluble fibers (i.e., inulin fiber) that are considered prebiotics. These studies demonstrate how dietary changes, such as including prebiotics, can modulate beneficial changes in the gut microbiome to protect against the detrimental effects of arsenic. They also remind us how drinking water containing toxins such as arsenic can alter the microbiome and lead to increased vulnerability to certain diseases.

CHLORINATION

Chlorinated water has been shown to change the gut microbiome, particularly by reducing *Clostridium perfringens, Clostridium difficile,* organisms of the family Enterobacteriaceae, and *Staphylococcus* species. These changes were associated with increased formation of colon tumors.[61] This raises the point that some commensal flora play a role in tumor formation, and exposures to certain chemicals such as chlorine can alter the composition of the gut microbiome and influence this process.

CADMIUM

Low-level cadmium exposure in water changes the composition of the gut microbiome. Exposure to cadmium may increase serum lipopolysaccharide levels and cause inflammation of the liver, which may subsequently lead to problems with energy homeostasis. When mice were exposed to low levels of cadmium for 10 weeks, they had increased levels of hepatic triacylglycerol and serum levels of free fatty acids and triacylglycerol.[77]

SUMMARY OF WATER CONTAMINATION

Good health can depend one's drinking water source. For example, emissions from nearby industries can impact the amounts of heavy metals in water. Arsenic has been found in more than one half of the hazardous waste sites proposed to be a part of the national priority list maintained by the Environmental Protection Agency (EPA). Approximately 2.3% of the U.S. population may have elevated urine levels of cadmium, and water is one of several sources of cadmium exposure.[68] In January 2016, the water crisis in Flint, Michigan, was uncovered, and the public discovered that the city's drinking water was contaminated with lead, a heavy metal that has toxic effects on many organ systems.

Certainly drinking water is important for your health, but taking measures to understand where the water comes from and what pollutants it might contain is also important. Information such as annual reports from municipal suppliers and results from testing of wells can help one determine whether to implement a home water filtration system to protect against contaminants (see Chapter 5).

Fertilizers and Pesticides

Perhaps as important as the type of food we eat, so too is the quality. Eating organic foods has health benefits because growers of those foods use the natural microflora of the soil as nutrients. Conventional agricultural techniques use chemically modified fertilizers and pesticides that pollute the water and soil. Disruption of the ecologic balance of the soil can affect the gut microbiome and put human health at risk.[3]

Some studies demonstrate that maternal exposure to farms, stables, and animals in utero can boost fetal immunity and decrease allergic and asthmatic reactions after birth.[48] Dr. Daphne Miller, in her book *Farmacology*, outlines this strategy and suggests spending time on a sustainable farm as a preventive strategy for allergies and asthma.[48] This drives home the concept that the soil is just as important as the food; although eating healthy plants is good, considering how they are grown and avoiding genetically modified foods is even better.

GLYPHOSATE

Glyphosate is the active ingredient in the most widely used herbicide as of 2016, Monsanto's Roundup.[50] Traces of this chemical have been found in sugar, corn, soy, and wheat. This dangerous substance inhibits the cytochrome P450 enzyme, which plays a significant role in detoxifying xenobiotics (i.e. foreign substances not usually made or present in the host). Disruption of this process works in synergy with disruption of the gut ecology and synthesis of aromatic amino acids and sulfate transport. The downstream sequelae are thought to contribute to the development of diabetes, obesity, depression, autism, Alzheimer's disease, cancer, and cardiovascular disease.[60]

The concept that environmental toxins cause disruption of homeostasis is known as *exogenous semiotic entropy*.[60] Understanding how nutrition and environmental chemicals interact additively or synergistically to affect the gut microbiome and health can help clinicians better understand various diseases and disorders.

The food chain is the primary route of exposure for chemicals known as endocrine disruptors. These chemicals include fertilizers, pesticides, and herbicides. Residues of these substances can be directly ingested, and they can alter natural phytoestrogen compounds in edible plants. There can be additive effects when multiple pesticide residues are ingested.[43] Persistent organic pollutants and pesticides have been associated with type 2 diabetes. The chemicals can undergo transformation with exposure to natural sunlight that can further increase their toxicity.[65] The gut microbiome is affected by these substances, and the resulting changes affect metabolomics and can alter the protective inner layer of the gut and lead to some of the conditions mentioned.

Food choices are important for maintaining good health. Considerations include whether fruits and vegetables are organically grown or grown with the aid of harmful pesticides and fertilizers. Food safety systems should be used to assess the risk of chemicals along the food chain and how they can affect target organs.[43] Without appropriate assessment in place, ingestion of contaminated food by children and adults can have serious health implications, especially during the prenatal development.

Genetically modified organisms (GMOs) contain genetic material that has been altered by the use of genetic engineering techniques. Most corn and soybean crops in the United States have been genetically engineered to withstand the application of herbicides for weed control. The use of herbicides in farming is thought to contribute to changes in the gut microbiome that select for resistance genes.[31] Antibiotic-resistant organisms may result from the genetic changes in foods that are transferred to the gut flora, subsequently impacting human health.

Glyphosate and 2,4-dichlorophenoxyacetic acid (2,4-D) have been classified as possible carcinogens.[50] Genetic transformation of foods has the potential to produce allergens or toxins that could alter the nutritional quality of the food.[36] In the gut microbiome, these ingested foods are processed by the commensal flora, and the toxic metabolic byproducts produced can cause a variety of pathologic conditions. Moreover, the gut microbiome changes as a result of exposure to these chemicals, allowing different populations of microbes to dominate and persist in the gut.

Dysbiosis is a key factor in the development of many health problems. Although herbicides have helped farmers with weed management without destroying the crop itself, genetic modification of crops poses a hazard to human health.[36,50] The emergence of glyphosate-resistant weeds raises another health concern because farmers are being forced to apply the herbicide multiple times, apply additional herbicidal chemicals, and alter their farming methods.[1,2] As problems with resistance escalate, further genetic modifications are needed within the food chain, affecting humans and animals that ingest these crops. With obesity reaching epidemic proportions in the United States and nonalcoholic fatty liver disease becoming one of the top indications for liver transplantation, the effects of growing and eating GMOs should be seriously considered.

Food Chemicals

The chemicals used to produce foods can be harmful to the gut microbiome and health. For example, the food industry has used chemicals called emulsifiers to help ensure long shelf life and good texture of its products, but data supporting the negative health effects of emulsifiers is mounting. Processed foods are thought to strongly contribute to the obesity epidemic. Obesity is associated with low-grade inflammation and altered gut microbiome, and emulsifiers promote dysbiosis and dysfunction of the gut barrier. These substances, also called obesogens, are thought to be associated with metabolic disorders and weight gain.[13]

POTASSIUM BROMATE

Potassium bromate is a food chemical that has substantial harmful effects. It has long been used in breads as an additive to strengthen the dough. Many countries have banned its use, but it continues to be allowed in the United States. It is considered to be a carcinogen, and it can cause oxidative damage to DNA,[78] which may contribute to breakdown of the protective barrier in the gut and lead to increased intestinal permeability.

EMULSIFIERS

Carboxymethylcellulose and polysorbate-80, two emulsifiers, were shown to contribute to low-grade inflammation, metabolic syndrome, and obesity in mice. In mice that were predisposed to colitis, these substances triggered significant colonic inflammation. The composition of the gut microbiome in the exposed mice was found to be different from that in controls, and inflammation increased as an effect of the emulsifiers.[16]

Carrageenan, another emulsifier, is made from red seaweed. It is often found in organic and nonorganic dairy products and is used in toothpaste to create a smooth texture. It activates a proinflammatory cascade and induces inflammation in colonic cells. The types of flora found in the colon as a result of exposure to carrageenan may affect the development of colonic neoplasia or inflammatory bowel disease.[4] Exposure to several different emulsifiers may alter the gut microbiome in such a way that a particular individual could become more susceptible to problems such as inflammatory bowel disease when also exposed to carrageenan.

Some authorities think that use of carrageenan should be reconsidered because degraded carrageenan is a known carcinogen in animal models, and undegraded carrageenan has cancer-promoting effects. Exposure to acid in the stomach can convert undegraded carrageenan to the degraded form, and food processing may allow for contamination of the food product with degraded carrageenan.[69] The impact this food additive has on the gut microbiome and the potential health hazards that can ensue are worthy of consideration.

ARTIFICIAL SWEETENERS

Another class of food chemicals that deserves attention is artificial sweeteners. Millions of people worldwide use artificial sweeteners with the hope that they will lose weight. However, data support the opposite finding; the sweeteners contribute to metabolic derangements and glucose intolerance by altering the gut microbiome.[67]

Various microbial communities are involved in several important processes in which the gut, diet, and metabolism are closely intertwined.[10] Studies have shown that nonnutritive sweeteners are associated with increased risk of diabetes, obesity, and metabolic syndrome. Some of the proposed mechanisms include interference with established responses to glucose and energy homeostasis and disruption of the gut microbiome, which leads to glucose intolerance and stimulation of the insulin response by interference with sweet-taste receptors found throughout the digestive tract.[55] When artificial sweeteners provoke an insulin response without the presence of a corresponding caloric load, the person may have increased cravings for sweet foods. In this way, diet soda and other foods that use artificial sweeteners can actually lead to a higher risk of obesity. The means by which nonnutritive sweeteners impact metabolism and energy homeostasis are complex and are probably related to a variety of peripheral and central mechanisms,[9] some of which still need to be elucidated.

The use of artificial sweeteners deserves attention as we look for ways to optimize patients' health and reduce factors that can contribute to the problems they are trying to avoid. Although the food industry and society have been attempting to move toward more natural sweeteners, such as those derived from *Stevia rebaudiana*, with the hope that health concerns would be reduced, one study has questioned whether this type of sweetener acts as an endocrine disruptor.[64] Although natural sweeteners are thought to be preferable to other nonnutritive sweeteners, further research is needed before more definitive recommendations can be made.

ANTIBIOTICS

The use of antibiotics in dairy products and meats is a concern. When oral antibiotics are taken for an infection, other microbes in the gut are also affected. Often overlooked are exposures of food products to antibiotics and the impact this may have on the gut microbiome, which can certainly be altered by antibiotics.[51]

In many farming practices, it is common to deliver antibiotics to animals in their feed to act as a growth promoter and to prevent disease. It is estimated that every individual in the United States consumes more than 27 g of antibiotics each year because of this practice.[51] Agricultural use has significantly contributed to the development of antibiotic resistance and severe infections worldwide.

Diversity of the gut microbiome is an important factor in modulating inflammation, diabetes, cardiovascular disease, obesity, and many other conditions. Exposure to antibiotics on a chronic basis decreases biodiversity and may be an important driver of inflammation. Reduced biodiversity of the gut microbiome can increase susceptibility to certain enteric infections, alter the microbiome after infection, and create more severe intestinal pathology.[63] The result is a vicious cycle of dysbiosis.

HORMONES

Use of hormones such as recombinant bovine growth hormone, which is used in the dairy industry to boost the milk production, is a controversial subject. This hormone may have a role in the development of obesity, although it would be an indirect one because the growth hormone is not thought to be active in humans.[65] Any foreign substance has the potential to change the microbiome and gut ecology. Even organic milk, which does not have added hormones, potentially has higher levels of estrogens in it because the cows that are producing the milk are kept in a constant state of pregnancy.

The amount of hormones that pass into milk and dairy products are a concern.[14] However, the data on the impact of hormones in dairy products on the gut microbiome and risk of malignancies such as prostate, breast, and endometrial cancer are controversial, and further investigation is warranted.

IRRADIATED FOODS

Some foods are irradiated to increase their shelf life and reduce foodborne illnesses. Meats are irradiated to eradicate gram-negative organisms that contribute to spoilage.[52] Irradiation is also used on mushrooms to prolong quality because their postharvest life is only a few days despite the use of drying techniques. Electron beam irradiation, an emerging technique, may be used. One study proposed that this method decontaminates mushrooms and improves their antioxidant activity.[27] Another study suggested that applying gamma irradiation with freezing or oven drying preserves the total tocopherols and could be a useful combination.[26]

Food irradiation is thought to be a safe practice that can improve community health issues.[25] If there are no major changes to the food itself and an improved chemical and nutrient profile results, there should not be a substantial negative impact on the gut microbiome, but further studies are necessary. The irradiation process does destroy microbes on foods, and the altered microbial profile may or may not have sequelae in the human gut. It is important to understanding to what degree particular foods should be irradiated so that they maintain their integrity.

MICROWAVED FOODS

Microwaving is a common method of heating and cooking. Although it is not possible to comment on the changes that every type of food undergoes when microwaved and what the sequelae on the gut microbiome may be, we offer a few examples. A study done by Lopez-Berenguer and colleagues showed that there was a general decrease in human bioactive compounds in broccoli, except for minerals, when it was microwaved. Vitamin C was degraded and leached, and phenolic compounds and glucosinolates were lost due to leaching in water. Longer cooking times and larger water volumes were associated with a greater degree of nutrient loss, and it was suggested that these methods should be avoided.[38]

Considering the safety of microwaved foods is important. Although the heat from microwaves may be capable of sterilization, heating and cooking of frozen food products in a microwave oven is not always even. Parts of the package may not be heated and cooked as well as others.[62] This could potentially make some foods unsafe and put consumers at risk for enteric infections.

Perhaps more important than the process of microwaving itself is the surface with which the foods are in contact during the process. Melamine is a chemical used to produce cooking utensils, plates, plastic products, and fertilizer in some countries. Plastic tableware from China is manufactured using a melamine-formaldehyde resin. The U.S. Food and Drug Administration (FDA) suggests that poisoning from melamine can cause kidney failure, nephrolithiasis, blood pressure problems, and death. A 2014 study strongly suggested that foods should not be microwaved with melamine-formaldehyde tableware. Microwaving can affect the overall migration of this substance into the food, especially with repeated cycles of heating.[56]

Although the FDA suggests that migration is most likely when heating acidic foods, the official suggestion for consumers is to avoid microwaving with melamine-formaldehyde plastic tableware. A discussion about microwaving foods, including infant formula, in various types of containers is beyond the scope of this chapter, but consumers should be aware of the effects of various cooking methods as well as the surface material of the containers in which the foods are heated.

Further studies regarding the effects of microwaving on the gut microbiome and disease are warranted, but it seems logical that ingesting foreign substances such as melamine and eating foods with a lower than usual nutrient profile can affect the microbiome, gut health, and overall nutrition. Studies show that microwaving foods causes a loss of valuable nutrients and vitamins. There also is concern that the process of heating may change the food's chemistry, contributing to free radical development and other negative health effects. This may be one of many factors influencing disease and health problems in the United States and worldwide.

Environmental Chemicals and Other Factors

Environmental chemicals and other factors can alter the gut microbiome and human health. Xenobiotics are exogenous foreign substances that are not naturally produced or found in an organism. Many environmental chemicals fall into this category, including pollutants, cosmetics, drugs, and dietary components.[33] An increasing body of evidence shows that interactions between xenobiotics and the gut microbiome modulate chemical toxicity and cause or exacerbate various diseases.

The gut microbiome helps to process nutrients, chemicals, and other substances. It plays an important role in metabolism and in sequestration and transformation of xenobiotics; the sequelae of these processes can lead to functional changes in the gut microbiome.[41] For example, there are arsenic-associated genes in *E. coli*, *Staphylococcus* spp., and *Bacteroides*. The gut microbiome may also play a role in metabolizing polycyclic aromatic hydrocarbons. In a similar way, the microbiome of the skin can metabolize toxins in air pollution before absorption.[22]

The emerging view of environmental toxins includes genetics, epigenetics, exposures, metabolism, and xenobiotic processing by the microbiota. Whether a toxin is considered an obesogen, diabetogen, airborne chemical, metal, or other exposure, there are important considerations when it comes to the environment and how it impacts the gut and overall health (Fig. 6.1).

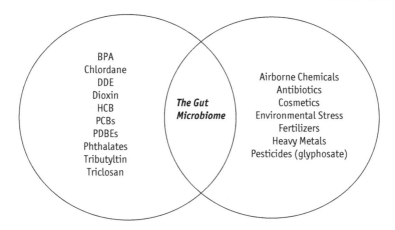

FIGURE 6.1. Environmental factors affecting the gut microbiome. The circle on the *left* lists specific toxins. The circle on the *right* lists specific categories of toxins. BPA = Bisphenol A; DDE = dichlorodiphenyldichloroethylene; HCB = hexachlorobenzene; PCBs = polychlorinated biphenyls; PDBEs = polybrominated diphenyl ethers.

OBESOGENS AND DIABETOGENS

Certain agents contribute to the development of obesity and diabetes mellitus. They are categorized as obesogens and diabetogens, respectively. Men with type 2 diabetes have reduced levels of organisms of the phylum Firmicutes. Blood glucose levels have been associated with altered ratios of Bacteroidetes to Firmicutes and *Bacteroides-Prevotella* to *Clostridium coccoides–Eubacterium rectale*. Diabetics also have more organisms of the class Betaproteobacteria.[66]

Understanding what factors contribute to the presence or absence of certain microbial strains has clinical significance. For more than a decade, experts have proposed that certain environmental toxins can contribute to obesity and diabetes.[32] Associations have been proposed for the following chemicals: dichlorodiphenyldichloroethylene (DDE), hexachlorobenzene (HCB), highly chlorinated polychlorinated biphenyls (PCBs), dioxin, and chlordane. Occupational exposures to insecticides and herbicides such as chlordane, heptachlor, chlorpyrifos, diazinon, alachlor, cyanazine, and trichlorfon have also been described.[66]

Agricultural chemicals such as DDE can be excreted in breast milk, which creates an exposure for the child. Although chemicals such as HCB, a carcinogenic fungicide, have been banned, it is possible that epigenetic marks made by exposure of prior generations could be passed down through generations.[74] The production of PCBs was banned in the United States, but waterways and buildings remain contaminated with these toxic, probably carcinogenic chemicals.

Compounds known as organotins are organic derivatives of tin, and they are used commonly to stabilize plastics. Tributyltin and related compounds can be transferred to the food supply through contact with materials such as parchment paper and food containers, and they can induce adipocyte differentiation.[65] Studies of how the various microbial communities in the gut respond to these exposures are needed to determine whether interactions with organotins favor development of obesity and diabetes.

Other common endocrine disruptors include bisphenol A (BPA) and other plastic components (see Chapter 2). BPA is commonly used in plastics and the lining of metal cans. Metabolites of this substance can be found in up to 90% of adults and children. BPA can impair the immune system and its responses. It can also contribute to the development of type 1 diabetes, at least in the mouse model.[6] This alteration in the immune system is a mechanism by which low-grade inflammation and dysbiosis contribute to the risk of metabolic syndrome and obesity.[15] One review demonstrated associations between BPA and adverse perinatal, childhood, and adult outcomes such as metabolic disease, reproductive disorders, and developmental defects.[59]

BPA has received a lot of attention, spurring the development of BPA-free containers and metal cans. This may help reduce the overall exposure to BPA, but it will not eliminate it given the widespread use of BPA in many other products. Moreover, manufacturers often replace BPA with similar chemicals, such as bisphenol S (BPS) and bisphenol F (BPF), which may have similar health concerns.[17] Further studies are needed to determine the health implications of topical exposure to BPA and related chemicals.

Triclosan is a common substance that can be found in cleaning supplies, toothpastes, and soaps (see Chapter 9). This environmental chemical has the potential to alter gut microbiota, endocrine function, and body mass index (BMI).[37] Triclosan can be found in personal care products, and a related compound called congener triclocarban can be found in numerous children's toys. The fact that triclosan can be detected in human blood and urine implies that it is absorbed systemically and can have more than just a topical effect.[37] Few epidemiologic studies directly link triclosan to type 1 and type 2 diabetes, but contact with this substance has been associated with rhinitis, food allergy, and low thyroid hormone levels.[6]

Flame retardants such as polybrominated diphenyl ethers (PDBEs) are widely used chemicals and are considered to be endocrine disruptors. Humans can be exposed by inhalation of indoor air and by food ingestion. In rats, this type of chemical can cause a variety of responses, including elevated tumor necrosis factor-α levels, hyperglycemia, and decreased insulin levels.[6]

Although good-quality epidemiologic studies in humans are lacking, this substance should at least be considered a risk factor for diabetes based on some of the physiologic responses it helps to propagate.

Phthalates are another group of compounds that are commonly used in cosmetics, pharmaceuticals, and food packaging as plasticizers.[6,65] They can contaminate food products, especially fatty foods, due to lipophilicity, and they have been associated with dysregulation of sex hormones, obesity, and insulin resistance.[65] Phthalates can induce oxidative stress and inflammation and have been associated with type 2 diabetes and asthma.[6]

This review has only touched on some of the environmental chemicals associated with obesity and diabetes, but we hope that it raises the awareness of clinicians about the many factors involved in the development of metabolic syndrome and its sequelae. Although caloric intake and food choices are important, they may not be the only driving factors in the obesity epidemic. Being cognizant of external factors, chemicals, and environmental exposures may help in managing the diversity of the gut microbiome and optimizing health.

SYSTEMIC NICKEL ALLERGY SYNDROME

Changes in the gut microbiome have been associated with allergy, and it is interesting to consider whether probiotics can modulate the allergic response and reduce symptoms. Systemic nickel allergy syndrome is a condition that may offer some insight. The syndrome can include symptoms of contact dermatitis and gastrointestinal symptoms with ingestion of nickel-containing foods. Those with this condition must follow a restrictive diet.

One study suggested that supplementation with *Lactobacillus reuteri* could help patients with this condition who must follow a low-nickel diet.[58] Supplementation helps to reduce the frequency and severity of symptoms. The study results suggested that the microbiome and particular microbial populations may play a significant role in the modulation of allergy and treatment of food allergy, at least for exposures to nickel.

Special Considerations

Other topics are pertinent to the discussion of gut dysbiosis. In addition to diet, nutrition and environmental toxins, various pathologic conditions underscore the significance of the microbiome in optimizing health through diet and toxin avoidance.

AUTISM

Autism is associated with gut dysbiosis with overgrowth of anaerobic organisms such as *Clostridium*, Bacteroidetes, and *Desulfovibrio*.[60] One hypothesis is that early in childhood infections and the use of antibiotics set the stage for an imbalance in gut flora. This impairs the immune system and allows for increased intestinal permeability. Subsequently, neurotoxic compounds, and xenobiotics are produced and absorbed, affecting the gut-brain axis.[47]

Delivery of intraventricular propionic acid and short-chain fatty acids (produced by the anaerobic bacteria found in those with autism spectrum disorders) to rats resulted in autistic-type behaviors such as abnormal movements, repetitive actions, cognitive deficits, and decreased social interactions.[42] This finding highlights how alterations in the gut microbiome can be a risk factor for autism. In the era of genomics, it is interesting to speculate whether the diet and environmental exposures of the mother in combination with inherited epigenomic modifications resulting from DNA methylation could impact the gut microbiome of the child and thereby predispose him or her to autism.

Environmental risk factors that have been proposed in susceptible individuals include diet, maternal diabetes, prenatal or perinatal stress, parental age, medications, zinc deficiency, supplements, pesticides, and infections.[35] There is likely a complex interplay among various factors, and the gut may be at the center. Use of this interplay to develop novel therapies or interventions could help management and avoid risk factors. One study suggested that treating high-risk infants with very high levels of lysozymes could suppress the growth rate of clostridia and reduce the risk of developing autism.[71] Although the answer to autism may not be in lysozyme therapy alone, this study raises the point that modulation of the gut microbiome by many of the previously described mechanisms may play an important role in prevention or treatment.

CANCER

At the center of any discussion of cancer is the epigenome, which includes the sleeve of chemical compounds overlying DNA that modulates actions of the genome. The gut microbiome interacts with the genome and epigenome, and all of these factors are affected by diet, nutrition, and environmental toxins. Changes in the intestinal environment have been associated with progression of adenomas and tumor formation in the colon. A study demonstrated that bacterial biofilms in the colon could make the colonic tissue more susceptible to carcinogenesis by upregulation of polyamine metabolites in the host tissues.[34]

Adding probiotics to a diet rich in cruciferous vegetables and green tea polyphenols is one way to bring about epigenetic changes in bacterial DNA or their target genes to help reduce the risk of colon cancer.[54] This approach addresses some of the proposed hypotheses regarding the causes of colon cancer, such as inflammation, bacterial toxins, and toxic microbial metabolites.[12] It certainly refines the concept behind the adenoma-carcinoma sequence and emphasizes that manipulation of the gut microbiota can have a therapeutic or preventive role in management of colonic neoplasia.[23]

Discussion of cancer and the microbiome is not limited to colon cancer. The microbiota influence the metabolism of estrogen and deconjugation reactions modulated by some bacterial species and could cause increased absorption of free estrogens. Elevated estrogen levels can promote development of breast, ovarian, and endometrial cancers.[54]

The development of liver and lung cancer may also be influenced by the gut microbiota. Toll-like receptors (e.g., TLR4) in the liver can be activated by microbial lipopolysaccharides and can result in injury and inflammation in liver tumors. Chronic inflammation and chromatin modifications are two proposed mechanisms involved in chronic obstructive pulmonary disease (COPD) and lung cancer.[54] Inflammation and alterations in the gut microbiome and the intestinal barrier are emerging as key concepts in the development of a variety of cancers, and exposures to environmental toxins and dietary factors drive these changes.

GUT-BRAIN AXIS

Research has demonstrated the key role that the gut microbiota play in a variety of neuropsychiatric conditions. The gut contains approximately 100 million neurons, more than the spinal cord, and it produces most of the body's serotonin.[18] It seems logical that there would be some connection between the gut and the nervous system. Studies using rodents have demonstrated that the gut influences emotion, stress, pain, and brain neurotransmitters. Some investigators suggest that the gut microbiota are involved in brain signaling and that the brain can alter the gut's microbial composition.[45]

Gut microbiota communicate with the central nervous system by several methods, including neural, endocrine, and immune pathways; this is how they influence brain function and behavior.[21] Understanding these mechanisms may improve our understanding of cognition, mood, personality, sleep, and many conditions ranging from autism to schizophrenia and may provide a platform on which to develop novel interventions and therapies.[10]

Chronic stress is a problem that plagues many people. A growing body of evidence supports the hypothesis that the gut microbiome plays a role in early programming and later responses to acute and chronic stress. Using this information to develop strategies to mitigate stress could prove helpful to many.[7]

Future of the Microbiome

Medicine is evolving at a rapid pace. Research into the gut microbiome's impact on human health is uncovering exciting findings and providing information never before considered. More research is needed to understand how the microbiome-gut-brain axis works and how interactions between the epigenome and the gut microbiome alter disease expression.

DNA methylation, the epigenetic process by which methyl groups are added to DNA to modify function, is proving to be one of the major factors in understanding disease because of the role it plays in epigenetic modulation of gene regulation. Fully understanding the role that nutrition and the gut play in this process is important. Educating patients about a healthy diet and lifestyle and empowering them to take command of their future by avoiding certain environmental toxins will prove to be one of the best interventions health care providers can offer. In the coming years, more refined diagnostic testing will likely become available. This will give patients and clinicians an idea of what health problems they have or may develop based on their microbial profile and degree of epigenomic alterations. Novel therapies and interventions aimed at modulating the gut microbiome will be developed to help prevent disease and detoxify the body to alter the disease course.

Conclusions

Interactions among diet, nutrition, and environmental toxins modulate the gut microbiome and affect a vast array of medical conditions. The purpose of reviewing these issues was not to create a sense of alarm but to raise awareness about the influences nutrition and environmental exposures can have on the gut microbiome and health. Exciting research is surfacing regarding the importance of gut health and the role of particular microbes in health, disease, and longevity.[5] We propose that for many conditions, from obesity to diabetes and cardiovascular disease to autism and schizophrenia, interactions among the gut microbiome and various complex pathways, including the endocrine, nervous, metabolic, and immune systems, will prove to be central to controlling inflammation, diminishing gut permeability, and healing patients.

It is not possible for humans to live in a bubble and avoid all environmental exposures. However, we hope that providing information about these issues will give clinicians the tools to educate and treat their patients. Using the power of the microbiome can allow health care providers to tailor prevention strategies and influence the course of disease.

Eating a well-balanced, healthy, antiinflammatory diet with plenty of colorful fruits and vegetables and probiotic foods is a great place to start. The key to gut health is biodiversity of the gut microbiome, and this type of diet can help to establish and maintain good health. We also suggest that consumers be aware of what they are buying and using on a regular basis. Reading the labels on foods is just as important as reading the labels on cosmetic products, soaps, tableware, and food containers. Eating organic foods whenever possible and making an effort to purchase products that are healthy and safe and do not contain harmful chemicals is a good practice to follow (see Chapters 8, 11 and 14).

- Many factors are involved in modulation of disease, and one of the central players is the gut microbiome. Giving patients current information and advising them about gut health can influence overall health outcomes and promote well-being. The following key points are emphasized:
- Intestinal permeability and inflammation are the root cause of many diseases, and the gut microbiome plays a vital role in this process.
- Understanding what constitutes a good diet is key to ensuring gut microbial health.
  - Avoid nonnutritive sweeteners and emulsifiers.
  - Drink filtered water.
  - Eat well-washed produce, and choose organic when possible.
  - Avoid processed foods, meat manufactured with antibiotics, and dairy products produced with hormones.
- Avoiding harmful environmental toxins can protect the gut microbiome and influence disease.
  - Use glass, ceramics, or stainless steel instead of plastics when cooking or heating foods to avoid BPA, BPS, BPF, and other harmful chemicals.
  - Use cosmetics and personal care items that are free from harmful chemicals such as triclosan and phthalates.
- Pregnant women should consider vaginal delivery and breast feeding if possible.

- Many conditions, including obesity, cancer, neurologic disease, autism, inflammatory bowel disease, irritable bowel syndrome, allergies, asthma, kidney disease, liver disease, and cardiac disease, are impacted by the composition of the gut microbiome.
- Understanding the factors that influence the gut microbiome is key to appreciating how to counsel patients to live healthy lifestyles.

REFERENCES

1. Benbrook, C.M. 2012. Impacts of genetically engineered crops on pesticide use in the U.S.: The first sixteen years. *Environ Sci Eur.* 24:24. doi: 10.1186/2190-4715-24-24.
2. Benbrook, C.M. 2016. Enhancements needed in GE crop and food regulation in the U.S. *Front Public Health.* 4:59. doi 10:3389/pubh.2016.00059.
3. Bhardwaj, D., Ansari, M.W., Sahoo, R.K., & Tuteja, N. 2014. Biofertilizers function as key player in sustainable agriculture by improving soil fertility, plant tolerance and crop productivity. *Microb Cell Fact.* 13: 66.
4. Bhattacharyya, S., Liu, H., Zhang, Z., et al. 2010. Carrageenan-induced innate immune response is modified by enzymes that hydrolyze distinct galactosidic bonds. *J Nutr Biochem.* 21:906–913.
5. Biagi, E., Franceschi, C., Rampelli, S., et al. 2016. Gut microbiota and extreme longevity. *Curr Biol.* 26:1480–1485.
6. Bodin, J., Stene, L.C., & Nygaard, U.C. 2015. Can exposure to environmental chemicals increase the risk of diabetes type 1 development? *Biomed Res Int.* 2015:208947.
7. Borre, Y.E., Moloney, R.D., Clarke, G., Dinan, T.G., & Cryan, J.F. 2014. The impact of microbiota on brain and behavior: mechanisms & therapeutic potential. *Adv Exp Med Biol.* 817:373–403.
8. Briskey, D., Tuckerb, P., Johnson, D., & Coombes, J. 2016. Microbiota and the nitrogen cycle: Implications in the development and progression of CVD and CKD. *Nitric Oxide.* 57:64–70.
9. Burke, M., & Small, D. 2015. Physiological mechanisms by which non-nutritive sweeteners may impact body weight and metabolism. *Physiol Behav.* 152:381–388.
10. Burokas, A., Moloney, R.D., Dinan, T.G., & Cryan, J.F. 2015. Microbiota regulation of the mammalian gut-brain axis. *Adv Appl Microbiol.* 91:1–62.
11. Camilleri, M., Lasch, K., & Zhou, W. 2012. Irritable bowel syndrome: Methods, mechanisms, and pathophysiology. The confluence of increased permeability, inflammation, and pain in irritable bowel syndrome. *Am J Physiol Gastrointest Liver Physiol.* 303:G775–G785.
12. Candela, M., Turroni, S., Biagi, E., et al. 2014. Inflammation and colorectal cancer: When microbiota-host mutualism breaks. *World J Gastroenterol.* 20:908–922.
13. Cani, P.D., & Everard, A. 2015. Keeping gut lining at bay: Impact of emulsifiers. *Trends Endocrinol Metab.* 6:273–274.

14. Cavaliere, C., Capriotti, A., Foglia, P., et al. 2015. Natural estrogens in dairy products: Determination of free and conjugated forms by ultra high performance liquid chromatography with tandem mass spectrometry. *J Separation Sci.* 38:3599–3606.
15. Chassaing, B., & Gewirtz, A.T. 2014. Gut microbiota, low-grade inflammation, and metabolic syndrome. *Toxicol Pathol.* 42:49–53.
16. Chassaing, B., Koren, O., Goodrich, J.K., et al. 2015. Dietary emulsifiers impact the mouse gut microbiota promoting colitis and metabolic syndrome. *Nature.* 519:92–96.
17. Chen, D., Kannan, K., Tan, H., et al. 2016. Bisphenol analogues other than BPA: Environmental occurrence, human exposure, and toxicity. A review. *Environ Sci Technol.* 50:5438–5453.
18. Chopra D, & Tanzi, R.E. 2015. *Super Genes: Unlock the Astonishing Power of Your DNA for Optimum Health and Well-Being.* New York, NY: Harmony Books.
19. Condette, J., Bach, V., Mayeur, C., Gay-Quéheillard, J., & Khorsi-Cauet, H. 2015. Chlorpyrifos exposure during perinatal period affects intestinal microbiota associated with delay of maturation of digestive tract in rats. *J Pediatr Gastroenterol Nutr.* 61:30–40.
20. Conlon, M.A., & Bird, A.R. 2015. The impact of diet and lifestyle on gut microbiota and human health. *Nutrients.* 7:17–44.
21. Cryan, J.F., & Dinan, T.G. 2012. Mind-altering microorganisms: The impact of the gut microbiota on brain and behaviour. *Nat Rev Neurosci.* 13:701–712.
22. Dietert, R.R., & Silbergeld, E.K. 2015. Biomarkers for the 21st century: Listening to the microbiome. *Toxicol Sci.* 144:208–216.
23. Dulal, S., & Keku, T.O. 2014. Gut microbiome and colorectal adenomas. *Cancer J.* 20:225–231.
24. Ferguson, J.F., Allayee, H., Gerszten, R.E., et al. 2016. Nutrigenomics, the microbiome, and gene-environment interactions. New directions in cardiovascular disease research, prevention, and treatment: A scientific statement from the American Heart Association. *Circ Cardiovasc Genet.* 9:291–313.
25. Fernandes, A., Antonio, A.L., Oliveira, M.B., Martins, A., & Ferreira, I.C. 2012. Effect of gamma and electron beam irradiation on the physico-chemical and nutritional properties of mushrooms: A review. *Food Chem.* 135:641–650.
26. Fernandes, A., Barreira, J.C., Antonio, A.L., Oliveira, M.B., Martins, A., & Ferreira, I.C. 2014. Effects of gamma irradiation on chemical composition and antioxidant potential of processed samples of the wild mushroom *Macrolepiota procera. Food Chem.* 149:91–98.
27. Fernandes, A., Barreira, J.C., Antonio, A.L., et al. 2015. How does electron beam irradiation dose affect the chemical and antioxidant profiles of wild dried *Amanita* mushrooms? *Food Chem.* 182:309–315.
28. Flint, H.J., Duncan, S.H., Scott, K.P., & Louis, P. 2015. Links between diet, gut microbiota composition and gut metabolism. *Proc Nutr Soc.* 74:13–22.
29. Gauguet, S., D'Ortona, S., Ahnger-Pier, K., et al. 2015. Intestinal microbiota of mice influences resistance to *Staphylococcus aureus* pneumonia. *Infect Immun.* 83:4003–4014.

30. Ghaisas, S., Maher, J., & Kanthasamy, A. 2016. Gut microbiome in health and disease: Linking the microbiome-gut-brain axis and environmental factors in the pathogenesis of systemic and neurodegenerative diseases. *Pharmacol Ther.* 158:52–62.

31. Gillings, M.R., Paulsen, I.T., & Tetu, S.G. 2015. Ecology and evolution of the human microbiota: Fire, farming and antibiotics. *Genes (Basel).* 6:841–857.

32. Heindel, J.J., Blumberg, B., Cave, M., et al. 2016. Metabolism disrupting chemicals and metabolic disorders. *Reprod Toxicol.*

33. Johnson, C., Patterson, A., Idle, J., & Gonzalez, F. 2012. Xenobiotic metabolomics: Major impact on the metabolome. *Annu Rev Pharmacol Toxicol.* 52:37–56.

34. Johnson, C.H., Dejea, C.M., Edler, D., et al. 2015. Metabolism links bacterial biofilms and colon carcinogenesis. *Cell Metab.* 21:891–897.

35. Koufaris, C., & Sismani, C. 2015. Modulation of the genome and epigenome of individuals susceptible to autism by environmental risk factors. *Int J Mol Sci.* 16:8699–8718.

36. Landrigan, P.J., & Benbrook, C.M. 2015. GMOs, herbicides, and public health. *N Engl J Med.* 373:693–695.

37. Lankester, J., Patel, C., Cullen, M.R., Ley, C., & Parsonnet, J. 2013. Urinary triclosan is associated with elevated body mass index in NHANES. *PLoS One.* 8:e80057.

38. López-Berenguer, C., Carvajal, M., Moreno, D.A., & García-Viguera, C. 2007. Effects of microwave cooking conditions on bioactive compounds present in broccoli inflorescences. *J Agric Food Chem.* 55:10001–10007.

39. Lu, K., Cable, P.H., Abo, R.P., et al. 2013. Gut microbiome perturbations induced by bacterial infection affect arsenic biotransformation. *Chem Res Toxicol.* 26:1893–1903.

40. Lu, K., Abo, R.P., Schlieper, K.A., et al. 2014. Arsenic exposure perturbs the gut microbiome and its metabolic profile in mice: An integrated metagenomics and metabolomics analysis. *Environ Health Perspect.* 122:284–291.

41. Lu, K., Mahbub, R., & Fox, J.G. 2015. Xenobiotics: Interaction with the intestinal microflora. *ILAR J.* 56:218–227.

42. Macfabe, D.F. 2012. Short-chain fatty acid fermentation products of the gut microbiome: Implications in autism spectrum disorders. *Microb Ecol Health Dis.* 23. doi: 10.3402/mehd.v23i0.19260.

43. Mantovani, A. 2015. Endocrine eisrupters and the safety of food chains. *Horm Res Paediatr.* Epub ahead of print.

44. Massey, V.L., Stocke, K.S., Schmidt, R.H., et al. 2015. Oligofructose protects against arsenic-induced liver injury in a model of environment/obesity interaction. *Toxicol Appl Pharmacol.* 284:304–314.

45. Mayer, E.A., Tillisch, K., & Gupta, A. 2015. Gut/brain axis and the microbiota. *J Clin Invest.* 125:926–938.

46. McDermott, A.J., & Huffnagle, G.B. 2014. The microbiome and regulation of mucosal immunity. *Immunology.* 142: 24–31.

47. Mezzelani, A., Landini, M., Facchiano, F., et al. 2015. Environment, dysbiosis, immunity and sex-specific susceptibility: A translational hypothesis for regressive autism pathogenesis. *Nutr Neurosci.* 18:145–161.
48. Miller, D. 2013. *Farmacology.* New York, NY: William Morrow.
49. Mulak, A., & Bonaz, B. 2015. Brain-gut-microbiota axis in Parkinson's disease. *World J Gastroenterol.* 21:10609–10620.
50. Myers, J.P., Antoniou, M.N., Blumberg, B., et al. 2016. Concerns over use of glyphosate-based herbicides and risks associated with exposures: A consensus statement. *Environ Health.* 15:19.
51. Nami, Y., Haghshenas, B., Abdullah, N., et al. 2015. Probiotics or antibiotics: future challenges in medicine. *J Med Microbiol.* 64:137–146.
52. O'Bryan, C.A., Crandall, P.G., Ricke, S.C., & Olson, D.G. 2008. Impact of irradiation on the safety and quality of poultry and meat products: A review. *Crit Rev Food Sci Nutr.* 48:442–457.
53. Parashar, A., & Udayabanu, M. 2016. Gut microbiota regulates key modulators of social behavior. *Eur Neuropsychopharmacol.* 26:78–91.
54. Paul, B., Barnes, S., Demark-Wahnefried, W., et al. 2015. Influences of diet and the gut microbiome on epigenetic modulation in cancer and other diseases. *Clin Epigenet.* 7:112.
55. Pepino, M.Y. 2015. Metabolic effects of non-nutritive sweeteners. *Physiol Behav.* 152:450–455.
56. Poovarodom, N., Junsrisuriyawong, K., Sangmahamad, R., & Tangmongkollert, P. 2014. Effects of microwave heating on the migration of substances from melamine formaldehyde tableware. *Food Addit Contam Part A Chem Anal Control Expo Risk Assess.* 31:1616–1624.
57. Quintana-Murci, L., Davenport, E.R., Mizrahi-Man, O., 2014. Seasonal variation in human gut microbiome composition. *PLoS One.* 9:e90731.
58. Randazzo, C.L., Pino, A., Ricciardi, L., et al. 2015. Probiotic supplementation in systemic nickel allergy syndrome patients: Study of its effects on lactic acid bacteria population and on clinical symptoms. *J Appl Microbiol.* 118:202–211.
59. Rochester, J. 2013. Bisphenol A and human health: A review of the literature. *Reprod Toxicol.* 42:132–155.
60. Samsel, A., & Seneff, S. 2013. Glyphosate's suppression of cytochrome P450 enzymes and amino acid biosynthesis by the gut microbiome: Pathways to modern diseases. *Entropy.* 15:1416–1463.
61. Sasada, T., Hinoi, T., Saito, Y., et al. 2015. Chlorinated water modulates the development of colorectal tumors with chromosomal instability and gut microbiota in Apc-deficient mice. *PLoS One.* 10:e0132435.
62. Schiffmann, R. 2013. Microwave ovens and food safety: Preparation of Not-Ready-to-Eat products in standard and smart ovens. *J Microw Power Electromagn Energy.* 47:46–62.
63. Sekirov, I., Tam, N.M., Jogova, M., et al. 2008. Antibiotic-induced perturbations of the intestinal microbiota alter host susceptibility to enteric infection. *Infect Immun.* 76:4726–4736.

64. Shannona, M., Rehfeld, A., Frizzella, C., et al. 2016. In vitro bioassay investigations of the endocrine disrupting potential of steviol glycosides and their metabolite steviol, components of the natural sweetener Stevia. *Mol Cell Endocrinol.* 427:65–72.

65. Simmons, A.L., Schlezinger, J.J., & Corkey, B.E. 2014. What are we putting in our food that is making us fat? Food additives, contaminants, and other putative contributors to obesity. *Curr Obes Rep.* 3:273–285.

66. Snedeker, S.M., & Hay, A.G. 2012. Do interactions between gut ecology and environmental chemicals contribute to obesity and diabetes? *Environ Health Perspect.* 120:332–339.

67. Suez, J., Korem,T., Zilberman-Schapira, G., Segal, E., & Elinav, E. 2015. Non-caloric artificial sweeteners and the microbiome: Findings and challenges. *Gut Microbes.* 6:149–155.

68. Tchounwou, P.B., Yedjou, C.G., Patlolla, A.K., & Sutton, D.J. 2012. Heavy metal toxicity and the environment. *EXS.* 101:133–164.

69. Tobacman, J.K. 2001. Review of harmful gastrointestinal effects of carrageenan in animal experiments. *Environ Health Perspect.* 109:983–994.

70. Turta, O., & Rautava, S. 2016. Antibiotics, obesity and the link to microbes: What are we doing to our children? *BMC Med.* 14:57.

71. Weston, B., Fogal, B., Cook, D., & Dhurjat, I.P. 2015. An agent-based modeling framework for evaluating hypotheses on risks for developing autism: Effects of the gutmicrobial environment. *Med Hypotheses.* 84:395–401.

72. Winglee, K., & Fodor, A.A. 2015. Intrinsic association between diet and the gut microbiome: Current evidence. *Nutr Dietary Suppl.* 7:69–76.

73. Wlodarska, M., Willing, B.P., Bravo, D.M., & Finlay, B.B. 2015. Phytonutrient diet supplementation promotes beneficial *Clostridia* species and intestinal mucus secretion resulting in protection against enteric infection. *Sci Rep.* 5:9253.

74. Xin, F., Susiarjo, M., & Bartolomei, M.S. 2015. Multigenerational and transgenerational effects of endocrine disrupting chemicals: A role for altered epigenetic regulation? *Semin Cell Dev Biol.* 43:66–75.

75. Yoo, J.Y., & Kim, S.S. 2016. Probiotics and prebiotics: Present status and future perspectives on metabolic disorders. *Nutrients.* 8:173.

76. Yoshifuji, A., Wakino, S., Irie, J., Tajima, T., Hasegawa, K., Kanda, T., et al. 2015. Gut *Lactobacillus* protects against the progression of renal damage by modulating the gut environment in rats. *Nephrol Dial Transplant.* 31:401–412.

77. Zhang, S., Jin,Y., Zeng, Z., Liu, Z., & Fu, Z. 2015. Subchronic exposure of mice to cadmium perturbs their hepatic energy metabolism and gut microbiome. *Chem Res Toxicol.* 28:2000–2009.

78. Zhang, Y., Jiang, L, et al. 2011. Possible involvement of oxidative stress in potassium bromate-induced genotoxicity in human HepG2 cells. *Chem Biol Interact.* 189:186–191.

7

Interaction of Pharmaceuticals with Environmental Chemicals

ANDERSON J. MARTINO-ANDRADE AND SHANNA H. SWAN

Key Concepts

- Commonly used pharmaceuticals, particularly mild analgesics, can act as endocrine disruptors.
- Acetaminophen (*N*-acetyl-*p*-aminophenol [APAP]) and other mild analgesics are widely used during pregnancy, and there is evidence of ubiquitous exposure from environmental sources.
- A pilot biomonitoring study found APAP in 100% of urine samples obtained from 111 U.S. pregnant women.
- Laboratory animal and *in vitro* studies indicate that many analgesics, including APAP, acetylsalicylic acid, and ibuprofen, can act as endocrine disruptors by inhibiting testicular production of prostaglandins, testosterone, and insulin-like growth factor 3.
- Epidemiologic studies suggest associations between prenatal exposure to some analgesics and cryptorchidism in humans, which are corroborated by the endocrine-mediated mechanisms described for these drugs.
- Mild analgesics and some environmental chemicals (e.g., phthalates) can disturb common endocrine pathways, raising the possibility of interactive effects.

Introduction

The most compelling evidence of prenatally induced endocrine-disrupting effects in humans comes from the unfortunate experience with the synthetic nonsteroidal estrogenic compound diethylstilbestrol (DES). The U.S. Food and Drug Administration (FDA) approved the use of this drug from 1947 to 1971 to prevent miscarriages and premature births.[9,51] However, DES proved ineffective, and it caused reproductive tract abnormalities in the daughters and sons of mothers who ingested the drug during their pregnancies, particularly during the first trimester. Of significant impact was the increased number of cases of vaginal adenocarcinoma in young women exposed *in utero* to DES.[22]

In the early 1990s, research in wildlife and laboratory animals revealed that exposure to environmental chemicals such as pesticides, components of plastics, and many other industrial chemicals could lead to developmental effects that were strikingly similar to those observed in humans exposed *in utero* to DES. Several of these environmental chemicals were demonstrated to be endocrine disruptors, with some acting as estrogenic or antiandrogenic compounds. The accumulating evidence of a decline in human reproductive health after World War II led to the hypothesis that the increasing human exposure to chemicals in the environment, particularly endocrine disruptors, could be associated with common male reproductive disorders of developmental origin, such as cryptorchidism, hypospadias, low sperm counts, and testicular cancer.[9,58]

In the past 2 decades, research on endocrine-disrupting chemicals has grown significantly. There has been an increase in the number of compounds identified as EDCs, but it also has become evident that chemicals can disrupt the endocrine system through multiple mechanisms. Although the strongest evidence of human endocrine disruption is linked to a pharmaceutical (i.e., DES), researchers have only recently turned their attention to the possibility of endocrine-disrupting effects of commonly used pharmaceuticals such as analgesics and antidepressants.[29,35,38] Analgesics are of special concern because of their common use worldwide, including by pregnant women.

In this chapter, we review data on prenatal exposure to analgesics, particularly to acetaminophen, which is the most commonly used analgesic by pregnant women. We also review *in vitro, in vivo*, and epidemiologic studies that report hormonal disturbances relevant to gonadal development and male genital abnormalities associated with developmental exposure to mild analgesics. Finally, we discuss the potential for interactions between analgesics and common environmental chemicals in light of their intertwined mechanisms of action.

Mild Analgesics and their Use in Pregnancy

Mild analgesics are among the most widely consumed medications worldwide, and they often are available as nonprescription (over-the-counter) drugs. This category includes nonsteroidal anti-inflammatory drugs

(NSAIDs); salicylates, a class of NSAIDs primarily represented by acetyl-salicylic acid (ASA); acetaminophen (*N*-acetyl-*p*-aminophenol [APAP]), also known as paracetamol; and dipyrone, whose use is restricted or banned in several countries. They are used to manage pain and often to control fever and inflammatory conditions. Table 7.1 shows the characteristics of commonly used mild analgesics, their main adverse effects, and their estimated prevalence of use in pregnancy.

Overall, studies from many parts of the world indicate substantial use of mild analgesics by pregnant women. In the United States, the estimated use of analgesics and other drugs by pregnant women was reported by two large multisite, case-control studies, the Slone Epidemiology Center's Birth Defects Study (BDS) and the National Birth Defects Prevention Study (NBDPS) coordinated by the Centers for Disease Control and Prevention (CDC).[56,63] A review of these studies focusing on early pregnancy use indicated that 56% of U.S. women used APAP at some point during the first trimester, whereas ibuprofen (IBP) and ASA were used by 24% and 5% of the women, respectively.[56]

A publication based on records of 20,251 BDS participants interviewed between 1976 and 2004 indicated that although ASA use declined in the late 1970s, APAP use increased and remained high.[63] From 1981 to 2004, 60% to 70% of interviewed women reported taking APAP at some point during pregnancy.[63] An increase in use was also observed for other analgesics as they became available as nonprescription drugs, such as IBP (1984) and naproxen (1994).[63] In Denmark, a study reported use of APAP by 50.3% of 88,142 pregnant women selected from the Danish National Birth Cohort.[43] Another Danish study reported that mild analgesics were used during pregnancy by 56.2% of 491 mothers.[29] In that study, APAP use was reported by 47.6% of participants, and IBP and ASA were used by 7.7% and 4.3%, respectively. A few women (2.05%) reported simultaneous use of more than one mild analgesic.

In a study conducted in the Netherlands with 3184 mother–male infant pairs, 29.9% of mothers reported use of mild analgesics during pregnancy.[49] The EDEN mother-child cohort conducted in Nancy and Poitiers, France, reported analgesic use by 81% of 895 women during the first or second trimester.[41] Dipyrone has been withdrawn from the U.S. market, but it is still used in parts of South America, Europe, Africa, and Asia as a prescription or over-the-counter drug. Studies report dipyrone use by 5% to 11% of pregnant women.[5,10]

Mild analgesics exert their therapeutic effects primarily through inhibition of the cyclooxygenase (COX) enzyme. This enzyme catalyzes the conversion of arachidonic acid to prostanoids (e.g., prostaglandins), which are mediators involved in the promotion of inflammation and pain.[7] In the general population and among pregnant women, the profile of therapeutic and toxic

Table 7.1. Characteristics of Over-the-Counter Mild Analgesics and Use in Pregnancy

Chemical Name	Trade Names	Type and Uses	Estimated Use (%) and Restrictions in Pregnancy*	Main Toxic Effects	Analgesic Mode of Action
Acetaminophen (APAP)	Tylenol, Panadol	Analgesic, antipyretic	First choice as a pain reliever in pregnancy (56%)	Liver toxicity	Reversible COX[†] inhibition and additional mechanisms
Acetylsalicylic acid (ASA)	Aspirin, Bayer Aspirin, Ecotrin	Salicylate, NSAID[‡]	Not recommended except for specific conditions (5.3%)	Gastrointestinal ulcers; acid-base balance disturbance; renal toxicity	Irreversible COX inhibition
Fenoprofen	Nalfon	NSAID	Restricted; not recommended in third trimester (NA)	Gastrointestinal ulcers, renal toxicity	Reversible COX inhibition
Ibuprofen (IBP)	Advil, Motrin	NSAID	Restricted; not recommended in third trimester (24%)	Gastrointestinal ulcers, renal toxicity	Reversible COX inhibition
Indomethacin	Indocin, Tivorbex	NSAID	Restricted; not recommended in third trimester except for treatment of preterm labor under medical supervision (NA)	Gastrointestinal ulcers, renal toxicity	Reversible COX inhibition

Ketoprofen	Orudis, Oruvail, Nexcede, Actron	NSAID	Restricted; not recommended in third trimester (NA)	Gastrointestinal ulcers, renal toxicity	Reversible COX inhibition
Naproxen	Aleve, Naprelan, Naprosyn, Flanax	NSAID	Restricted; not recommended in third trimester (4.3%)	Gastrointestinal ulcers, renal toxicity	Reversible COX inhibition

*According to Thorpe, P.G., Gilboa, S.M., Hernandez-Diaz, S., et al. 2013. Medications in the first trimester of pregnancy: most common exposures and critical gaps in understanding fetal risk. *Pharmacoepidemiol Drug Saf.* 22:1013–1018.

†Therapeutic and classic toxic effects depend on the selectivity for cyclooxygenase (i.e., COX-2 and COX-1).

‡Nonsteroidal anti-inflammatory drugs (NSAIDs) typically are used as analgesics, anti-inflammatories, and in the treatment of arthritis.

NA = not available or unknown.

responses exerted by mild analgesics depends strongly on the site of action and on the selectivity of the drug by the two main COX isoforms, COX-1 and COX-2. Inflammatory responses are mostly mediated by prostanoids formed after COX-2 expression; COX-1 is expressed constitutively in most cells to generate prostanoids that modulate numerous physiologic processes, such as gastric epithelial cytoprotection and renal blood flow.[44]

The mode of action of APAP is not completely elucidated, but it is agreed that it reduces prostaglandin synthesis through inhibition of COX-1 and COX-2, particularly when low levels of arachidonic acid and peroxides are available; this could explain the reduced anti-inflammatory activity of APAP compared with NSAIDs[18] Evidence also suggests that APAP activates the endocannabinoid system directly or through its metabolite *N*-(4-hydroxyphenyl)-arachidonoylethanolamide (AM404).[15,40] ASA is thought to irreversibly inhibit COX-1 ad COX-2, but the inhibition produced by other NSAIDs is reversible.

Among NSAIDs, the range of therapeutic and toxic responses varies according to pharmacokinetic characteristics and COX selectivity. Dipyrone has limited anti-inflammatory effects, and the analgesic mode of action is credited to several effects of dipyrone metabolites, including COX inhibition and interaction with the endocannabinoid system.[14]

ASA and other NSAIDs are usually contraindicated during pregnancy because they have been associated with increased risk of early pregnancy loss and particularly because administration during late gestation can affect the physiology of the pregnancy and the fetus. The systemic inhibition of prostaglandin synthesis during the third trimester can cause constriction of the ductus arteriosus and critically reduce renal blood flow.[42] The premature closure of the fetal ductus arteriosus—a blood vessel connecting the fetal pulmonary artery and descending aorta that allows blood to bypass pulmonary circulation—can cause pulmonary hypertension in newborns. Reduced renal blood flow induced by anti-inflammatory drugs may result in diminished fetal urine output and consequent deficiency of amniotic fluid (i.e., oligohydramnios). ASA may increase the risk of peripartum hemorrhage because the drug can irreversibly bind to COX and therefore permanently inhibit platelet activation.[42]

APAP has been accepted as the first-choice mild analgesic for pregnant women because it is not a typical anti-inflammatory drug and does not cause the previously mentioned problems.[3,42] However, as with any other drugs, APAP is not free of toxicity, and its widespread use by pregnant women has raised concerns about possible adverse effects to the developing fetus.[1,27,29,49] Several studies indicate that prenatal exposure to APAP and other mild analgesics is associated with adverse health consequences for infants, including increased risk of asthma, attention deficit hyperactivity disorder (ADHD), and endocrine and reproductive disorders, particularly cryptorchidism.[29,33,50]

This chapter presents new data on APAP exposure during pregnancy and review the evidence of possible endocrine and reproductive alterations associated with prenatal exposure to mild analgesics, with particular focus on male reproductive development and genital defects. Also discussed are some of the mechanisms of endocrine disruption by mild analgesics and the possibility of interactive effects with environmental endocrine disruptors that target similar hormonal systems.

HUMAN BIOMONITORING STUDIES OF ACETAMINOPHEN

Few studies have obtained biomarkers of mild analgesics in general populations or in specific groups such as children and pregnant women[36] To investigate prenatal APAP exposure, we analyzed urinary concentrations of this drug in a subset ($n = 111$) of pregnant women enrolled in the Study for Future Families (SFF). The SFF is a multicenter pregnancy cohort study conducted at prenatal clinics in California (Harbor, University of California–Los Angeles, and Cedars-Sinai medical centers), Minnesota (University of Minnesota Health Center, Minneapolis), and Missouri (University Physicians, Columbia) from September 1999 through August 2002 and in Iowa (University of Iowa, Iowa City) from September 2002 to February 2005 and has been described elsewhere.[52,54]

APAP concentrations in urine were measured at the Institute for Prevention and Occupational Medicine of the German Social Accident Insurance (Institute of the Ruhr-Universität Bochum, Bochum, Germany) by high-performance liquid chromatography and isotope dilution tandem mass spectrometry (HPLC-MS/MS), as described elsewhere.[13,36] APAP was measured in spot urine samples taken at a median of 27 weeks' gestation, and the main results are shown in Table 7.2.

APAP was detected in all 111 SFF urinary samples analyzed, confirming the ubiquitous exposure of pregnant women to this drug. A total of 24 (21.6%) of 111 women had urinary concentrations greater than 4000 µg/L, a cutoff value used to indicate recent APAP use (36 to 48 hours). This cutoff value was set based on the drug elimination kinetics and empirical evidence indicating that concentrations of approximately 4000 µg/L are found in urine spot samples 36 to 48 hours after the administration of a single tablet of APAP (500 mg).[36] Values lower than this cutoff level can indicate past intentional use (>48 to 36 hours) or unintentional (background) exposure. Considering the short half-life of this drug and the fact that only spot urine samples were

Table 7.2.   Urinary Concentrations of Acetaminophen in a Subset of Pregnant Women Enrolled in the Study for Future Families

Parameter	Background Exposure*	Possible Intentional Use[1]	Total
N (%)	87 (78.4%)	24 (21.6%)	111 (100%)
Mean (SD)	562 (923)	87,919 (165,188)	19,450 (83,732)
Median	75.9	21,468	261.3
Minimum	4.06	4354	4.06
Maximum	3927	767,518	767,518
25th percentile	21.8	7916	33.9
75th percentile	719.9	83,058	2839

*A cutoff value of 4000 µg/L was used to differentiate users and nonusers of acetaminophen. This value was based on the drug elimination kinetics as previously published (Modick, H., Weiss, T., Dierkes, G., Bruning, T., & Koch, H.M. 2014. Ubiquitous presence of paracetamol in human urine: Sources and implications. *Reproduction*. 147:R105–R117; Dierkes, G., Weiss, T., Modick, H., Kafferlein, H.U., Bruning, T., & Koch, H.M. 2014. N-Acetyl-4-aminophenol (paracetamol), N-acetyl-2-aminophenol and acetanilide in urine samples from the general population, individuals exposed to aniline and paracetamol users. *Int J Hyg Environ Health*. 217:592–599).

analyzed, it is surprising that recent intentional use of APAP was identified in more than 20% of pregnant women.

In 2014, Modick and colleagus[36] reported concentrations of APAP in spot urine samples of 2098 adults from the general German population who were presumably not pregnant and not occupationally exposed to aniline, a chemical compound that is converted *in vivo* into APAP. The median concentration of APAP was 61.7 µg/L (range, 0.65 µg/L to 2274 mg/L). A total of 106 individuals (5% of the study population) had urinary concentrations greater than the cutoff level used to indicate recent use. Nielsen and colleagues[39] investigated the urinary concentrations of APAP in 145 Danish school children between the ages of 6 and 11 years and their mothers. APAP was detected in all mothers, with concentrations ranging from 4.9 µg/L to 3.0 g/L (median, 120 µg/L), and 23 mothers (15.9%) had concentrations greater than the cutoff value of 4000 µg/L. All children except one had measurable levels of APAP (median, 27 µg/L; maximum, 2.0 g/L), and nine children (6.2%) had concentrations greater than 4000 µg/L. However, as reported by Modick and coworkers,[36] the use of this cutoff value is arbitrary and can result in overestimations or underestimations of intentional use. For instance, occupational exposure to aniline can produce urinary concentrations greater than this value, and the therapeutic use of APAP can result in urinary concentrations lower than 1000 µg/L 2 days after administration, depending on the dose used.[13,36]

Despite limitations, human biomonitoring data can be useful to document human exposure to mild analgesics. It is remarkable that urinary concentrations of APAP are found ubiquitously among different groups and that pregnant women, as indicated by the SFF data, are those with the highest proportion of individuals with recent intentional use. This may reflect the fact that APAP is often recommended by doctors during all stages of pregnancy and is therefore perceived by pregnant women as a medication without risks, leading to overuse. Studies using larger sample sizes are needed to more accurately document human exposure during pregnancy and associated health outcomes.

SOURCES OF ACETAMINOPHEN EXPOSURE

In addition to intentional or therapeutic use of APAP, the ubiquitous detection of urinary concentrations of this drug indicates the existence of possible unintentional (background) sources of exposure. Unintentional exposure may occur by direct ingestion of APAP residues in food and water or through exposure to aniline, an important source material in the chemical industry that is converted *in vivo* to APAP.[28,37] According to human data, 56% to 69% of an oral aniline dose is excreted as unconjugated APAP in urine and additional 2.5% to 6.1% is excreted as its mercapturic acid conjugate.[37]

To address the question of intentional, background, and occupational APAP exposure, Dierkes and coworkers[13] measured the urinary concentrations of APAP and acetanilide, a biomarker of aniline exposure, in three groups: 31 volunteers not occupationally exposed to aniline and not using APAP for at least 1 week before urine collection (i.e., group 1); 6 subjects occupationally exposed to aniline but with no recent use of APAP (i.e., group 2); and 2 volunteers who used APAP the day before sampling but who had no known occupational exposure to aniline (i.e., group 3). All participants in group 1, with no intentional use of APAP and no occupational exposure to aniline, had detectable urinary concentrations of APAP, ranging from 8.4 to 2263 µg/L, but no measurable levels of acetanilide. Subjects from group 2 had detectable concentrations of both chemicals, although APAP levels were about 100 times higher than levels of acetanilide, which is consistent with results from animal studies and estimated excretion ratios in humans exposed to aniline. In this group, the median (range) concentration of APAP was 5720 µg/L (4150 to 10,885 µg/L). In the two volunteers who used APAP 1 day before urine sampling, the concentrations of APAP were in the milligram per liter range (159 and 275 mg/L), 70 to 120 and 15 to 25 times higher than the maximum levels detected in groups 1 and 2, respectively. Similar to group 1, the volunteers taking APAP had no measurable concentrations of acetanilide, suggesting no exposure to aniline.

The ubiquitous detection of APAP in urine samples of subjects in group 1 indicates the existence of important sources of background exposure other than aniline, possibly through direct exposure to APAP in water and diet. As pointed out by Dierkes and coworkers,[13] APAP is used in veterinary medicine in many countries with no specific regulations in regard to holding time and maximal residue levels in food products obtained from animals receiving this drug. Therefore, animal products provide possible sources of exposure, although this and other sources deserve further scrutiny. Hong and colleagues[25] detected concentrations of APAP in wastewater in South Korea at concentrations greater than 1 μg/L.

Developmental Exposure to Mild Analgesics and Male Reproductive Disorders

Several *in vitro* and *in vivo* studies indicate that mild analgesics can alter the testicular development and lead to endocrine disturbances and reproductive tract defects.[1,29,31,35,61] Prostaglandins regulate several functions in the reproductive system, including ovulation, luteolysis, and parturition in females and modulation of immune responses and spermatogenesis in males.[17,47,60] In the developing testis, prostaglandin D_2 (PGD2) is involved in seminiferous cord formation by maintaining continued expression of SOX9, a key regulator of Sertoli cell differentiation and subsequent testis development and masculinization of the reproductive tract.[26,64] Table 7.3 summarizes the main *in vitro* and *in vivo* effects of common mild analgesics on endocrine end points associated with male reproductive development.

Early studies conducted by Gupta and coworkers[19] indicated that *in utero* exposure of B10.A mice to COX inhibitors (i.e., ASA and indomethacin) could induce antiandrogenic effects in male offspring, expressed as reduced anogenital distance (AGD), a well-known marker of prenatal androgen insufficiency in males.[19] In other studies, urogenital ducts from CD-1 mice cultured *in vitro* and treated with ASA and indomethacin failed to complete wolffian duct differentiation.[20] These compounds also prevented wolffian duct differentiation in female explants treated with exogenous testosterone.[20]

Kristensen and colleagues[29] reported reduced AGDs in male Wistar rats exposed *in utero* to APAP at doses of 150, 250, and 350 mg/kg/day from gestation days 13 to 21, which is consistent with an antiandrogenic mode of action.

Table 7.3. Summary of *In Vitro*, *Ex Vivo*, and *In Vivo* Studies on Endocrine and Reproductive Effects of Mild Analgesics

Study	Model	Time and Route of Dosing	Substance and Dose Levels	Hormonal Changes	Main Reproductive Effects
In Vitro and *Ex Vivo* Models					
Gupta and Bentlejewski, 1992	Urogenital explants of CD-1 mice	Culture of mouse ducts and urogenital sinus (gestation day 13) for 5 days	Indomethacin: 1, 10, and 50 µg/mL	Not available	Incomplete wolffian duct development at 10 and 50 µg/mL
			ASA: 10, 100, and 1000 µg/mL	Not available	Incomplete wolffian duct development at 100 and 1000 µg/mL
Han et al., 2010	H295R human adrenocortical carcinoma cell line	48-hr exposure by culture medium	IBP: 0.02–20 mg/L	T production: decreased (significant trend) Estradiol production: increased at 2 and 20 mg/L and an overall significant trend	Not available
Kristensen et al., 2011	*Ex vivo* fetal rat testis organotypic culture	Culture of fetal testes (gestation day 14.5) for 3 days	APAP: 1 µM	T production: decreased PGD2: decreased	Not available
			ASA: 1 and 10 µM	T production: decreased (10 µM)PGD2: decreased (10 µM)	Not available
Kristensen et al., 2012	*Ex vivo* fetal rat testis organotypic culture	Culture of fetal testes (gestation day 14.5) for 3 days	APAP: 0.1–100 µM	T production: decreased (0.5–100 µM)PGD2: increased (only at 100 µM) INSL3: no effect	No effects on testis morphology No effects on Leydig cell number No effect on percentage of apoptotic gonocytes

Table 7.3. Continued

Study	Model	Time and Route of Dosing	Substance and Dose Levels	Hormonal Changes	Main Reproductive Effects
			ASA: 0.1–100 µM	T production: decreased (10 and 100 µM)PGD2: no effect INSL3: not measured	No effects on testis morphology No effects on Leydig cell number No effect on percentage of apoptotic gonocytes
			Indomethacin: 1 and 10 µM	T production: decreased PGD2: decreased (1 and 10 µM) INSL3: not measured	Not available
Albert et al., 2013	Organotypic culture of adult human testis	Culture adult human testes for 24–48 hr	APAP: 10 and 100 µM	T production: decreased (10 and 100 µM)PGD2: decreased (100 µM) PGE2: decreased (100 µM) INSL3 not altered	No effects on testis morphology
			ASA: 10 and 100 µM	T production: decreased (10 and 100 µM)PGD2: decreased (10 and 100 µM) PGE2: decreased (10 µM) INSL3: decreased (10 and 100 µM)	No effects on testis morphologyIncreased number of Leydig cells (100 µM)

Study	Model	Treatment	Effects	Morphology
		Indomethacin: 10 and 100 µM	T production: decreased (10 and 100 µM)PGD2: decreased (10 and 100 µM) PGE2: decreased (10 and 100 µM) INSL3: decreased (100 µM)	No effects on testis morphologyIncreased number of Leydig cells (10 µM)
Mazoud-Guittot et al., 2013	Organotypic culture of fetal human testis and luciferase reporter gene cells for nuclear receptor–mediated agonistic or antagonistic activity of AR/ER/PPARγ	Culture fetal human testes (gestation weeks 7–12) incubated for 24–72 hr; AR/ER/PPAR-sensitive luciferase cells incubated for 16 hr — APAP and AM404 (APAP metabolite): 10 µM (APAP 0.1–100 µM for INSL3);	T production: decreased INSL3: decreased (dose dependent) AMH: no effect PGD2: no effect PGE2: decreased AR/ER/PPARγ: no activation	No effects of testis morphology or Sertoli cell number
		ASA: 10 µM (0.1–100 µM for testosterone)	T production: increased (dose-dependent)INSL3: no effect AMH: increased PGD2: no effect PGE2: decreased AR/ER/PPARγ: no activation	No effects of testis morphology or Sertoli cell number
		Indomethacin: 10 µM	T production: increased INSL3: no effect AMH: no effect PGD2: no effect PGE2: decreased AR/ER/PPARγ: no effect, except for PPARγ agonistic activity	No effects of testis morphology or Sertoli cell number

(continued)

Table 7.3. Continued

Study	Model	Time and Route of Dosing	Substance and Dose Levels	Hormonal Changes	Main Reproductive Effects
Tinwell et al., 2013	H295R human adrenocortical carcinoma cell line	48-hr exposure by culture medium	APAP: 250–1000 µM	T production: decreased (500 and 1000 µM)Estradiol production: increased (25–1000 µM)	Not available
			IBP: 12.5–50 µM	T production: no effect Estradiol production: no effect	
Van den Driesche et al., 2015	Human xenografted fetal testis	Host mice treated orally once daily for 7 days	APAP: 350 mg/kg	Serum T 1 hr after last treatment: no effect	Seminal vesicle weight: reduced
		Host mice treated orally 3 times daily for 7 days	APAP: 20 mg/kg	Serum T 1 hr after last treatment: no effect	Seminal vesicle weight: reduced
		Host mice treated orally 3 times daily for 1 day	APAP: 20 mg/kg	Serum T 1 hr after last treatment: no effect	Seminal vesicle weight: no effect

Study	Model	Exposure	Dose	Hormone/PGE2 effects	Other effects
Holm et al., 2015	H295R human adrenocortical carcinoma cell line	48-hr exposure by culture medium	APAP: 0.1, 0.314, 1, 3.14, 10, 31.4, 100, 314, and 1000 µM	Pregnenolone: increased (EC_{50} = 146 µM) 17α-hydroxyprogesterone: decreased (EC_{50} = 437 µM) Androstenedione: decreased (EC_{50} = 289 µM) Testosterone: decreased (EC_{50} = 97 µM) Estrone: increased (EC_{50} = 182 µM) β-Estradiol: increased (EC_{50} = 373 µM)	Not available
In Vivo Studies					
Gupta and Goldman, 1986	B10.A mice	Gestation day 11–14, subcutaneous injections	ASA 150 and 400 mg/kg/day	Not available	AGD: reduced (150 and 400 mg/kg)
			Indomethacin 1 mg/kg/day	Not available	AGD: reduced
Gupta, 1989	CD-1 mice	Gestation day 13–17, subcutaneous injections	ASA 100 mg/kg/day	PGE2 in fetal genital tract: reduced	Not available
			Indomethacin 1 mg/kg/day	PGE2 in fetal genital tract: reduced	Not available
Wise et al., 1991	Sprague-Dawley rats	Gestation day 11–19, oral gavage	ASA: 75, 150, and 300 mg/kg/day	Not available	AGD: no effects Preputial separation: no effects Testicular descent: no effects

(continued)

Table 7.3. Continued

Study	Model	Time and Route of Dosing	Substance and Dose Levels	Hormonal Changes	Main Reproductive Effects
Little et al, 1995	Balb/c mice	Gestation day 12–18; subcutaneous injections	Indomethacin: 1 mg/kg/day	- PGE2 in fetal genital tract: reduced - PGE2 in bulbourethral gland: reduced	AGD: no effect
Kristensen et al., 2011	Wistar rats	Gestation day 13–21; oral gavage	APAP: 150, 250 and 350 mg/kg/day	T testosterone content/ production: no effect	AGD: reduced (absolute and relative) in all doses
			ASA: 150, 200, and 250 mg/kg/day	T testosterone content/ production: no effect	AGD: reduced (but not after body weight correction)
Dean et al., 2013	Wistar rats	Gestation day 15–18; subcutaneous injections	Indomethacin 1 mg/kg/day	T testosterone: no effect PGE2 in fetal testis: reduced	AGD: no effect Reduced fetal testis weight, but no effects on juvenile and adult testis Penis length: reduced only in adult rats
Axelstad et al., 2014	Wistar rat	Gestation day 13–19 and lactation day 14–22; oral gavage	APAP: 350 mg/kg/day	Not available	Nipple retention (day 13) LABC weight: reduced (day 16) AGD: no effect

Van den Driesche et al., 2015	Wistar rat	Gestation day 13–17 (or 20); oral gavage	APAP 350 mg/kg/day (once daily)	Intratesticular testosterone 3 hr after last treatment: on day 17 reduced; reduced mRNA expression of steroidogenic enzymes CYP17A1 and CYP11A1	AGD: reduced
		Gestation day 13–17; oral gavage	APAP 20 mg/kg (3 times daily)	Intratesticular testosterone 3 hr after last treatment on day 17: unchanged	Not available
Holm et al., 2015	Mice C57BL/6JBomTac	Gestation day 7 to delivery; oral gavage	APAP: 50 and 150 mg/kg/day	Not available	AGD: reduced (150 mg/kg/day in 10 week-old-mice)

AGD = anogenital distance; AMH = antimullerian hormone; APAP = acetaminophen; AR = androgen receptor; EC_{50} = half maximal effective concentration; ER = estrogen receptor; IBP = ibuprofen; INSL3 = insulin-like factor 3; LABC = levator ani/bulbocavernosus muscle; PGD2 = prostaglandin D_2; PGE2 = prostaglandin E_2; PPARγ = peroxisome proliferator–activated receptor-γ; SA = acetylsalicylic acid; T = testosterone.

Van den Driesche and coworkers[61] confirmed these results by showing a significant suppression of intratesticular testosterone content in rat fetuses exposed *in utero* to 350 mg/kg/day of APAP, which also resulted in shortened AGDs. In pregnant mice, administration of APAP at 150 mg/kg/day or aniline at 93 mg/kg/day from gestation day 7 to delivery induced short AGDs in male[23] and female offspring.[24] It was also shown that aniline is rapidly converted into APAP in the mouse liver.[23] However, some studies reported a lack of effects on the AGD after *in utero* exposure to mild analgesics in different animal models, including Sprague-Dawley rats exposed to ASA,[65] Balb/c mice and Wistar rats exposed to indomethacin,[11,34] and Wistar rats exposed to APAP.[4]

In the study by Axelstad and colleagues,[4] nipple retention and reduced weight of levator ani/bulbocavernosus muscle, effects associated with prenatal androgen deficiency, were observed in male Wistar rats exposed *in utero* to APAP (350 mg/kg/day), despite the lack of effects on the AGD. Results of two studies also indicated that *in utero* exposure to APAP and indomethacin can deplete germ cells in the ovaries of mice and rats, leading to reduced follicle reserves and impaired fertility.[12,24]

The changes in male reproductive tract development in laboratory animals are further supported by mechanistic *in vitro* studies and rat and human testis *ex vivo* culture systems. A series of these studies found that mild analgesics could induce multiple hormonal disturbances, including inhibition of testosterone production and insulin-like factor 3 (INSL3), a testicular hormone involved in gubernacular development and abdominal descent of the testis.[1,29,31,35,61] Culture systems of fetal rat testicular explants have shown inhibition of testosterone production by APAP, ASA, and indomethacin, as well as reduction of INSL3 levels by APAP.[29,31]

Organotypic cultures of adult testes have also indicated interference of mild analgesics with hormonal production in humans. Using adult human testicular explants, Albert and coworkers[1] demonstrated that APAP, ASA, and indomethacin inhibited testosterone production *in vitro* (10^{-5} to 10^{-4} M). However, in human fetal testis explants, the hormonal disturbances observed were more varied, with unexpected stimulatory effects of ASA (10^{-7} to 10^{-4} M) and indomethacin (10^{-5}M) on testosterone synthesis.[35] In this *ex vivo* model system, APAP and its metabolite AM404 induced no changes in testosterone production in the fetal testis but significantly reduced INSL3 production.

Mazaud-Guittot and colleagues[35] investigated possible estrogen, androgen, and peroxisome proliferator-activated receptor-γ (PPARγ) agonistic and antagonistic activities of APAP and ASA by *in vitro* reporter gene assays. The results were negative for all receptor-mediated agonistic or antagonistic responses, indicating that the endocrine modulation exerted by these compounds involves other hormonal signaling pathways or alternative mechanisms, such as interference with gonadal function and hormonal production.

Tinwell and coworkers[57] tested APAP and IBP *in vitro* using the human estrogen receptor transcriptional activation (hERTa) and the H295R (human adrenocortical carcinoma cell) steroidogenesis assays. Both compounds tested negative in the hERTa assay, indicating absence of intrinsic estrogenic activity. In the H295R steroidogenesis assay, APAP but not IBP significantly reduced the production of testosterone and increased the production of estradiol.

Holm and colleagues[23] also found that APAP disrupted steroidogenesis in H295R cells by decreasing hormone concentrations downstream of progesterone, including pregnenolone, androstenedione, and testosterone, suggesting impairment of CYP17A1 (17α-hydroxylase/17,20 lyase/17,20 desmolase) and other downstream enzymes, while also increasing the concentrations of estrone and estradiol, possibly by augmented CYP19 (aromatase) activity. Han and associates[21] reported similar results for IBP: decreased testosterone and increased estradiol concentrations in H259R cell media after IBP exposure (see Table 7.3). In this study, aromatase activity was significantly increased after preincubation of H295R cells with IBP. In the study by Albert and colleagues[1], testosterone production in H295R cells was inhibited by APAP, ASA, and indomethacin.

In their study, van den Driesche and colleagues[61] provided another piece of evidence for the endocrine-disruptive properties of APAP, with possible repercussions for the developing fetus. The study showed inhibition of testosterone production by this drug in a xenograft model of human fetal testis. In this model, fragments of second-trimester human fetal testis were transplanted to castrated, human chorionic gonadotrophin (hCG)-treated host mice, which were subsequently exposed to APAP (20 mg/kg) three times daily for 7 days. This human-relevant dose regimen reduced plasma testosterone concentrations and seminal vesicle weights compared with vehicle controls. These effects were not observed when host mice were treated for a short term (1 day) with this dose (3 × 20 mg/kg), indicating that prolonged exposure may be needed for the manifestation of testosterone insufficiency in the human xenografted fetal testis. The results obtained in this study contrast with the findings reported by Mazaud-Guittot and coworkers,[35] who used an *ex vivo* culture system and showed reduced levels of INSL3 but no effects on testosterone production. However, the *ex vivo* culture system[35] used testes at gestation weeks 7 to 12 and exposure times restricted to 1 to 3 days, whereas the xenograft study used testes at 14 to 17 weeks' gestation and up to 7 days of exposure. These differences in the age window of exposure and duration of treatment may explain, in part the discrepancy between the study findings.

The study by van den Driesche and colleagues[61] also investigated the effects of APAP in a rat model. In addition to suppressed fetal intratesticular testosterone content and reduced AGD, a treatment dose of 350 mg/kg/day reduced the expression of two key steroidogenic enzymes in the rat fetal testis, CYP17A1 and CYP11A1 (cytochrome P-40scc/cholesterol 20-22-desmolase), but expression of INSL3 and transcription factor SOX9 were unchanged. However, repeated-dose treatment of rat dams (gestation day 13 to 17) with the same dosage used in the human xenograft study (i.e., three daily doses of 20 mg/kg) did not change fetal intratesticular testosterone content.

Overall, the *in vitro* and *in vivo* studies of mild analgesics indicate potential endocrine-disrupting effects, which are in agreement with epidemiologic studies suggesting associations between prenatal exposure to some of these drugs and genital defects, particularly cryptorchidism, in humans.

ASSOCIATIONS BETWEEN MATERNAL EXPOSURE TO MILD ANALGESICS AND MALE GENITAL OUTCOMES IN HUMANS

The first association between mild analgesics and genital malformations was made in 1996 by Berkowitz and Lapinski,[6] who reported a relationship between the use of analgesics during pregnancy and increased risk of cryptorchidism (adjusted odds ratio [OR] = 1.93; 95% confidence interval [CI], 1.03 to 3.62), although the type of analgesic and timing of exposure were not described. This study remained largely unrecognized until three epidemiologic studies reported on the same topic (Table 7.4).

Jensen and coworkers[27] investigated the associations between maternal use of APAP, IBP, and ASA and the risk of cryptorchidism in 47,700 liveborn singleton sons of mothers enrolled in the Danish National Birth Cohort during 1996 and 2002. Exposure to these drugs was assessed by self-report through a questionnaire at enrollment in early pregnancy and a series of telephone interviews. Gestational exposure was defined by use of these drugs at least once during pregnancy, but information on trimester-specific and repeated (cumulative) exposure was also obtained. Information on cryptorchidism was obtained from the Danish National Patient Registry and included all diagnoses of cryptorchidism and information on patients undergoing orchiopexy, which indicates more severe and persistent cases.

Exposures to APAP, IBP, and ASA were analyzed separately and combined. For APAP, the sample size allowed analyses by trimester or combined trimesters. APAP was used by 22,449 mothers (47%) at some point during

Table 7.4. Epidemiologic Studies on Prenatal Exposure to Mild Analgesics and Cryptorchidism

Study	Study Type	Population and Sample Size	Exposure Assessment	Outcome and Associations
Jansen et al., 2010	Prospective birth cohort	47,700 mother–male infant pairs from the Danish National Birth Cohort	Self-reported use of medications through questionnaires and telephone interviews	Increased risk of cryptorchidism in sons of mothers reporting: first- and second-trimester APAP use (HR = 1.33 [CI, 1.00–1.77]); APAP use in all three trimesters (HR = 1.17 [CI, 0.94–1.46]); cumulative APAP use (4 wk) during gestation weeks 8–14 (i.e., male programming window) (HR =1.38 [CI, 1.05–1.83]). No associations reported for IBP or ASA.
Kristensen et al., 2011	Prospective birth cohort	1040 Danish mother–male infant pairs* and 1463 Finnish mother–male infant pairs	Self-reported use of medications through questionnaires and/or telephone interviews	Increased risk of cryptorchidism in sons of Danish mothers reporting: use of more than one analgesic simultaneously at any time during pregnancy (OR = 7.55 [CI, 1.94–29.30]); second-trimester use of any analgesic (OR = 2.30 [CI, 1.12–4.73]). ASA only (OR = 3.73 [CI, 1.15–12.30]). IBP only (OR = 4.59 [CI, 1.10–19.00]), or simultaneous use of more than one analgesic (OR = 16.10 [CI, 3.29–78.60]). In the Finnish cohort, the use of analgesics was not associated with cryptorchidism.

(continued)

Table 7.4. Continued

Study	Study Type	Population and Sample Size	Exposure Assessment	Outcome and Associations
Snijder et al., 2012[†]	Prospective birth cohort	3184 mother-male infant pairs from the Generation R Study, the Netherlands	Self-reported use of medications through questionnaires	Increased risk of cryptorchidism in sons of mothers reporting: midgestation (weeks 14–22) use of any mild analgesic (OR = 2.12 [CI, 1.17–3.83]), APAP (OR = 1.89 [CI, 1.01–3.51]), or other painkillers (OR = 8.93 [CI, 1.84–43.24]). No associations with hypospadias

[*]Analyses in the Danish cohort included only the data from the telephone interviews (N = 491).

[†]Snijder, C.A., Kortenkamp, A., Steegers, E.A., et al. 2012. Intrauterine exposure to mild analgesics during pregnancy and the occurrence of cryptorchidism and hypospadia in the offspring: The Generation R Study. *Hum Reprod.* 27:1191–1201 also examined possible associations between maternal analgesic use and hypospadias.

APAP = acetaminophen; ASA = acetylsalicylic acid; CI = 95% confidence interval; HR = adjusted hazard ratio; IBP = ibuprofen; OR = adjusted odds ratio.

pregnancy. IBP and ASA were used by 7% and 5% of women, respectively. Among mothers using IBP and ASA, 57% and 50%, respectively, also used APAP. Sons of women reporting use of APAP in the first and the second trimesters had an increased risk of cryptorchidism (hazard risk [HR] = 1.33; 95% CI, 1.00 to 1.77) but less so for orchiopexy (HR = 1.26; 95% CI, 0.86 to 1.84). The associations were weaker but also seen in sons of mothers reporting APAP use in all three trimesters or only during gestation weeks 8 to 14, the suggested masculinization programming window in humans.

Exposure to IBP or ASA was not consistently associated with cryptorchidism. Similarly, combined exposure to more than one drug did not increase the risk of cryptorchidism. No clear dose-response relationship was associated with cumulative use of APAP (i.e., weeks of use), but more than 4 weeks of use was associated with hazard risk point estimates above 1.0. Exposure to APAP during more than 4 weeks within the masculinization programming window increased the risks of cryptorchidism (HR = 1.38; 95% CI, 1.05 to 1.83) and orchiopexy (HR= 1.44; 95% CI, 1.00 to 2.06).

Kristensen and colleagues[29] investigated the associations between mild analgesics and cryptorchidism in prospective birth cohorts in Copenhagen, Denmark, and Turku, Finland. In the Danish cohort, 1040 mothers of boys were enrolled. Pharmaceutical use in pregnancy was assessed through self-administered written questionnaires ($n = 834$) and by telephone interviews ($n = 491$). A total of 285 mothers participated in both the telephone interview and the questionnaire assessment. The written questionnaire assessed medication use in general, and the telephone interview specifically addressed the use of analgesics. In the Danish cohort, 26.1% (218 of 834) of mothers who completed the questionnaire reported use of analgesics during pregnancy. Among mothers who were interviewed by telephone, 56.2% (276 of 491) reported use of analgesics, suggesting that analgesic use was strongly underreported in the self-administered questionnaire. Analyses in the Danish cohort were therefore performed only with the data collected by telephone interviews. In the Finnish cohort ($N = 1463$), 42.3% of participants reported use of analgesics during pregnancy, but only self-administered questionnaires were available for this group of women.

In the Danish cohort, the risk of cryptorchidism was significantly increased for boys of mothers reporting simultaneous use of more than one analgesic at some time during pregnancy (adjusted OR = 7.55; 95% CI, 1.94 to 29.30; $P = .007$). In the second-trimester, use of any analgesic increased the risk of cryptorchidism (OR = 2.30; 95% CI, 1.12 to 4.73; $P = .032$), as did the individual use of IBP (OR = 4.59; 95% CI, 1.10 to 19.00; $P = .047$) and ASA (OR = 3.76; 95% CI, 1.15 to 12.30; $P = .01$). For APAP, the trend was similar but not statistically significant (OR = 1.97; 95% CI, 0.94 to 4.12; $P = .099$). The risk was further increased with simultaneous use of more than one analgesic during the second trimester (OR = 16.10; 95% CI, 3.29 to 78.60; P = .001).

In the Finnish cohort, no significant associations were seen between cryptorchidism and the use of analgesics during pregnancy. Although the analysis of the Finnish cohort used only data from questionnaires, 42.3% of Finnish mothers reported use of mild analgesics during pregnancy, suggesting that underreporting may not be as severe as in Denmark. However, in agreement with previous data, the birth prevalence of cryptorchidism was much lower in Finland (2.4%) than in Denmark (9.0%), and larger cohorts are needed in Finland to obtain a similar number of cases.

In the Generation R Study conducted in Rotterdam, The Netherlands, information on maternal use of medications was obtained through self-administered questionnaires at different time points during pregnancy for a total of 3184 mothers of boys.[49] Cryptorchidism or hypospadias was assessed during routine pediatric examinations at the child health care centers. The prevalence of cryptorchidism and hypospadias over 30 months of follow-up was 2.1% and 0.7%, respectively. A total of 29.9% of mothers used mild analgesics during pregnancy. The use of analgesics during midgestation (weeks 14 to 22) was significantly associated with the risk of cryptorchidism (adjusted OR = 2.12; 95% C; 1.17 to 3.83). This risk remained statistically significant for exposure to APAP (OR = 1.89; 95% CI, 1.01 to 3.51) or "other painkillers" (OR = 8.93; 95% CI, 1.84 to 43.2). No significant associations were observed at other time points, including early and late gestation. Maternal use of analgesics at any point was not associated with hypospadias.

Concerns about Drug and Environmental Chemical Interactions

Accumulating data suggest that pregnant women are exposed passively to APAP through exposure to aniline or other unknown sources. This is concerning because the proposed mechanisms of action and cellular targets of APAP are remarkably similar to those of common environmental endocrine-disrupting chemicals, particularly phthalate esters.

Phthalates are among the endocrine disruptors that cause most significant health concerns due to their widespread use as plasticizers and additives in consumer products such as toys, food packaging, medical devices, cosmetics, and formulations of pharmaceuticals and pesticides (see Chapter 2). In laboratory rats, certain phthalates target the fetal Leydig and Sertoli cells and induce multiple hormonal disturbances, which result in a cluster of male reproductive tract abnormalities known as the *phthalate syndrome*.

The syndrome is characterized by cryptorchidism, hypospadias, short AGD, malformed or small sex accessory organs, and histopathologic changes in the testis. Androgen deficiency has been described as a key event in the induction of effects that comprise the rat phthalate syndrome.[16,59]

Several epidemiologic studies support the hypothesis that phthalates impair prenatal androgen action in humans, as demonstrated by associations between maternal exposure to certain phthalates and short AGD in newborn males.[8,52,53,55] Experimental data indicate that in addition to androgen suppression by the fetal testis, phthalates can inhibit the production of INSL3, a peptide hormone produced by Leydig cells to support testicular descent.

In vitro and *in vivo* studies have demonstrated that mild analgesics can inhibit androgen and INSL3 production in rat and human fetal testis.[29,35,61] It has also been hypothesized that the testicular effects of phthalates are the result of imbalances in the androgen-to-estrogen ratio,[62] an endocrine effect that has also been described *in vitro* for some mild analgesics.[21,23,57] Some phthalates share structural similarities with salicylates and can to some extent inhibit prostaglandin synthesis, which is the pharmacologic target of mild analgesics.

Studies by Kristensen and associates[30] demonstrated that mild analgesics, certain phthalates, some estrogenic endocrine disruptors (e.g., ultraviolet filter component benzophenone-3), and some parabens used as preservatives in cosmetics and food, and bisphenol A (BPA) inhibit PGD_2 secretion in a mouse juvenile Sertoli cell lineage (SC5) without causing any signs of cytotoxicity. Overall, inhibition was independent of PPAR receptor binding and occurred without significant changes in the expression of COX genes (*PTGS1* and *PTGS2*), providing evidence for direct inhibition of the COX enzymes.

The compounds that displayed the most potent inhibition of prostaglandin synthesis in SC5 cells were di-isobutyl and di-n-butyl phthalate, benzophenone 3 (BP3), and isobutylparaben (iBPa). These compounds were predicted to induce the most potent inhibition of the COX-2 enzyme in a modeling system that simulated the affinity of compounds to the binding in the hydrophobic part of COX-2's binding site. In this model, the strength of the interactions between COX and phthalate esters is related to the size of the side chain of the ester molecule. The interaction and therefore COX inhibition increases with increasing length and branching of the side chain, although only to a certain extent. The simulation modeling predicts lower affinity for phthalates with longer side chains, such as di-2-ethylhexyl phthalate (DEHP) and di-isononyl phthalate (DINP), which is corroborated by the experimental data showing less potent prostaglandin inhibition by these compounds.

DEHP and its monoester metabolite MEHP were unable to inhibit PGD_2 production by SC5 mice cells. These results differ from the known potency of antiandrogenic phthalates in animal and human studies, which reveal that DEHP metabolites are among the most potent antiandrogenic and reproductive toxic phthalates. However, *ex vivo* exposure of fetal rat testes to MEHP significantly reduced PGD2 and testosterone production, suggesting species differences in susceptibilities to MEHP and different metabolic capabilities.[30] For example, it has been speculated that generation of secondary oxidized metabolites, such as 5-OH-MEHP, might occur in rat fetal explants but not in SC5 cells and that this step would be necessary for inhibition of PGD2 and testosterone synthesis.[30] The primary monoester metabolite (MEHP) and several secondary oxidized metabolites of DEHP (e.g., 5-OH-MEHP) are commonly found in human urine samples, and negative associations were found between the concentrations of these metabolites in maternal urine samples and the AGD of human male newborns.

Although it is difficult to establish a clear link between prostaglandin inhibition and antiandrogenic effects, there is increasing concern about the impact of drugs or chemicals that may interact through these pathways. Kugathas and coworkers[32] demonstrated that several commonly used pesticides also could bind to the COX-2 active site and inhibit PGD2 synthesis in SC5 mice cells.

PGD2 is part of a regulatory loop responsible for the continuing expression of SOX9, a key regulator of Sertoli cell differentiation and testis development. However, the linkage between inhibition of prostaglandins and suppression of testosterone production and other hormonal disturbances is unclear.[1,35] It is likely that mild analgesics, phthalates, pesticides, and other EDCs that induce male reproductive disorders work through multiple mechanisms.

Figure 7.1 shows some of the common targets of mild analgesics and phthalates in the developing fetal testis that may contribute to induction of male reproductive tract abnormalities in laboratory animals and humans. It is proposed that these chemicals may inhibit the synthesis of PGD2 in the developing testis, leading to abnormal Sertoli cell differentiation. This effect could result in a series of cellular and hormonal perturbations in the fetal testis, particularly inhibition of INSL3 and testosterone production by Leydig cells.

There is evidence that mild analgesics and phthalates can disrupt the normal balance between androgens and estrogens by altering the expression or activity of steroidogenic enzymes such as CYP17A1 (17α-hydroxylase/17,20 lyase/17,20 desmolase) and CYP19 (aromatase). However, it has been suggested that analgesics and phthalates may impair Leydig cell function by mechanisms that are independent of prostaglandin suppression.

No single event may be able to explain the full spectrum and severity of observed effects induced by these chemicals; a combination of multiple

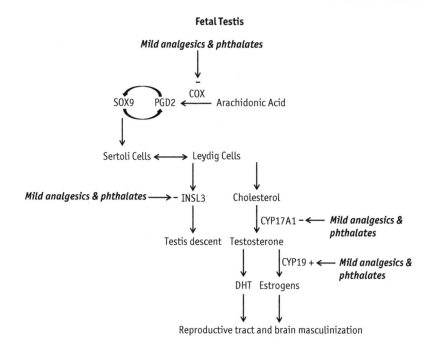

FIGURE 7.1. Mechanisms of endocrine disruption by mild analgesics and phthalates in the fetal testis. Mild analgesics and certain phthalates can target the cyclooxygenase enzyme (COX), which is involved in the synthesis of prostaglandin D$_2$ (PGD2), a mediator that promotes continuing expression of SOX9, a key regulator of Sertoli cell differentiation and testis development. In addition, these compounds can directly target the fetal Leydig cells and induce multiple hormonal disturbances, including suppression of insulin-like factor 3 (INSL3) and testosterone production. Mild analgesics and phthalates can disrupt the normal balance between androgens and estrogens by altering the expression of steroidogenic enzymes such as CYP17A1 and CYP19 (aromatase). DHT = dihydrotestosterone; + = stimulation; – = inhibition.

mechanisms may instead be operative. For example, abnormal Sertoli cell differentiation may result in poor Leydig cell development and aggravate the hormonal perturbations (e.g., inhibition of steroidogenesis) induced directly by these compounds. Different hormones may be involved in the same physiologic events, as is the case of the cooperative action of INSL3 and androgens in testis descent, and several other processes, including testis development itself, may depend on appropriate hormonal balance, such as normal androgen-to-estrogen ratios.[48,62]

The hormonal changes induced by these compounds may also affect brain sexual differentiation. Androgens play a critical role in brain masculinization in many species, and at least in rodents, these effects largely depend on the local conversion of androgens into estrogens by aromatase enzyme. Estradiol-induced brain masculinization is partially mediated by prostaglandin E_2 (PGE2) through COX-2 activation, which may represent an additional target for analgesics and environmental chemicals.[2]

Conclusions

Persuasive data indicate that mild analgesics and common environmental endocrine disruptors, particularly phthalates, share many mechanisms of action inhibiting collectively testosterone, INSL3, and prostaglandins, which result in phenotypic changes in experimental animals and possibly in humans. However, many details of these intricate pathways, including the initial molecular events and species differences, are not completely elucidated and deserve further investigation.

It remains to be determined whether prenatal exposure to APAP and other mild analgesics is associated with short AGD in humans and whether co-exposures of phthalates and these drugs have amplified effects. Prior animal studies have demonstrated that antiandrogenic compounds with similar and dissimilar mechanisms of action (e.g., androgen receptor antagonists and inhibitors of testosterone biosynthesis) produce cumulative dose-additive effects on male reproductive development.[45,46]

Axelstad and colleagues[4] investigated the effects of co-administration of antiandrogenic chemicals in rats, including phthalates and APAP. Overall, APAP was not able to aggravate the antiandrogenic effects of a mixture of environmental antiandrogens, although only two dose levels of the mixture and one APAP dose have been tested. Additional evidence from epidemiologic and experimental animal studies is needed to fully characterize the potential interactions between antiandrogenic environmental chemicals and mild analgesics.

Mild analgesics are widely used by pregnant women, with APAP still considered the first choice during pregnancy. Our analysis of APAP concentrations in urine of SFF participants confirms the pervasive use of this drug by pregnant women and indicates widespread unintentional exposure to this drug or its metabolic precursors, such as aniline. Observational epidemiologic studies revealed important and consistent associations between self-reported maternal exposure to APAP and other mild analgesics and cryptorchidism. These results are supported by biologically plausible mechanisms demonstrated in animal studies and *in vitro* experiments, particularly inhibition of testosterone and INSL3 production.

Mild analgesics and common environmental endocrine disruptors such as phthalates share many of the mechanisms of action that result in reproductive disorders in animal models and possibly in humans. These mechanisms involve multiple cellular and molecular targets, and future animal and epidemiologic studies should focus on possible interactive effects of these chemicals. Overall, the evidence that mild analgesics, similar to common environmental endocrine disruptors, can cause hormonal disturbances and potentially lead to male genital defects after *in utero* exposure should be taken into account in the examination of the risk-benefit balance of taking these drugs during pregnancy.

Because persistent pain and inflammatory conditions may be harmful to the expecting mother and developing fetus, the use of mild analgesics may still be advisable. However, pregnant women should be educated to avoid unnecessary use of analgesics and to adopt healthy lifestyle habits to decrease exposure to phthalates and other environmental chemicals, such as by reducing the consumption of processed foods, choosing fragrance-free cosmetics and personal care products, avoiding plastic containers for storing or warming food, and buying organic products whenever possible.

REFERENCES

1. Albert, O., Desdoits-Lethimonier, C., Lesne, L., et al. 2013. Paracetamol, aspirin and indomethacin display endocrine disrupting properties in the adult human testis in vitro. *Hum Reprod.* 28:1890–1898.
2. Amateau, S.K., & McCarthy, M.M. 2004. Induction of PGE2 by estradiol mediates developmental masculinization of sex behavior. *Nat Neurosci.* 7:643–650.
3. Aminoshariae, A., & Khan, A. 2015. Acetaminophen: Old drug, new issues. *J Endodont.* 41:588–593.
4. Axelstad, M., Christiansen, S., Boberg, J., et al. 2014. Mixtures of endocrine-disrupting contaminants induce adverse developmental effects in preweaning rats. *Reproduction.* 147:489–501.
5. Banhidy, F., Acs, N., Puho, E., & Czeizel, A.E. 2007. A population-based case-control teratologic study of oral dipyrone treatment during pregnancy. *Drug Saf.* 30:59–70.
6. Berkowitz, G.S., & Lapinski, R.H. 1996. Risk factors for cryptorchidism: a nested case-control study. *Paediatr Perinat Epidemiol.* 10:39–51.
7. Bloor, M., & Paech, M. 2013. Nonsteroidal anti-inflammatory drugs during pregnancy and the initiation of lactation. *Anesth Analg.* 116:1063–1075.
8. Bornehag, C.G., Carlstedt, F., Jonsson, B.A., et al. 2015. Prenatal phthalate exposures and anogenital distance in Swedish boys. *Environ Health Perspect.* 123:101–107.
9. Colborn, T., vom Saal, F.S., & Soto, A.M. 1993. Developmental effects of endocrine-disrupting chemicals in wildlife and humans. *Environ Health Perspect.* 101:378–384.

10. da Silva Dal Pizzol, T., Schuler-Faccini, L., Mengue, S.S., & Fischer, M.I. 2009. Dipyrone use during pregnancy and adverse perinatal events. *Arch Gynecol Obstet.* 279:293–297.

11. Dean, A., Mungall, W., McKinnell, C., & Sharpe, R.M. 2013. Prostaglandins, masculinization and its disorders: Effects of fetal exposure of the rat to the cyclooxygenase inhibitor indomethacin. *PloS One.* 8:e62556.

12. Dean, A., van den Driesche, S., Wang, Y., et al. 2016. Analgesic exposure in pregnant rats affects fetal germ cell development with inter-generational reproductive consequences. *Sci Rep.* 6:19789.

13. Dierkes, G., Weiss, T., Modick, H., Kafferlein, H.U., Bruning, T., & Koch, H.M. 2014. *N*-Acetyl-4-aminophenol (paracetamol), *N*-acetyl-2-aminophenol and acetanilide in urine samples from the general population, individuals exposed to aniline and paracetamol users. *Int J HygEnviron Health.* 217:592–599.

14. dos Santos, G.G., Dias, E.V., Teixeira, J.M., et al. 2014. The analgesic effect of dipyrone in peripheral tissue involves two different mechanisms: Neuronal K(ATP) channel opening and CB(1) receptor activation. *Eur J Pharmacol.* 741:124–131.

15. Fu, J., Bottegoni, G., Sasso, O., et al. 2012. A catalytically silent FAAH-1 variant drives anandamide transport in neurons. *Nat Neurosci.* 15:64–69.

16. Furr, J.R., Lambright, C.S., Wilson, V.S., Foster, P.M., & Gray, L.E. Jr. 2014. A short-term in vivo screen using fetal testosterone production, a key event in the phthalate adverse outcome pathway, to predict disruption of sexual differentiation. *Toxicol Sci.* 140:403–424.

17. Gaytan, M., Bellido, C., Morales, C., Sanchez-Criado, J.E., & Gaytan, F. 2006. Effects of selective inhibition of cyclooxygenase and lipooxygenase pathways in follicle rupture and ovulation in the rat. *Reproduction.* 132:571–577.

18. Graham, G.G., Davies, M.J., Day, R.O., Mohamudally, A., & Scott, K.F. 2013. The modern pharmacology of paracetamol: Therapeutic actions, mechanism of action, metabolism, toxicity and recent pharmacological findings. *Inflammopharmacology.* 21:201–232.

19. Gupta, C., & Goldman, A.S. 1986. The arachidonic acid cascade is involved in the masculinizing action of testosterone on embryonic external genitalia in mice. *Proc Natl Acad Sci U S A.* 83:4346–4349.

20. Gupta, C., & Bentlejewski, C.A. 1992. Role of prostaglandins in the testosterone-dependent wolffian duct differentiation of the fetal mouse. *Biol Reprod.* 47:1151–1160.

21. Han, S., Choi, K., Kim, J., et al. 2010. Endocrine disruption and consequences of chronic exposure to ibuprofen in Japanese medaka (*Oryzias latipes*) and freshwater cladocerans *Daphnia magna* and *Moina macrocopa*. *Aquatic Toxicol.* 98:256–264.

22. Herbst, A.L., Ulfelder, H., & Poskanzer, D.C. 1971. Adenocarcinoma of the vagina: Association of maternal stilbestrol therapy with tumor appearance in young women. *N Engl J Med.* 284:878–881.

23. Holm, J.B., Chalmey, C., Modick, H., et al. 2015. Aniline is rapidly converted into paracetamol impairing male reproductive development. *Toxicol Sci.* 148:288–298.

24. Holm, J.B., Mazaud-Guittot, S., Danneskiold-Samsoe, N.B., et al. 2016. Intrauterine exposure to paracetamol and aniline impairs female reproductive development by reducing follicle reserves and fertility. *Toxicol Sci.* 150:178–189.

25. Hong, Y., Sharma, V.K., Chiang, P.C., & Kim, H. 2015. Fast-target analysis and hourly variation of 60 pharmaceuticals in wastewater using UPLC-high resolution mass spectrometry. *Arch Environ Contam Toxicol.* 69:525–534.

26. Jakob, S., & Lovell-Badge, R. 2011. Sex determination and the control of Sox9 expression in mammals. *FEBS J.* 278:1002–1009.

27. Jensen, M.S., Rebordosa, C., Thulstrup, A.M., et al. 2010. Maternal use of acetaminophen, ibuprofen, and acetylsalicylic acid during pregnancy and risk of cryptorchidism. *Epidemiology.* 21:779–785.

28. Kao, J., Faulkner, J., & Bridges, J.W. 1978. Metabolism of aniline in rats, pigs and sheep. *Drug Metab Dispos.* 6:549–555.

29. Kristensen, D.M., Hass, U., Lesne, L., et al. 2011. Intrauterine exposure to mild analgesics is a risk factor for development of male reproductive disorders in human and rat. *Hum Reprod.* 26:235–244.

30. Kristensen, D.M., Skalkam, M.L., Audouze, K., et al. 2011. Many putative endocrine disruptors inhibit prostaglandin synthesis. *Environ Health Perspect.* 119:534–541.

31. Kristensen, D.M., Lesne, L., Le Fol, V., et al. 2012. Paracetamol (acetaminophen), aspirin (acetylsalicylic acid) and indomethacin are anti-androgenic in the rat foetal testis. *Int J Androl.* 35:377–384.

32. Kugathas, S., Audouze, K., Ermler, S., et al. 2015. Effects of common pesticides on prostaglandin D2 (PGD2) inhibition in SC5 mouse sertoli cells, evidence of binding at the COX2 active site, and implications for endocrine disruption. *Environ Health Perspect.* 124:452–459.

33. Liew, Z., Ritz, B., Rebordosa, C., Lee, P.C., & Olsen, J. 2014. Acetaminophen use during pregnancy, behavioral problems, and hyperkinetic disorders. *JAMA Pediatr.* 168:313–320.

34. Little, J.S. Jr., Goode, R.L., & Neubauer, B.L. 1995. Prenatal in vivo bulbourethral gland development is not affected by prostaglandin E2 inhibition. *J Androl.* 16:5–11.

35. Mazaud-Guittot, S., Nicolas Nicolaz, C., Desdoits-Lethimonier, C., et al. 2013. Paracetamol, aspirin, and indomethacin induce endocrine disturbances in the human fetal testis capable of interfering with testicular descent. *J Clin Endocrinol Metab.* 98:E1757–E1767.

36. Modick, H., Weiss, T., Dierkes, G., Bruning, T., & Koch, H.M. 2014. Ubiquitous presence of paracetamol in human urine: Sources and implications. *Reproducton.* 147:R105–R117.

37. Modick, H., Weiss, T., Dierkes, G., et al. 2015. Human metabolism and excretion kinetics of aniline after a single oral dose. *Arch Toxicol.* 90:1325–1333.

38. Muller, J.C., Imazaki, P.H., Boareto, A.C., et al. 2012. In vivo and in vitro estrogenic activity of the antidepressant fluoxetine. *Reprod Toxicol.* 34:80–85.

39. Nielsen, J.K., Modick, H., Morck, T.A., et al. 2015. *N*-acetyl-4-aminophenol (paracetamol) in urine samples of 6-11-year-old Danish school children and their mothers. *Int J Hyg Environ Health.* 218:28–33.

40. Ottani, A., Leone, S., Sandrini, M., Ferrari, A., & Bertolini, A. 2006. The analgesic activity of paracetamol is prevented by the blockade of cannabinoid CB1 receptors. *Eur J Pharmacol.* 531:280–281.

41. Philippat, C., Giorgis-Allemand, L., Chevrier, C., et al. 2011. Analgesics during pregnancy and undescended testis. *Epidemiology.* 22:747–749.

42. Rathmell, J.P., Viscomi, C.M., & Ashburn, M.A. 1997. Management of nonobstetric pain during pregnancy and lactation. *Anesth Analg.* 85:1074–1087.

43. Rebordosa, C., Kogevinas, M., Sorensen, H.T., & Olsen, J. 2008. Pre-natal exposure to paracetamol and risk of wheezing and asthma in children: A birth cohort study. *Int J Epidemiol.* 37:583–590.

44. Ricciotti, E., & FitzGerald, G.A. 2011. Prostaglandins and inflammation. *Arterioscler Thromb Vasc Biol.* 31:986–1000.

45. Rider, C.V., Furr, J., Wilson, V.S., & Gray, L.E. Jr. 2008. A mixture of seven antiandrogens induces reproductive malformations in rats. *Int J Androl.* 31:249–262.

46. Rider, C.V., Furr, J.R., Wilson, V.S., & Gray, L.E. Jr. 2010. Cumulative effects of in utero administration of mixtures of reproductive toxicants that disrupt common target tissues via diverse mechanisms of toxicity. *Int J Androl.* 33:443–462.

47. Sales, K.J., & Jabbour, H.N. 2003. Cyclooxygenase enzymes and prostaglandins in reproductive tract physiology and pathology. *Prostaglandins Other Lipid Mediat.* 71:97–117.

48. Sharpe, R.M. 2006. Pathways of endocrine disruption during male sexual differentiation and masculinization. *Best Pract Res Clin Endocrinol Metab.* 20:91–110.

49. Snijder, C.A., Kortenkamp, A., Steegers, E.A., et al. 2012. Intrauterine exposure to mild analgesics during pregnancy and the occurrence of cryptorchidism and hypospadia in the offspring: The Generation R Study. *Hum Reprod.* 27:1191–1201.

50. Sordillo, J.E., Scirica, C.V., Rifas-Shiman, S.L., et al. 2015. Prenatal and infant exposure to acetaminophen and ibuprofen and the risk for wheeze and asthma in children. *J Allergy Clin Immunol.* 135:441–448.

51. Swan, S.H. 2000. Intrauterine exposure to diethylstilbestrol: Long-term effects in humans. *APMIS* 108:793–804.

52. Swan, S.H., Main, K.M., Liu, F., et al. 2005. Decrease in anogenital distance among male infants with prenatal phthalate exposure. *Environ Health Perspect.* 113:1056–1061.

53. Swan, S.H. 2008. Environmental phthalate exposure in relation to reproductive outcomes and other health endpoints in humans. *Environ Res.* 108:177–184.

54. Swan, S.H., Liu, F., Hines, M., et al. 2010. Prenatal phthalate exposure and reduced masculine play in boys. *Int J Androl* 33:259–269.

55. Swan, S.H., Sathyanarayana, S., Barrett, E.S., et al. 2015. First trimester phthalate exposure and anogenital distance in newborns. *Hum Reprod.* 30:963–972.

56. Thorpe, P.G., Gilboa, S.M., Hernandez-Diaz, S., et al. 2013. Medications in the first trimester of pregnancy: Most common exposures and critical gaps in understanding fetal risk. *Pharmacoepidemiol Drug Saf.* 22:1013–1018.

57. Tinwell, H., Colombel, S., Blanck, O., & Bars, R. 2013. The screening of everyday life chemicals in validated assays targeting the pituitary-gonadal axis. *Regul Toxicol Pharmacol.* 66:184–196.

58. Toppari, J., Larsen, J.C., Christiansen, P., et al. 1996. Male reproductive health and environmental xenoestrogens. *Environ Health Perspect.* 104(Suppl 4):741–803.

59. Toppari, J., Virtanen, H.E., Main, K.M., & Skakkebaek, N.E. 2010. Cryptorchidism and hypospadias as a sign of testicular dysgenesis syndrome (TDS): Environmental connection. *Birth Defects Re A Clin Mol Teratol.* 88:910–919.

60. Uzun, B., Atli, O., Perk, B., Burukoglu, D. & Ilgin, S. 2014. Evaluation of the reproductive toxicity of naproxen sodium and meloxicam in male rats. *Hum Exp Toxicol.* 34:415–429.

61. van den Driesche, S., Macdonald, J., Anderson, R.A., et al. 2015. Prolonged exposure to acetaminophen reduces testosterone production by the human fetal testis in a xenograft model. *Sci Transl Med.* 7:288ra280.

62. Veeramachaneni, D.N., & Klinefelter, G.R. 2014. Phthalate-induced pathology in the foetal testis involves more than decreased testosterone production. *Reproduction.* 147:435–442.

63. Werler, M.M., Mitchell, A.A., Hernandez-Diaz, S., & Honein, M.A. 2005. Use of over-the-counter medications during pregnancy. *Am J Obstet Gynecol.* 193:771–777.

64. Wilhelm, D., Hiramatsu, R., Mizusaki, H., et al. 2007. SOX9 regulates prostaglandin D synthase gene transcription in vivo to ensure testis development. *J Biol Chem.* 282:10553–10560.

65. Wise, L.D., Vetter, C.M., Anderson, C.A., Antonello, J.M., & Clark, R.L. 1991. Reversible effects of triamcinolone and lack of effects with aspirin or L-656,224 on external genitalia of male Sprague-Dawley rats exposed in utero. *Teratology.* 44:507–520.

8

Pesticides and Neurodegenerative Disorders

JOHN W. MCBURNEY

Key Concepts

- Parkinson disease (PD), Alzheimer disease (AD), and amyotrophic lateral sclerosis (ALS) are common neurologic conditions that likely are caused by complex interactions of genetic vulnerabilities and environmental insults.
- Pesticides, which are widely applied in the environment, are intended to kill living organisms and are also toxic to humans.
- Epidemiologic evidence suggests that exposure to a variety of pesticides increases the risk of neurodegenerative disease.
- Environmental toxins, including pesticides, are thought to play the major causative role in PD and a lesser, although important, role in AD and ALS.
- Neurodegeneration is most clearly linked to inhibition of the mitochondrial electron transport chain, especially complex 1, with increased levels of reactive oxygen species resulting in accumulation of insoluble, misfolded protein polymers (i.e., Lewy bodies and neurofibrillary tangles).
- Integrative pest management (IPM) seeks to minimize the use of pesticides in agriculture, and its principles are applicable to the home and landscape.
- Because predicting individual genetic susceptibility to neurodegeneration is technically and economically unfeasible, primary prevention by limiting or eliminating exposure is the only reasonable option.

Introduction

Neurodegenerative diseases are chronic conditions characterized by death and degeneration of groups of neurons in the nervous system. Clinical manifestations of these conditions are determined by the function of the lost neurons. The incidence of these disorders increases dramatically with age. With aging populations, especially in the developed world, dramatic increases in the prevalence of neurodegenerative disease is anticipated.[72] Current concepts of the pathogenesis of neurodegenerative disease involve complex interactions between genetically based vulnerability and environmental toxins.

Pesticides are compounds that are applied to broad areas to control living organisms and are potentially toxic to humans.[73] Since 1950, pesticide use has increased by 50%, and pesticide toxicity has increased by 10-fold.[50] The burgeoning development of multiple chemicals in use in our environment exceeds our ability to effectively screen them for toxicity. In 2002, the U.S. Environmental Protection Agency (EPA) reported, "In the United States, more than 18,000 products are licensed for use … each year 2 billion pounds of pesticides are applied to crops, homes, schools, parks, and forests."[25]

Most toxins' roles in causing degenerative disease have been identified only in retrospect. This chapter examines the role that pesticides play in the complex causation of these most challenging and increasingly important conditions and outlines practical steps that individuals can take to decrease their risk.

Parkinson Disease

Parkinson disease (PD) is the second most prevalent neurodegenerative disorder, with a prevalence of 500 cases per 100,000 people and an annual incidence of 20 cases per 100,000.[57,71] It affects as many as 1.5 million people in the United States, with about 70,000 new cases diagnosed annually.[68] Multiple robust lines of evidence link a series of complex interactions of environmental toxins, including pesticides, with genetic susceptibility factors in the pathogenesis of this disorder.[13,68]

James Parkinson, a London physician, originally described this disorder in 1817.[56] Before his description of the characteristic clinical features of tremor, rigidity of the extremities, and postural instability, the disorder had not been clearly differentiated from other neurologic disorders, suggesting that before the industrial revolution, it was a rare disease, and the emergence was a reflection of increasing industrialization.[55] Subsequently, PD was associated with selective loss of pigmented neurons from the pars compacta of the substantia nigra (SN) and protein inclusions in surviving neurons.[3] Replacement with L-dopa, a dopamine precursor, reversed the principal motor manifestations of the disorder, confirming that the clinical manifestations were due the loss of function of degenerated SN dopaminergic neurons.[17]

EPIDEMIOLOGY

Epidemiologic studies have provided vital clues about the factors contributing to the pathogenesis of PD. PD demonstrates marked age dependence. It is rare before the age of 50 and dramatically increases in incidence with advancing age beyond the seventh decade.[18] PD is more common in industrialized than developing societies.[75] In developed societies, it is more common among rural dwellers and agricultural workers.[70]

Examination of temporal trends in age-adjusted annual incidence from Olmsted County, Minnesota, show that the annual incidence increased from 11.4 cases per 100,000 people from 1935 to 1944 to 18.2 cases per 100,000 for the period between 1967 and 1979.[18,57,75] Subsequent analysis from Olmstead County for the period between 1976 and 2005 showed an increase in the incidence of PD, with an increase in relative risk of 1.24 per decade. The effect was most marked in the cohort of men older than 70, with an increased relative risk of 1.35 per decade. Among women, there was trend toward increase that did not reach statistical significance. The overall age-adjusted incidence rate for PD in men increased from 38.8 cases per 100,000 people to 56 cases per 100,000 during the 30-year period.[65]

Multiple epidemiologic studies have linked rural living, employment in agriculture, and well water consumption with an increased risk of PD.[18,70] Workers regularly exposed to pesticides are also at increased risk.[23]

GENETICS

Genetic factors do not contribute directly to the pathogenesis of typical idiopathic PD. Familial PD is rare, accounting for no more than 10% of cases. In a large, comprehensive twin registry of 70,000 twin pairs, only 3 were concordant for PD.[71]

Nonetheless, multiple genes have been linked to increased risk for sporadic idiopathic PD, including *PARK7* (formerly *DJ1*), *PINK1*, *PARK2* (encodes parkin), *SNCA* (encodes α-synuclein), and *LRRK2* (encodes dardarin).[20] The gene products probably determine vulnerability to other factors such as environmental toxins and susceptibility to accumulation of α-synuclein, a protein that is abundant in the brain.

SNCA-environment interactions affecting the risk of PD have been evaluated. Individuals who are homozygous or heterozygous for the *SNCA* REP1 259 variant had a lower risk of developing PD after pesticide exposure, whereas those with the REP1 263 genotype had a higher risk, especially of early-onset PD.[33] In a study that looked at the role of genetic variants of the dopamine transporter (DAT) locus, the risk of PD was increased threefold for carriers of one susceptibility allele and fourfold for those with two or more alleles.[58]

VULNERABILITY OF SUBSTANTIA NIGRA DOPAMINERGIC NEURONS

Dopaminergic neurons are vulnerable to insult due to their size and bioenergetics.[53] Under physiologic conditions, SN neurons are under oxidative stress because metabolism of dopamine generates reactive oxygen species (ROS).[20,34] The SN cell body sends forth a long, unmyelinated axon to the striatum, where it extensively arborizes.[51] Nigral dopamine neurons have a higher basal rate of oxidative phosphorylation than dopamine neurons in the ventral tegmental area, which have different cytoarchitectonics.[53] The metabolism of dopamine by monoamine oxidase type B (MAO-B) forms ROS, produces oxidative stress, and renders SN dopamine neurons susceptible to further increases in ROS.[20]

Interest in the role of toxins in the pathogenesis of PD increased dramatically in the early 1980s as a result of a small epidemic of sudden-onset, severe parkinsonism in people who injected meperidine, a synthetic opioid, contaminated with 1-methy-4-phenyl-1,2,3,6-tetrahydropyridine (MPTP).[48] The victims, who were very young and at low risk for PD, developed signs and symptoms indistinguishable from those of severe PD over a few days after injection of the contaminated drug.[45]

The neurotoxicology of MPTP was extensively investigated, and it was subsequently developed as an animal model of PD. Animals exposed to MPTP develop clinical signs of PD. Pathologically, MPTP-induced parkinsonism is associated with selective loss of dopaminergic neurons from the SN but not the accumulation of Lewy bodies. On injection, MPTP, which is highly lipophilic, diffuses rapidly into the brain, where it is rapidly metabolized to a quaternary derivative (MPP+) by MAO-B. It is then transported into dopaminergic neurons by a dopamine transporter protein. In the neuron, the unstable MPP+ binds covalently to complex 1 of the electron transport system, resulting in a failure of ATP formation and increased formation of ROS, dysregulation of mitochondrial calcium regulation, and neuronal death.[45]

MECHANISMS OF DISEASE

The discovery that acute exposure to MPTP produced parkinsonism through inhibition of complex 1 of the electron transport chain led to the search for other complex 1 toxins. Rotenone is a compound that is found in the roots of several tropical plants. It is tasteless, colorless, and odorless. It has been used as an insecticide since the mid-19th century and was marketed to home gardeners in the United States as a broad-spectrum, "natural" insecticide beginning in the 1950s. It has been used in commercial agriculture and as a piscicide (i.e., fish killer) for removal of nuisance and invasive fish. The California Department of Pesticide regulation reported 15,000 pounds of rotenone was used in state in 2007.[67] It was withdrawn from use in the European Union (EU) in 2007, and use was voluntarily limited in the United States starting in 2008.

Rotenone is highly lipophilic and readily crosses the blood-brain barrier, where it is distributed throughout the central nervous system. In neurons, it inhibits the function of complex 1. Although it affects complex 1 diffusely in the brain, the unique bioenergetics of SN dopamine neurons makes them vulnerable to effects of disruption of the electron transport chain. Acute administration of very high doses of rotenone (10 to 18 mg/kg/day) does not result in selective loss of SN dopaminergic neurons.[13,30,63] With chronic low-level administration, gradual accumulation of ROS and deregulation of intra-mitochondrial calcium result in selective SN dopaminergic neuronal death.[34] Chronic rotenone exposure causes selective loss of SN dopaminergic neurons and, unlike in MPTP models, Lewy body accumulation in surviving neurons. The typical features of PD are reversible with administration of the dopamine precursor L-dopa.[34]

INSECTICIDES AND HERBICIDES LINKED
TO PARKINSON DISEASE

Rotenone is unlikely to be an important cause of PD because it has poor oral bioavailability, breaks down quickly due with exposure to moisture and ultraviolet light (preventing environmental accumulation), and has never been widely used in commercial agriculture, thereby sparing exposure of large neighboring populations.[34] However, rotenone does demonstrate the role that mitochondrial complex 1 toxins may play in the pathogenesis of the condition.

Many other pesticides are toxic to complex 1, including benzimidazole, bullatacin, 2-amino-6-chlorobenzothiadiazole, cyhalothrin, fenazaquin, fenpyroximate, Hoe 110779, pyridaben, pyrimidifen, Sandoz 547A, tebufenpyra, and D-thiangazole.[34] Permethrin is a synthetic analogue of pyrethrum a natural insecticide that is derived from dried chrysanthemum flower petals, and is a complex 1 inhibitor in common use as an insect repellant, including use in permethrin-impregnated fabric for military uniforms and recreational cloth-ing.[67] Several naturally occurring complex 1 toxins are orders of magnitude more potent than rotenone.[34]

Complex 1, the largest component of the respiratory chain enzymes, is composed of at least 43 subunits. It has important functions beyond its oxi-doreductive role, including regulation of the mitochondrial permeability transition pore (PTP). The PTP is a calcium-dependent channel in the inner mitochondrial membrane. It permits the passage of large (>1.5 kD) molecules and is associated with mitochondrial depolarization as a step in apoptosis and programmed cell death.[34] Under pathologic conditions, PTP opening is a step in the loss of calcium regulation, mitochondrial dysfunction, and cell necrosis.[34]

Complex 1 function is also compromised by polymerized accumulation of α-synuclein. Synuclein's role in mitochondrial function is incompletely understood, but it resides in the outer mitochondrial membrane and has important roles in stabilizing electron transport and in the secretory func-tion of the endoplasmic reticulum and Golgi apparatus. When α-synuclein accumulates, it polymerizes and forms β sheets, resulting in the formation of Lewy bodies, a common feature of idiopathic, inherited, and rotenone-induced forms of PD.[7]

Paraquat. One of the most commonly used herbicides in the world, paraquat was withdrawn from use in the EU in 2007 due to its potential to cause PD.[28] It is restricted to licensed applicators in the United States.[23]

Paraquat has extreme acute toxicity, especially through inhalational expo-sure, and it is classified by the EPA as a category 1 toxin by inhalation (high-est category), category 2 by ingestion, and category 3 by dermal contact.[23] It kills plants on contact by interfering with photosynthesis. It interferes with electron transfer, which results in generation of ROS. In animals, this affects mitochondrial function and increases oxidative stress through the generation of ROS, including superoxide and hydrogen peroxide.[11] Paraquat is subject to redox recycling, in which it is regenerated with the generation of ROS. Paraquat is similar structurally to MPP^+.[21]

In rodents, paraquat administration results in loss of dopaminergic neu-rons and lesions in the SN.[6] Exposure to paraquat is linked to a twofold increased risk of PD.[67] The risk of PD is increased when paraquat exposure is combined with maneb exposure.[16,68]

Maneb. Manganese ethylene bisdithiocarbamate (i.e., maneb) is a fungicide used in the United States since 1962. It is marketed under a variety of trade names and is used to prevent crop damage in the field and to protect harvested crops from damage during storage or transport. It controls a broader range of diseases than any other fungicide. It is in a class of pesticides called ethylene bisdithiocarbamates (EDBCs) that are notable for instability in the field; they break down into many biologically active and potentially injurious compounds. The EPA requires protective garments and a 24-hour reentry period for agricultural workers using maneb.

Cooking vegetables contaminated with maneb can result in the formation of ethylene thiourea, which is carcinogenic.[29] Approximately 2.5 million pounds of maneb are used annually, mostly on almonds, lettuce, peppers, and walnuts.[24] Key systemic toxicity of maneb causes depressed thyroxine production, goiter, and follicular hyperplasia and peripheral neuropathy.[61]

In a case-control study that looked at PD and exposure to paraquat or maneb, exposure to maneb increased the risk of PD (odds ratio [OR] = 2.27), whereas exposure to paraquat and maneb was associated with an even greater risk (OR = 4.17), especially if the exposure occurred at an early age.[16]

Manganese, a key constituent of maneb, is linked to parkinsonism in manganese miners and welders. Manganese-caused parkinsonism or manganism is different from idiopathic PD in several characteristics. The main site of effect of manganese in the brain is in the striatum, especially in the globus pallidus, where it accumulates. The striatum is the target of dopaminergic innervation from the midbrain. Replacement of dopamine with the dopamine precursor L-dopa is ineffective.[46] Manganism is an important cause of disability among manganese miners in China, where it is the second most common industrial disease. In the United States, welders have filed multibillion class action lawsuits because of manganese toxicity.[46]

Alzheimer Disease

AD is the most common neurodegenerative disease[59] and the most common cause of dementia, affecting more than 5 million people in the United States.[15] Dementia increases dramatically with advancing age, affecting 2% to 3% of those between 70 and 75 years of age and 20% to 25% of those 85 years or older. Worldwide, the number of people with dementia is projected to increase sharply in coming years.[1,31]

VASCULAR DEMENTIA VERSUS ALZHEIMER DISEASE

In developing countries where hypertension is uncontrolled, vascular dementia predominates, whereas in developed countries where there is good detection and control of hypertension, AD is the predominant cause of dementia.[59] Vascular dementia progresses in a stepwise fashion and is associated with deregulation of control of affect (i.e., pseudobulbar state). Memory deficits often occur later and often improve with cuing. In AD, memory problems occur early and are continuously progressive. Associated cortical deficits such as aphasia and apraxia are prominent.

AD and vascular dementia often occur together, and pure AD and pure vascular dementia may represent extremes of a spectrum.[59,64] Socioeconomic risk factors for AD and vascular dementias include obesity, sedentarism, diabetes, hypertension, hyperlipidemia, and metabolic syndrome.[59] With the decline in death due to cardiovascular disease and cerebrovascular disease, there has been an increase in life expectancy worldwide.[60] Because the risk of dementia increases sharply with age, there has been a dramatic increase in the prevalence of dementia. However, the age-specific incidence of dementia has not declined,[60] even as vascular dementia has, suggesting that there has been an increase in nonvascular dementia (i.e., dementia due to neurodegenerative diseases), principally AD.

Two main pathologic features characterize AD: amyloid plaques and neurofibrillary tangles. Amyloid is composed of extracellular aggregates of $\alpha\beta$ amyloid precursor protein, whose proteolysis generates β amyloid, the primary component of plaques found in the brains of AD patients. Neurofibrillary tangles are intraneuronal polymers of the neurotubule protein tau in a hyperphosphorylated form.

The predominant role of amyloid accumulation versus tangles in understanding the pathogenesis of AD is an unresolved problem. Amyloid and tau aggregates are thought to compromise neuronal energy supply, antioxidant response, and synaptic function.[12] In particular, neurofibrillary tangles are postulated to compromise axonal transport. Mitochondrial dysfunction with resultant increases in oxidative stress, increased generation of ROS, and neuroinflammation are key pathogenic steps in AD.[74]

PESTICIDES AND ALZHEIMER DISEASE

Genetics are thought to account for up to 70% of the risk of AD, especially apolipoprotein E-4 (*APOE**E4) allele status,[73] although only 0.1% results from autosomal dominant factors. However, the increasing prevalence and incidence of AD has resulted in renewed interest of the role that pesticides play in the increase in age-specific incidence.[1]

Several epidemiologic studies have examined the risk that exposure to pesticides, particularly insecticides, may play in the risk for developing dementia and AD. Pesticides can affect cognitive status in acute and short-term exposure,[8,62] but an even more important issue is whether exposure to pesticides leads to increased risk of dementia and AD.[4,5] Paroxenase 1 (PON1) is an arylesterase that is involved in the hydrolysis of organophophates. Polymorphisms in the *PON1* gene are associated with an increased risk of AD and PD.[26,27]

The PAQUID study was one of the largest studies to look at occupational pesticide exposure as a risk factor for development of PD and AD. The odds ratio for developing AD was elevated for men occupationally exposed (OR = 2.39; 95% confidence interval [CI], 1.02 to 5.63) but not for women. An even greater risk was seen for development of PD.[4]

The PHYTONER study was a study of the effects of pesticide exposure on 929 vineyard workers in France between 1997 and 1998. They were classified according to their long-term pesticide exposure as directly exposed, indirectly exposed, or nonexposed. Educational status, age, gender, alcohol consumption, smoking, psychotropic drug use, and depressive symptoms were controlled for in the data analysis. At 4 years, 614 subjects were available for follow-up evaluation. The relative risk of having a 2-point decline in the Mini-Mental State Examination score was 2.15 for exposed subjects.[5]

The Cache County Study on Memory Health was a prospective study of the development of dementia among subjects 65 years of age or older performed in Cache County, Utah.[36] More than 3000 subjects completed detailed occupational history questionnaires that included information about exposure to various forms of pesticides. Cognitive status was assessed using standardized measures at baseline and at 3, 7, and 10 years. The 572 exposed individuals were compared prospectively with nonexposed subjects for development of dementia. After controlling for multiple factors, including *APOE*E4* allele status and baseline cognitive status, exposed individuals were shown to be at increased risk for development of dementia. Risk was increased for all-cause dementia (hazard ratio [HR] = 1.38) and AD (HR = 1.42). The risk of AD was associated with organophosphate exposure (HR = 1.53) and organochlorine exposure (HR = 1.49).[36]

MECHANISM OF TOXICITY

In contrast to PD, the pathophysiology of AD and the cellular mechanisms that affect neurotoxicity and risk of AD are less well understood. As in PD, pesticides may cause neurotoxicity by affecting mitochondrial electron transport, resulting in increased production of ROS.

Organophosphates and carbamates work through inhibition of acetylcholinesterase, resulting in enhanced levels and prolonged action of acetylcholine.[73] This may cause chronic overstimulation of acetylcholine receptors, resulting in downregulation and decreased numbers of receptors, leading to dysfunction in cholinergic neurotransmission. A study of mechanisms of the neurotoxicology of organophophates suggested that they caused dysregulation of glutaminergic and dopaminergic neurotransmission, producing excitotoxic neuronal injury. Organophosphates lead to hyperactivity of cyclin-dependent kinase 5 (CDK5), causing tau hyperphosphorylation.[69] Increased accumulation of insoluble phosphorylated tau polymers impairs axonal function and stimulates formation of neurofibrillary tangles, a hallmark of AD.[13,69,73]

Amyotrophic Lateral Sclerosis

ALS is a devastating neurodegenerative disease characterized principally by degeneration of motor neurons in the cerebral cortex, brainstem, and spinal cord. It is the most common of the motor neuron diseases, with an annual incidence of 1 or 2 cases per 100,000 people and affecting between 20,000 and 30,000 individuals in the United State.[50] Increasing incidence rates for ALS have been reported in Scandinavia, France, and the United States in recent decades.[39] The peak incidence for ALS is between 58 and 63 years of age, with a decline after age 75.[41] Men are 1.2 to 1.56 times more likely to develop ALS than women.[39]

The disease is uniformly fatal, with median survival after diagnosis of less than 2 years. Survival beyond 10 years is reported but is rare. Death usually results from respiratory failure and inanition. Increasing recognition of nonmotor system features, including tremor, rigidity, and dementia, has led to the concept of a PD--dementia-ALS complex. Clusters of increased ALS prevalence are reported in several regions of the world, especially in Guam and the Kii peninsula of Honsho Island, Japan.[39]

GENETICS AND LIFESTYLE

Risk factors for ALS include genetics. Twin studies estimate that 61% of the risk of ALS is genetic.[2] Specific genetic risk factors are mutations of the chromosome 9 open reading frame 72 *(C9ORF72)*, the Cu-Zn superoxide dismutase *(SOD1)*, and the TAR DNA-binding protein *(TARDBP)* genes. Lifestyle risk factors include smoking, dietary factors, and athleticism. Exposures to electromagnetic fields, heavy metal intoxication, and occupations have also been considered risks for ALS.[39]

PESTICIDE EXPOSURES

Case reports and small case series have linked ALS and exposure to a variety of pesticides, including dithiocarbamate, organochlorines, pyrethroids, and methyl bromide.[32,37,54] A case-control study of workers at Dow Chemical between 1945 and 1994 found a relative risk of 3.45 of dying of ALS among workers exposed to 2,4-dichlorophenoxyacetic acid (2,4-D) based on 3 cases of 1517 workers who worked with the agent compared with no ALS cases in the 40,000 employees who worked at the same location who did not have contact with the agent.[10] Indirect evidence suggesting an increase of ALS due to exposure to carbamates has emerged from increased rates of ALS among veterans of Operation Desert Storm, when the carbamate pharmaceutical pyridostigmine was widely used by armed forces to prevent nerve gas poisoning.[38]

Two comprehensive reviews and meta-analyses of pesticide exposure and ALS were published in 2012.[41,50] Malek and colleagues examined 10 studies of pesticide exposure and development of ALS.[50] The studies had different ascertainment of the diagnosis of ALS and the methods used to characterize pesticide exposure. Two studies were cohort studies, and eight were case-control studies. The two cohort studies identified 2673 ALS deaths and 1,026,630 controls. The case-control studies included 1223 cases and 1904 controls. Results were expressed as odds ratios. An association was found between pesticide exposure and ALS among male subjects (OR = 1.88; 95% CI, 1.36 to 2.61) but not among female subjects, possibly due to a small number of female subjects included in the meta-analysis.[50]

Kamel and coworkers also investigated the association of ALS with specific pesticides using data from the Agricultural Health Study (AHS), a cohort of 84,739 licensed pesticide applicators and their spouses enrolled from 1993 through 1997.[39] Mortality data were collected through February 2010. ALS was recorded on the death certificates of 41 subjects. ALS was not associated with pesticide exposure as a group, but it was associated with organochlorine insecticides, pyrethroids, herbicides, and fumigants. Odds ratios were highest for aldrin (2.1), dieldrin (2.6), DDT (2.1), and toxaphene (2.0). Because of the small numbers affected, odds ratios did not reach statistical significance.[41] The investigators found that the most vigorous association appeared to be with organochlorines.

Alternative Methods for Pest Control

We have examined the extensive scientific evidence that pesticides contribute to the pathogenesis of the neurodegenerative disorders PD, AD, and ALS. No curative treatment exists for these conditions, nor is any likely in the near future. By the time each of these conditions are clinically evident, extensive and irreversible neuronal loss has occurred. The role that environmental toxins play in causing these conditions is not apparent acutely, and reducing exposure to these toxins is crucial for primary prevention.

The advent of the organochlorine insecticide DDT in 1939 and the broad-spectrum herbicide 2,4-D in the 1940s ushered in the chemical era of pest management. After World War II, DDT was in widespread use over large portions of the United States, especially in the southeast region, where aerial spraying was credited with elimination of malaria.[42] DDT was also used on a widespread basis on croplands.[40,44,47]

One of the first published demonstrations of the principles of integrated pest management (IPM) was outlined in control of the alfalfa aphid in 1959.[66] This study demonstrated that by using a process employing sound cultural practices, detailed knowledge of pest threats, flexible use of biologic and chemical agents, and goals of pest control rather eradication, decreased use of pesticides was possible and economically advantageous.

Around the same time, Rachael Carson, the leading science writer of her era, brought the dangers that widespread and indiscriminate use of pesticides, especially DDT, posed to light with the publication of *Silent Spring*.[14] The book ignited a social movement that resulted in congressional hearings in 1963 and formation of the EPA in 1970.[49] It has been widely credited with creating the environmental movement.[35] DDT was withdrawn from use in the United States in 1972.

In 1979, land grant universities were given funds to promote the environmental and economic benefits of IPM in the home and on farms. By 1993, Vice–President Al Gore announced an initiative that by 2000, 75% of all crop acreage would be grown under IPM principles.[40]

KEY POINTS OF INTEGRATED PEST MANAGEMENT USED TO CONTROL SINGLE PESTS OR PEST COMPLEXES

- **Pest:** an organism detrimental to humans, including invertebrates, vertebrates, and pathogens
- **Management:** decisions based on ecologic principles and on economic and social considerations

IPM is a multidisciplinary endeavor calling on expertise in agronomy (i.e., crop and soil science), entomology (i.e., pest and beneficial insects), plant pathology, economics, agricultural engineering, and climatology.[43]

Three important components of IPM are economic injury level (i.e., the lowest population density that causes economic damage), economic threshold (i.e., population size large enough to trigger an action to prevent increasing pest population from reaching the economic injury level), and general equilibrium position (i.e., average density over time).[66]

Benefits of IPM include decreased emergence of resistant organisms, decreased emergence of secondary infestations, lower costs, fewer environmental effects, and lower health impacts among workers and the general public.[44] The principles of IPM in the plant nursery are based on prevention, the use of the least toxic chemicals as a last resort, a systems-based (rather than incident-based) approach, prompt and accurate identification of pests, careful monitoring and record keeping, strict sanitation, maintenance of healthy crops, encouragement of beneficial organisms, and timely and effective control measures.[47]

URBAN INTEGRATED PEST MANAGEMENT

The principles of IPM that were originally for use in agriculture and commercial plant nurseries have been applied to the control of pests in the urban setting, including homes and schools. A strategy of prevention of infestations by making the home environment inhospitable to pests through good architectural controls (i.e., sealing cracks and crevices, window screens), controlling entry, and accumulation of moisture and eliminating sources of food is essential to minimize the need for pesticides. Accurate identification of household pests and use of the most appropriate and least toxic pesticide are essential to minimize toxic exposure.

All pesticides are by their nature designed to kill living organisms, and all pesticides should be used with care and respect. Careful consideration of the risks and benefits of any pesticide should be done. Chemical pesticides that interfere with neurotransmitter systems that are common to pests and humans have the greatest risk of toxicity and should be used only as last resorts. Many pesticides that are not licensed for use in the home can be found in household dust and in the yards where children play. Pesticides with prolonged duration of action may accumulate and cause lasting ecologic effects. Many older pesticides, currently limited to licensed applicators or withdrawn from market (e.g., Dursban [chlorpyrifos], carbaryl, nicotine) often lurk in garden sheds. They should not be used and should be disposed of responsibly. Mitochondrial toxins such as rotenone should also be avoided.

Potentially safer pesticides are derived from natural products. Some are specified for indoor use:

Plant-based oils. Plants make specialized (essential) oils in glands to defend themselves from insect attack. Examples include peppermint, clove, citrus, lavender, and thyme essential oils. They are available in aerosols, dusts, and wettable powders that often are combined with pyrethrum. They are highly effective and have extremely low toxicity. Formulations are available to control cockroaches, stink bugs, carpenter bees, yellow jackets, and a wide variety of household pests.[19]

Natural dusts. Silica dusts and diatomaceous earth are insecticides that are used in cracks and crevices to kill insect pests. They work by disrupting the insects' waxy outer covering, leading to desiccation and death. They are sometimes combined with pyrethrum.[20]

Boric acid. Boric acid or borate is highly toxic to insects. The mechanisms are unknown, but it exerts its effect after ingestion. It is available as a dust or as sprays. It is nontoxic to humans and animals, but care should be taken to avoid breathing the dust. It is also toxic to plants.[19]

Some safer alternatives are specified for garden and home landscape use:

Plant-based oils. Neem oil is a natural oil derived from the neem tree (*Azadirachta indica*), an evergreen tree native to India and cultivated in many areas of the tropics. Its oil is a complex mixture of polyunsaturated fatty acids and triglycerides. The main active ingredient in neem oil is azadirachtin, a triterpenoid. It is an insect repellant that exerts insecticidal activity by reducing feeding, and it is a growth regulator. It is active against a wide variety of insect pests, including aphids, armyworms, leafminers, thrips, and root weevil adults and larvae. It has a slightly foul odor and needs to be applied once or twice each week. It is certified organic and can be applied on fruit trees up until the day before harvest.[52]

Insecticidal soap. The soap is composed of fatty acids derived from plants and animals. It is used as a 1% or 2% aqueous solution to control soft-bodied insects such as aphids, spider mites, scale insects, and thrips. Household detergents and soaps are not acceptable substitutes. The concentrates can go bad and damage foliage and should be applied immediately after preperation.[19]

Other options are available:

Spinosad. This natural substance, which is formed by soil bacteria, can be toxic to insects. It is composed of two active ingredients, spinosad-A and spinosad-D. It is useful in controlling thrips, leafminers, spider mites, mosquitoes, ants, and fruit flies. It can be used on agricultural crops and ornamental plants. It is certified organic.[52]

Pyrethrum. This natural insecticide is derived from chrysanthemum flowers. It has been used for hundreds of years. The main source of pyrethrum was in Japan, which led to shortages with the outbreak of WWII. A synthetic analogue, permethrin, was developed in response to the shortage. It has a longer half-life, is more toxic, and should not be confused with natural pyrethrum. Pyrethrum breaks down in sunlight and does not accumulate in the environment. It can be used up until the date of harvest. It is often combined with other botanical insecticides such as neem oil.[19]

Diatomaceous earth. This natural dust can be used in the garden and home landscape and as a crack and crevice insecticide inside the home to control a wide variety of garden pests.

REDUCING PESTICIDE INGESTION

Foods are an important additional potential source of exposure to pesticides. Although epidemiologic studies directly linking the risk of neurodegenerative disorders with pesticide exposure through food is lacking, indirect evidence of this risk exists. Groundwater contamination with pesticides and consumption of well water are linked to increased risk of PD, demonstrating that oral ingestion is a means of exposure.[9]

Avoidance of exposure through food is prudent. Carefully cleaning fruits and vegetables to reduce pesticide residues is important to minimize pesticide exposure. Washing with a vinegar solution is more effective in removing residues than water alone. Peeling is another effective strategy to reduce exposure.

Although it is unclear whether organically grown food is more nutritious, organically grown produce does not carry pesticide residues and is preferable. Fruits and vegetables that are conventionally grown with heavy applications of pesticides and are difficult to clean or peel, such as the Environmental Working Group's *Dirty Dozen* should be organic. The environmental effects of widespread use of pesticides in conventional agriculture should be considered in making purchasing decisions.

REDUCING INSECTICIDE AND HERBICIDE EXPOSURE

- Prevent or eliminate causes of infestations.
- Avoid sprays in the home. Baits and gels are more effective and less likely to contaminate the home environment.
- Effective approaches to pests require accurate identification. IPM centers at land grant colleges, county extension agents, master gardener programs, and websites listed in the next section are good resources for pest identification.
- Pests such as termites, carpenter ants, and powderpost beetles are best left to professionals. Individuals can usually control many other pests with low-toxicity interventions.
- Read all labels before use!
- When using pesticides, wear personal protective equipment, including gloves, long sleeves, eye protection, closed shoes, and hats. Wash in hot water after use.
- Do not wear outside shoes inside the house to avoid tracking outside toxins such as pesticide residues inside.
- Vacuum with a high-efficiency particulate arrestance (HEPA) vacuum, and dust regularly. Household dust is not benign.

Resources

- National Pesticide Information Center (http://www.npic.orst.edu) is a cooperative venture between the EPA and Oregon State University. Information on pesticides is available with downloadable handouts.
- Bugs (www.livingwithbugs.com) is a great resource for information and advice on do-it-yourself pest management.
- University of California Statewide IPM Program (http://www.ipm.ucdavis.edu/PDF/PESTNOTES/index.html) is an extensive library of information on IPM for the home. Downloadable PDFs are effective as patient handouts.

REFERENCES

1. Abdulrahman, G.O. 2014. Alzheimer's disease: Current trends in Wales. *Oman Med J.* 29:280–284.

2. Al-Chalabi, A., Fang, F., Hanby, M.F., et al. 2010. An estimate of amyotrophic lateral sclerosis heritability using twin data. *J Neurol Neurosurg Psychiatry.* 81:1324–1326.

3. Alvord, E.C. Jr., Forno, L.S., Kusske, J.A., Kauffman, R.J., Rhodes, J.S., & Goetowski, C.R. 1974. The pathology of parkinsonism: A comparison of degenerations in cerebral cortex and brainstem. *Adv Neurol.* 5:175–193.

4. Baldi, I., Lebailly, P., Mohammed-Brahim, B., Letenneur, L., Dartigues, J.F., & Brochard, P. 2003. Neurodegenerative diseases and exposure to pesticides in the elderly. *Am J Epidemiol.* 157:409–414.

5. Baldi, I., Gruber, A., Rondeau, V., Lebailly, P., Brochard, P., & Fabrigoule, C. 2011. Neurobehavioral effects of long-term exposure to pesticides: Results from the 4-year follow-up of the PHYTONER study. *Occup Environ Med.* 68:108–115.

6. Berry, C., La Vecchia, C., & Nicotera, P. 2010. Paraquat and Parkinson's disease. *Cell Death Differ.* 17:1115–1125.

7. Bobela, W., Aebischer, P., & Schneider, B.L. 2015. Alpha-Synuclein as a mediator in the interplay between aging and Parkinson's disease. *Biomolecules.* 5:2675–2700.

8. Bosma, H., van Boxtel, M.P., Ponds, R.W., Houx, P.J., & Jolles, J. 2000. Pesticide exposure and risk of mild cognitive dysfunction. *Lancet.* 356:912–913.

9. Breckenridge, C.B., Berry, C., Chang, E.T., Sielken, R.L. Jr., & Mandel, J.S. 2016. Association between Parkinson's disease and cigarette smoking, rural living, well-water consumption, farming and pesticide use: Systematic review and meta-analysis. *PLoS One.* 11:e0151841.

10. Burns, C.J., Beard, K.K., & Cartmill, J.B. 2001. Mortality in chemical workers potentially exposed to 2,4-dichlorophenoxyacetic acid (2,4-D), 1945–1994: An update. *Occup Environ Med,* 58:24–30.

11. Bus, J.S., & Gibson, J.E. 1984. Paraquat: Model for oxidant-initiated toxicity. *Environ Health Perspect.* 55:37–46.

12. Cabezas-Opazo, F.A., Vergara-Pulgar, K., Perez, M.J., Jara, C., Osorio-Fuentealba, C., & Quintanilla, R.A. 2015. Mitochondrial dysfunction contributes to the pathogenesis of Alzheimer's disease. *Oxid Med Cell Longev.* 2015:509654.

13. Cannon, J.R., & Greenamyre, J.T. 2011. The role of environmental exposures in neurodegeneration and neurodegenerative diseases. *Toxicol Sci.* 124:225–250.

14. Carson, R. 1962. *Silent spring.* Greenwich, CN: Fawcett.

15. Centers for Disease Control and Prevention. 2013. Alzheimer's disease. http://www.cdc.gov/aging/aginginfo/alzheimers.htm.

16. Costello, S., Cockburn, M., Bronstein, J., Zhang, X., & Ritz, B. 2009. Parkinson's disease and residential exposure to maneb and paraquat from agricultural applications in the central valley of California. *Am J Epidemiol.* 169:919–926.

17. Cotzias, G.C. 1968. L-Dopa for Parkinsonism. *N Engl J Med.* 278:630.

18. de Lau, L.M., & Breteler, M.M. 2006. Epidemiology of Parkinson's disease. *Lancet Neurol.* 5:525–535.

19. DeAngelis, J. 2016. Living with Bugs. http://www.livingwithbugs.com/index.html.

20. Dias, V., Junn, E., & Mouradian, M.M. 2013. The role of oxidative stress in Parkinson's disease. *J Parkinsons Di.s* 3:461–491.
21. Drechsel, D.A., & Patel, M. 2008. Role of reactive oxygen species in the neurotoxicity of environmental agents implicated in Parkinson's disease. *Free Radic Biol Med.* 44:1873–1886.
22. Elbaz, A., Clavel, J., Rathouz, P.J., et al. 2009. Professional exposure to pesticides and Parkinson disease. *Ann Neurol,* 66:494–504.
23. Environmental Protection Agency. 1997. Reregistration Eligibility Decision. R.E.D. Facts: Paraquat dichloride. http://www3.epa.gov/pesticides/chem_search/reg_actions/reregistration/fs_PC-061601_1-Aug-97.pdf.
24. Environmental Protection Agency. 2001. The grouping of a series of dithiocarbamate pesticides based on a common mechanism of toxicity. http://archive.epa.gov/scipoly/sap/meetings/web/pdf/dithiofinal_aug17.pdf.
25. Environmental Protection Agency, Office of Pesticide Programs. 2002. Promoting safety for America's future. http://nepis.epa.gov/Exe/ZyNET.exe/2000JJFJ.txt?ZyActionD=ZyDocument&Client=EPA&Index=2000%20Thru%202005&Docs=&Query=&Time=&EndTime=&SearchMethod=1&TocRestrict=n&Toc=&TocEntry=&QField=&QFieldYear=&QFieldMonth=&QFieldDay=&UseQField=&IntQFieldOp=0&ExtQFieldOp=0&XmlQuery=&File=D%3A%5CZYFILES%5CINDEX%20DATA%5C00THRU05%5CTXT%5C00000009%5C2000JJFJ.txt&User=ANONYMOUS&Password=anonymous&SortMethod=h%7C-&MaximumDocuments=1&FuzzyDegree=0&ImageQuality=r75g8/r75g8/x150y150g16/i425&Display=p%7Cf&DefSeekPage=x&SearchBack=ZyActionL&Back=ZyActionS&BackDesc=Results%20page&MaximumPages=1&ZyEntry=1. Accessed: June 30, 2016
26. Erlich, P.M., Lunetta, K.L., Cupples, L.A., 2006. Polymorphisms in the PON gene cluster are associated with Alzheimer disease. *Hum Mol Genet.* 15:77–85.
27. Erlich, P.M., Lunetta, K.L., Cupples, L.A., et al. 2012. Serum paraoxonase activity is associated with variants in the PON gene cluster and risk of Alzheimer disease. *Neurobiol Aging.* 33:1015.e7–e23.
28. European Court of Justice. 2007, July 11. Judgment of the Court of First Instance in Case T-229/04. Kingdom of Sweden v Commission of the European Communities. http://curia.europa.eu/juris/liste.jsf?language=en&num=T-229/04.
29. EXTOXNET. 1993. Maneb: Pesticide information profile. http://pmep.cce.cornell.edu/profiles/extoxnet/haloxyfop-methylparathion/maneb-ext.html.
30. Ferrante, R.J., Schulz, J.B., Kowall, N.W., & Beal, M.F. 1997. Systemic administration of rotenone produces selective damage in the striatum and globus pallidus, but not in the substantia nigra. *Brain Res.* 753:157–162.
31. Ferri, C.P., Prince, M., Brayne, C., et al. 2005. Global prevalence of dementia: A Delphi consensus study. *Lancet.* 366:2112–2117.
32. Fonseca, R.G., Resende, L.A., Silva, M.D., & Camargo, A. 1993. Chronic motor neuron disease possibly related to intoxication with organochlorine insecticides. *Acta Neurol Scand.* 88:56–58.

33. Gatto, N.M., Rhodes, S.L., Manthripragada, A.D., et al. 2010. Alpha-Synuclein gene may interact with environmental factors in increasing risk of Parkinson's disease. *Neuroepidemiology.* 35:191–195.

34. Greenamyre, J.T., Sherer, T.B., Betarbet, R., & Panov, A.V. 2001. Complex I and Parkinson's disease. *IUBMB Life.* 52:135–141.

35. Griswold, E. 2012. How "Silent Spring" ignited the environmental movement. http://www.nytimes.com/2012/09/23/magazine/how-silent-spring-ignited-the-environmental-movement.html.

36. Hayden, K.M., Norton, M.C., Darcey, D., et al. 2010. Occupational exposure to pesticides increases the risk of incident AD: The Cache County study. *Neurology.* 74:1524–1530.

37. Hoogenraad, T.U. 1988. Dithiocarbamates and Parkinson's disease. *Lancet.* 1:767.

38. Horner, R.D., Kamins, K.G., Feussner, J.R., et al. 2003. Occurrence of amyotrophic lateral sclerosis among Gulf War veterans. *Neurology.* 61:742–749.

39. Ingre, C., Roos, P.M., Piehl, F., Kamel, F., & Fang, F. 2015. Risk factors for amyotrophic lateral sclerosis. *Clin Epidemiol.* 7:181–193.

40. Integrated Pest Management Program. 2016. *Introduction to Integrated Pest Management (IPM).* Iowa State University. http://www.ipm.iastate.edu/files/01 IPM Introduction.pdf.

41. Kamel, F., Umbach, D.M., Bedlack, R.S., et al. 2012. Pesticide exposure and amyotrophic lateral sclerosis. *Neurotoxicology.* 33:457–462.

42. Kinkela, D. 2011. *DDT and the American Century: Global Health, Environmental Politics, and the Pesticide That Changed the World.* Chapel Hill, NC: University of North Carolina Press.

43. Kogan, M. 1998. Integrated pest management: Historical perspectives and contemporary developments. *Annu Rev Entomol.* 43:243–270.

44. Kogan, M. 2013. Integration and integrity in IPM. *Am Entomol.* 59:150–160.

45. Kopin, I.J. 1987. MPTP: An industrial chemical and contaminant of illicit narcotics stimulates a new era in research on Parkinson's disease. *Environ Health Perspect.* 75:45–51.

46. Kwakye, G.F., Paoliello, M.M., Mukhopadhyay, S., Bowman, A.B., & Aschner, M. 2015. Manganese-induced parkinsonism and Parkinson's disease: Shared and distinguishable features. *Int J Environ Res Public Health.* 12:7519–7540.

47. Landis, T.D., & Dumroese, R.K. 2014. Integrated Pest Management—an Overview and Update. *Forest Nursery Notes* Summer 2014:16–26.

48. Langston, J.W., Ballard, P., Tetrud, J.W. & Irwin, I. 1983. Chronic Parkinsonism in humans due to a product of meperidine-analog synthesis. *Science* 219: 979–980.

49. Lytle, M.H. 2007. *The Gentle Subversive: Rachel Carson, Silent Spring, and the Rise of the Environmental Movement.* New York, NY: Oxford University Press.

50. Malek, A.M., Barchowsky, A., Bowser, R., Youk, A., & Talbott, E.O. 2012. Pesticide exposure as a risk factor for amyotrophic lateral sclerosis: A meta-analysis of epidemiological studies. *Environ Res.* 117:112–119.

51. Matsuda, W., Furuta, T., Nakamura, K.C., et al. 2009. Single nigrostriatal dopaminergic neurons form widely spread and highly dense axonal arborizations in the neostriatum. *J Neurosci.* 29:444–453.

52. National Pesticide Information Center. 2012. Neem oil general fact sheet. http://npic.orst.edu/factsheets/neemgen.pdf.

53. Pacelli, C., Giguere, N., Bourque, M.J., Levesque, M., Slack, R.S., & Trudeau, L.E. 2015. Elevated mitochondrial bioenergetics and axonal arborization size are key contributors to the vulnerability of dopamine neurons. *Curr Biol.* 25:2349–2360.

54. Pall, H.S., Williams, A.C., Waring, R., & Elias, E. 1987. Motoneurone disease as manifestation of pesticide toxicity. *Lancet.* 2:685.

55. Pan-Montojo, F., & Reichmann, H. 2014. Considerations on the role of environmental toxins in idiopathic Parkinson's disease pathophysiology. *Transl Neurodegener.* 3:10.

56. Parkinson, J. 2002. An essay on the shaking palsy. [1817]. *J Neuropsychiatry Clin Neurosci.* 14:223–236; discussion 222.

57. Rajput, A.H., Offord, K.P., Beard, C.M., & Kurland, L.T. 1984. Epidemiology of parkinsonism: Incidence, classification, and mortality. *Ann Neurol.* 16:278–282.

58. Ritz, B.R., Manthripragada, A.D., Costello, S., et al. 2009. Dopamine transporter genetic variants and pesticides in Parkinson's disease. *Environ Health Perspect.* 117:964–969.

59. Rizzi, L., Rosset, I., & Roriz-Cruz, M. 2014. Global epidemiology of dementia: Alzheimer's and vascular types. *Biomed Res Int.* 2014:908915.

60. Rocca, W.A., Petersen, R.C., Knopman, D.S., et al. 2011. Trends in the incidence and prevalence of Alzheimer's disease, dementia, and cognitive impairment in the United States. *Alzheimers Dement.* 7:80–93.

61. Roede, J.R., Hansen, J.M., Go, Y.M., & Jones, D.P. 2011. Maneb and paraquat-mediated neurotoxicity: Involvement of peroxiredoxin/thioredoxin system. *Toxicol Sci.* 121:368–375.

62. Rohlman, D.S., Lasarev, M., Anger, W.K., Scherer, J., Stupfel, J., & McCauley, L. 2007. Neurobehavioral performance of adult and adolescent agricultural workers. *Neurotoxicology.* 28:374–380.

63. Rojas, J.C., Simola, N., Kermath, B.A., Kane, J.R., Schallert, T., & Gonzalez-Lima, F. 2009. Striatal neuroprotection with methylene blue. *Neuroscience.* 163:877–889.

64. Roman, G. 2001. Diagnosis of vascular dementia and Alzheimer's disease. *Int J Clin Pract Suppl.* (120):9–13.

65. Savica, R., Grossardt, B.R., Bower, J.H., Ahlskog, J.E., & Rocca, W.A. 2016. Time trends in the incidence of Parkinson disease. *JAMA Neurol.* 73:981–989.

66. Stern, V., Smith, R, van den Bosch, R. 1959. The integration of chemical and biological control of the spotted alfalfa aphid: The integrated control concept. *Hilgardia.* 29:81–101.

67. Tanner, C.M., Kamel, F., Ross, G.W., et al. 2011. Rotenone, paraquat, and Parkinson's disease. *Environ Health Perspect.* 119:866–872.

68. Tanner, C.M., Goldman, S.M., Ross, G.W., & Grate, S.J. 2014. The disease intersection of susceptibility and exposure: Chemical exposures and neurodegenerative disease risk. *Alzheimers Dement.* 10:S213–S225.

69. Torres-Altoro, M.I., Mathur, B.N., Drerup, J.M., et al. 2011. Organophosphates dysregulate dopamine signaling, glutamatergic neurotransmission, and induce neuronal injury markers in striatum. *J Neurochem.* 119:303–313.

70. Wan, N., & Lin, G. 2016. Parkinson's disease and pesticides exposure: New findings from a comprehensive study in Nebraska, USA. *J Rural Health.* 32:302–313.

71. Wirdefeldt, K., Gatz, M., Bakaysa, S.L., et al. 2008. Complete ascertainment of Parkinson disease in the Swedish Twin Registry. *Neurobiol Aging.* 29:1765–1773.

72. World Health Organization. 2006. *Neurological Disorders: Public Health Challenges.* Geneva, Switzerland: World Health Organization.

73. Zaganas, I., Kapetanaki, S., Mastorodemos, V., et al. 2013. Linking pesticide exposure and dementia: What is the evidence? *Toxicology.* 307: 3–11.

74. Zhang, F., & Jiang, L. 2015. Neuroinflammation in Alzheimer's disease. *Neuropsychiatr Dis Treat.* 11:243–256.

75. Zhang, Z.X., & Roman, G.C. 1993. Worldwide occurrence of Parkinson's disease: An updated review. *Neuroepidemiology.* 12:195–208.

9

Disinfection in the 21st Century: Is There Harm in Being Clean?

PATRICIA A. HUNT, TERRY C. HRUBEC, AND VANESSA E. MELIN

Key Concepts

- The addition of antimicrobials to household and personal care products has resulted in intimate daily contact with a wide array of chemicals designed to indiscriminately kill good and bad microbes.
- Rapid adoption of these chemicals for use in consumer products has resulted in extensive environmental contamination and ubiquitous exposure.
- Because some biocides are endocrine-disrupting chemicals, they can induce adverse developmental, reproductive, neurological, and immunological effects in humans and wildlife.
- Parabens are used as preservatives in personal care products, and all widely used forms appear to be physiologically estrogenic. Their widespread use and extensive environmental contamination constitute a serious confounder to assessments of the health effects of this class of chemicals.
- The broad-spectrum antimicrobials triclosan and triclocarban are used in a wide range of cleaning supplies and personal care products. Evidence that they disturb thyroid homeostasis makes their widespread contamination in wildlife and the environment a concern.
- Quaternary ammonium compounds (QACs) are commercial disinfectants whose efficacy has resulted in their extensive use in consumer applications. Although the toxicity of these compounds has been insufficiently evaluated, heavy use of QACs has produced widespread environmental contamination.

Introduction

Long before germs were linked to disease, cleanliness in operating and hospital environments was key to reducing illness. The concept of *clean* has evolved into a societal quest for a germ-free environment. Despite attempts to kill them, the amazing adaptive ability of microorganisms twists our weapons of destruction into an evolutionary accelerant that generates superbugs with resistance to the chemicals used against them. Human exposure to the antimicrobial residues in the environment diminishes natural immunity, impairs reproductive health, and may have other serious human health consequences.

Although the study of the human microbiome is in its infancy, a fascinating and growing body of evidence implicates good microbes in metabolic, nutritional, and immunologic homeostasis. Microorganisms likely play a major role in human disease and human health.[36] The recognition that our lives are so intimately intertwined with microbiota that we cannot live happily without them suggests that devising new and better ways of sanitizing our environment is not without peril.

The post-WWII era brought a rapid influx of chemicals into the lives of people living in developed countries, with the United States leading the charge in production and consumption. The rapid pace of product development was accompanied by improved marketing strategies. This cycle has continued and increased in voracity, and we are faced with a ceaseless barrage of advertisements for antibacterial soap, germ-killing cleaners, and hand sanitizers on the Internet, radio, television, billboards, and receipt papers. In the quest for germ-free lives, we have inadvertently welcomed a host of chemicals designed to indiscriminately kill good and bad microbes into the most intimate aspects of our lives.

Controlling Microorganisms: Defining the Approaches

Defining the approaches taken to control, prevent, or destroy microorganisms is an essential first step. Although the general term *biocide* is used for chemical agents that control microorganisms, an important distinction is made with respect to where they are used and whether they destroy or inhibit growth: *Antiseptics* are applied to living tissue, whereas *disinfecting agents* are applied to the surface of inanimate objects to control microorganisms. Disinfecting agents are antimicrobial pesticides used to control harmful microorganisms, including bacteria, viruses, and fungi. They are regulated by the U.S. Environmental Protection Agency (EPA) and can be broadly classified as sanitizers, disinfectants, and sterilants.

Sanitizers reduce but do not completely eliminate microorganisms. *Disinfectants* destroy or inactivate most microorganisms and some viruses, but they may not eliminate spores. *Sterilants* physically or chemically destroy or eliminate all forms of life, including spores.

SOME BIOCIDES ARE ENDOCRINE-DISRUPTING CHEMICALS

The National Institutes of Health (NIH) National Institute of Environmental Health Sciences (NIEHS) defines endocrine-disrupting chemicals (EDCs) as chemicals that may interfere with the body's endocrine system and produce adverse developmental, reproductive, neurologic, and immunologic effects in humans and wildlife. EDCs can be naturally occurring (e.g., phytoestrogens) or man-made chemicals. Man-made EDCs include a diverse range of compounds with many applications, including pesticides, industrial chemicals, pharmaceuticals, and personal care products.

EDCs tend to be stable, which makes them suitable for industrial applications. It can also make them persist in the environment for years, resulting in exposure long after chemical use has been discontinued or banned.[26] The dependence of human physiology and male and female reproduction on carefully orchestrated hormonal cues makes EDCs a threat to human health. This review of the environmental and biological effects of biocides focuses on their potential endocrine-disrupting effects.

Four common classes of biocides—parabens, triclosan, triclocarbon, and quaternary ammonium compounds (QACs)—are reviewed because adverse health effects have been ascribed to them and because their prevalence in household and personal care products makes them ubiquitous environmental contaminants. The properties, uses, and potential environmental and biological effects are summarized for each. These biocides illustrate the potential hazards of the 21st century approach to controlling microorganisms in daily life.

Parabens

WHAT ARE THEY AND WHAT ARE THEIR
ENDOCRINE-DISRUPTING PROPERTIES?

Parabens are synthetic alkyl esters of p-hydroxybenzoic acid that were first used as preservatives in pharmaceuticals in the mid-1920s but rapidly expanded for use in a wide range of consumer products.[40]

The most commonly used parabens are methylparaben, ethylparaben, n-propylparaben, n-butylparaben, isobutylparaben, isopropylparaben, and benzylparaben. The most common metabolite of these parabens is *p*-hydroxybenzoic acid (PHBA), which can be conjugated to *p*-hydroxyhippuric acid (PHHA). Parabens are effective against gram-positive bacteria, yeast, and molds, but they have little effect on bacterial spores and no effect on viruses, mycobacteria, or prions.

Like many EDCs, the potential effects of parabens have been dismissed by many on the grounds that their low affinity for the classic estrogen receptors makes them only weakly estrogenic and unlikely to induce biological effects. However, data from the in vitro estrogen receptor assay and the in vivo utero-trophic assay suggest that all widely used parabens are physiologically estrogenic.[8] Other mechanisms of action consistent with an endocrine-disrupting role have been reported, including binding to the androgen, thyroid hormone, and peroxisome proliferator-activated-γ (PPARγ) receptors; inhibition of the sulfotransferase enzyme; and mitochondrial toxicity.[8,21,87]

WHERE AND HOW ARE WE EXPOSED?

Due to their low cost, high water solubility, and stability, parabens are used as preservatives in a wide range of cosmetics and personal care products such as shampoos and facial and skin cleansers and lotions. Methylparaben and n-propylparaben are the most common parabens in consumer products, and they are often used together. Amounts of less than 0.3% are typical in these products, although mixtures of parabens of up to 0.8% are allowed. Parabens are also used as antimicrobials in some processed foods, in food packaging, as preservatives in pharmaceuticals (http://www.cdc.gov/BIOMONITORING/Parabens_BiomonitoringSummary.html), and in industrial products such as varnishes, glue, and animal feed.[40]

Exposure is thought to occur orally from the consumption of food and pharmaceuticals and transdermally from the use of paraben-containing products on the skin. However, parabens have also been detected in air, dust, and soil,[6] and biomonitoring data are consistent with widespread exposure. In analyses of 2548 urine samples collected from the general population of the United States in 2005 and 2006 as part of the annual National Health and Nutrition Examination Survey (NHANES), methylparaben and n-propylparaben were detected in more than 90% of samples and ethylparaben and butylparaben in more than 40%. Levels were higher in adolescent and adult women than in men, and these variations and those observed among racial and ethnic groups were ascribed to differences in the use of personal care products.[12] Similarly, a screen of Danish men found methylparaben and n-propylparaben in urine from 98% of subjects and in most serum samples.[34]

Since the publication of these initial studies, data from studies too numerous to cite have reported widespread exposure in different populations of children and adults around the world. In addition to underscoring the pervasiveness of exposure, the combined data from these studies provide evidence that exposure is related to lifestyle. Paraben levels in men and women have been correlated with their use of personal care products.[6,9] A 3-day intervention study involving Latina girls provides compelling evidence that exposure is influenced by consumer choices and documents reductions in exposure levels within days of discontinuing paraben-containing products[41] (see Chapter 14).

HOW PERSISTENT ARE THEY IN THE ENVIRONMENT?

Parabens are thought to be rapidly metabolized and eliminated from the body, and biomonitoring suggests that parabens are detectable in the urine of almost everyone in developed countries. They are a significant water contaminant[40] due to discharge from factories producing parabens and urban wastewater that contains residue from consumer products. Wastewater treatment is effective in removing parabens, but effluent from treatment facilities releases them into the environment.

Parabens are readily biodegradable under aerobic conditions, but they remain stable over time in anaerobic sludge.[40] Parabens also are highly reactive with chlorine, raising concern that chlorination of wastewater effluent produces halogenated parabens that may be especially persistent contaminants.[40] A study of marine mammals in U.S. coastal waters provided sobering evidence of a high prevalence of parabens (predominantly methylparaben) in eight species of marine mammals and astonishingly high levels in some individuals.[96]

WHAT ARE THE CURRENT HEALTH CONCERNS?

Most attention has focused on two health concerns: effects on reproductive health and breast cancer.

Male Reproductive Effects. Epidemiologic data on the effects of parabens on male reproduction are limited to two studies from infertility clinics. An association between the levels of butylparaben in paternal urine and

DNA damage in sperm in male partners attending an infertility clinic was reported.[60] A subsequent study focused on in vitro fertilization (IVF) outcomes, and although based on a very small sample size, it found a slight decrease in the odds of live birth associated with paternal urinary levels of methylparaben and propylparaben.[27]

As has been seen for other extensively studied EDCs (e.g., BPA[73]), experimental findings for the effects of parabens on male reproductive health have varied. This in part reflects differences in the species and strains of animals used; the timing, duration, and route of exposure; and the end points evaluated.

The doses in most studies were designed to correspond to the acceptable daily intake dose of 10 mg/kg/day. Although no effect on male rodents exposed during fetal development has been reported in several studies,[24,49,86] others have reported reduced sperm counts or testosterone levels in association with exposure during prenatal and early postnatal development or postnatal exposure alone to butylparaben[49,68,101] or n-propylparaben.[69] One study examined the effect of butylparaben on spermatogenesis in the rat and found a significant increase in spermatogenic cell apoptosis several hours after the administration of a single dose.[3] Based on the available data, there is substantial evidence that exposure during early postnatal development can adversely impact male reproductive health, but data on the effects of prenatal exposure are insufficient.

Female Reproductive Effects. Epidemiologic data on female reproductive health are extremely limited and confined to studies of infertility patients. An initial study reported an inverse association between urinary levels of propylparaben and diminished ovarian reserve.[83] A subsequent analysis by the same group, however, found no association between urinary paraben levels and IVF outcome for women undergoing infertility treatment.[64]

Experimental data are also limited. The most comprehensive analysis of the effects of prepubertal exposure on sexual maturation in the female rat found morphologic changes in the uterus and ovary and changes in the timing of sexual maturation and estrus cycle length with high doses of methylparaben and isopropylparaben.[90] Studies of exposure during fetal development are limited. No effects were reported in an industry study,[24] but altered gene expression in the ovary[86] and decreased leptin levels[7] have been reported in female rat fetuses exposed to butylparaben.

Breast Cancer. The clinical use of diethylstilbestrol (DES) in the 1940s through the 1970s to treat high-risk pregnancies has provided compelling evidence that developmental exposure to synthetic estrogens increases the risk of breast cancer in adult women,[47] and concern that environmental exposure to EDCs may be affecting the incidence of female cancers is growing.[77]

Widespread use of parabens in cosmetics and personal care products and reports of detectable levels of parabens in human breast tissue, milk, and tumors[22] raise many concerns. Data directly bearing on the issue, however, are largely confined to in vitro studies, in which parabens have been reported to stimulate the proliferation or alter expression profiles of MCF-7 breast cancer cells.[13,20,70,74,94] The in vitro nature of these studies does not diminish their importance. The inherent difficulty of conducting meaningful epidemiologic studies of pervasive chemicals and the lack of a suitable animal model for human breast cancer make these essential studies. For example, one study demonstrating that epidermal growth factor receptor ligands enhance oncogene expression in butylparaben-primed breast cancer cells illustrates how in vitro models can be used to gain important insight into the mechanisms of action in vivo.[71]

PARABENS: THE TAKE-HOME MESSAGE

The use of parabens in a wide range of personal care products has made them significant environmental contaminants. Like other EDCs originally categorized as weakly estrogenic, recent data suggest that the endocrine-disrupting properties of these chemicals are likely to be complex. Their pervasiveness makes establishing harmful effects in humans virtually impossible, but the data suggest that savvy consumers can significantly reduce their exposure by avoiding personal care products containing parabens.

Triclosan

WHAT IS IT AND WHAT ARE ITS ENDOCRINE-DISRUPTING PROPERTIES?

Triclosan is an antimicrobial agent that has been used for more than 40 years as a disinfectant and preservative. It is incorporated in medical and household cleaning products and in personal care products. Triclosan is also incorporated in plastics, fabrics, toys, paints, medical devices, and kitchen utensils that are designed such that they leach the chemical for extended periods.

Triclosan, or 5-chloro-2-(2,4-dichlorophenoxy)-phenol, is classified as a halogenated aromatic hydrocarbon and is structurally similar to polychlorinated biphenyls (PCBs), polybrominated diphenyl ethers (PBDEs), and dioxin.[19] Production estimates from 2007 found yearly global production to be more than 1500 tons, with more than 300 tons produced in the United States[38] and more than 450 tons produced in Europe.[80] In Europe, about 85% of the total volume of triclosan is used in personal care products, 5% in textiles, and 10% in plastics and food contact materials.[80]

As an antimicrobial, triclosan is active against most gram-negative and gram-positive bacteria and some fungi.[48] It is bacteriostatic (i.e., stops bacteria from reproducing) at low concentrations and bactericidal (i.e., kills bacteria) at higher concentrations. At sublethal concentrations, it acts by inhibiting bacterial lipid biosynthesis.[42] At bactericidal concentrations, it permeates the bacterial cell wall and targets multiple cytoplasmic and membrane sites, including RNA synthesis and the production of marcomolecules.[19] In addition to bacteria, triclosan is toxic to many other organisms in the ecosystem, including aquatic plants, invertebrates, fish, frogs, and mammals. Triclosan has low acute toxicity and for a long time was considered safe,[48] but there is increasing evidence that triclosan alters the endocrine and reproductive systems and interferes with neural and immune function.

Triclosan has thyroid hormone and gonadotropic hormone activity[93] and is structurally similar to thyroid hormone. Thyroid hormones play a pivotal role in regulating adult metabolism, and during development, they are essential for cell differentiation and neural development. Environmentally relevant concentrations (i.e., relevant to human exposures) of triclosan have been reported to alter the thyroid hormones T_3 and T_4 in male and female rats,[18,85,102] and exposure is thought to induce hepatic enzymes involved in T_4 metabolism, thereby reducing circulating levels.[72] In frogs, triclosan interferes with thyroid hormone–mediated limb development and decrease expression of thyroid receptor mRNA.[89] In vitro studies of rat and human cells suggest that triclosan affects a number of different biochemical processes important for thyroid hormone homeostasis.[18] If triclosan also perturbs the thyroid axis in humans, the implications for developmental processes could be profound.[19]

The effect of triclosan on gonadotropic hormones is less clear. It is structurally similar to known estrogenic and androgenic EDCs, including PCBs, PBDEs, and bisphenol A.[19] Triclosan can bind estrogen and androgen receptors and can exert estrogenic, weak androgenic, and antiandrogenic effects.[93] It also acts as an antiandrogen by inhibiting testosterone production at a number of steps in the synthetic pathway. The available evidence suggests that triclosan acts at multiple steps in the pathways for estrogen and androgen signaling.[52,53]

Adverse effects have been reported in several species and in cell lines, and the combined data suggest that the biological effects of triclosan exposure likely depend on the tissue, developmental stage, and level of exposure.

Triclosan that enters the body is metabolized, and the impact of these metabolites is likely to be species-specific but has not been studied in detail.[19]

WHERE AND HOW ARE WE EXPOSED?

Triclosan is contained in a wide range of personal care products, including toothpaste, deodorant, shampoo, soaps, detergents, and cosmetics.[78] In 2010, use in personal care products and cosmetics was estimated to account for 99% of triclosan use.[80] It is also incorporated in manufactured goods, including medical devices, children's toys, carpets, kitchen utensils, and food storage containers, and an increasing number of clothes and fabrics are treated with triclosan to reduce odors and impart antibacterial properties to the material.[80]

Human exposure is common, and triclosan residues can be measured in human blood, urine, tissue, and breast milk.[15] Triclosan is detected in 75% of urine samples[11] and 97% of breast milk samples in the United States and Sweden.[1,4,25] Human exposure occurs through oral ingestion (e.g., toothpaste, mouthwashes, dental treatments), and infants can be exposed through breast milk. Triclosan in personal care products can be absorbed through the skin. In humans, the primary route of excretion is in the urine, and urinary concentrations are a good measure of exposure.

HOW PERSISTENT IS IT IN THE ENVIRONMENT?

An estimated 95% of the triclosan in consumer products is washed off the skin and ends up in residential wastewater. Removal of triclosan through wastewater treatment ranges from no removal to 100%.[19] Incomplete removal results in the release of triclosan into rivers, streams, and lakes, but an estimated 50% of triclosan in wastewater partitions into and remains in biosolid sludge. Through spreading of sludge onto soil, triclosan contaminates soils and surface waters. Triclosan is widely detectable in surface waters and wastewater effluent in the United States, Canada, Europe, Australia, Japan, and China[80] and is one of the top 10 most frequently encountered contaminants in U.S. rivers and streams.[51]

Triclosan is lipophilic, moderately water soluble, and relatively persistent in the environment, with a half-life of at least 11 days in river water.[5] In aerobic soils, biodegradation occurs with a half-life of 18 days,[99] but under anaerobic conditions (i.e., sediment and sewage sludge), triclosan can persist for years. Triclosan and its breakdown products have been measured in 30-year-old sediment from Lake Greifensee in Switzerland and in 40-year-old sediments from fresh and estuarine water in the United States.[19]

In personal care products, concentrations are typically in the range of 0.1% to 0.3%. After wastewater treatment, concentrations can reach 0.01 to 2.7 μg/L in effluent and 5 to 55 mg/kg in sewage sludge (i.e., biosolids). In surface water, triclosan concentrations up to 2.3 μg/L have been reported, with 0.8 mg/kg found in freshwater and estuarine sediments.[19]

Although these environmental levels may seem low compared with the concentrations used in consumer products, they have profound effects on the ecosystem. For example, triclosan in biosolids applied to soils can alter nitrogen cycling and inhibit plant growth, and levels in surface water are sufficient to disrupt development in amphibians and fish.[19]

In addition to direct toxic effects on organisms in the ecosystem, the formation of toxic byproducts in the environment is a concern. Triclosan breaks down into lipophilic, stable, and persistent compounds—most notably dioxins and chloroform—that accumulate and may be more toxic than triclosan itself.[19] Chloroform forms through the reaction of triclosan with chlorine or chloramine added during wastewater processing and in drinking water treatment. Although environmental concentrations of triclosan react with chlorine to form chloroform during purification of drinking water, the amount formed is low and unlikely to pose a health risk. However, significant amounts of chloroform are formed when treated drinking water is combined with triclosan-containing products, such as when washing dishes or showering.[19] Chronic exposure to chloroform can cause liver damage and possibly cancer.[59] Additionally, 2,4-dichlorophenol (2,4-DCP) and 2,4,6-trichlorophenol (2,4,6-TCP) are produced by the degradation of triclosan, and the U.S. EPA has flagged both as priority pollutants due to their higher stability, well-known toxicity, and endocrine-disrupting activity.[19]

WHAT ARE THE CURRENT HEALTH CONCERNS?

The potential health issues of triclosan include endocrine disruption, altered immune and skeletal muscle function, antibiotic resistance, and the formation of carcinogenic byproducts.[19] Although not a direct health concern, triclosan alters many components of the ecosystem, endangering its stability and indirectly threatening human health.

The known health effects caused by triclosan include disruption of thyroid hormone homeostasis and gonadotropic hormones. These effects are significant, and recent evidence suggests effects on other organ systems. Using data from the 2003–2006 NHANES, urinary triclosan levels were compared with serum cytomegalovirus (CMV) antibody levels and diagnosis of allergies or hay fever in adults and children older than 6 years of age in the United States. Triclosan levels were positively associated with allergy and hay fever, suggesting that triclosan exposure could affect immune function and be associated with other inflammatory diseases.[15]

A subsequent epidemiologic study based on NHANES data found a positive association between urinary triclosan concentration and increased body mass index (BMI),[54] strengthening support for an effect of triclosan on immune function. Experimentally, triclosan has been reported to alter contractility in skeletal and cardiac muscle, reducing grip strength of mice and swimming ability of fish,[14] and it has been identified as a hepatic tumor promoter in mice.[100]

TRICLOSAN: THE TAKE-HOME MESSAGE

Triclosan is a serious environmental contaminant. It is pervasive and stabile in the environment, has endocrine-disrupting ability, is toxic to plants and aquatic organisms, is degraded to toxic byproducts, and has potential for creating antimicrobial resistance. The increased use of triclosan in personal care products stems from relaxed regulation combined with aggressive and widespread advertising that reinforces fears of microbial infection.

Although soaps containing less than 1% are no more efficacious than non-antimicrobial soap,[80] concentrations in hand and dish soaps marketed as antibacterial are typically 0.3%. In 2005, an FDA panel determined that there was a lack of data demonstrating evidence of the benefits of triclosan use.[39] One concern is that serious damage to the environment and potential harm to human health is occurring through the use of a chemical that provides little or no obvious benefit.

Triclocarban

WHAT IS IT AND WHAT ARE ITS ENDOCRINE-DISRUPTING PROPERTIES?

Triclocarban, or N-(4-chlorophenyl)-N-(3,4-dichlorophenyl)urea, is a non-phenolic carbanilide with use and properties similar to those of triclosan. Triclocarban is also a broad-spectrum antimicrobial and is added to a wide range of medical products, household cleaning supplies, and personal care products at levels of 0.5% to 5% by weight.[38]

It is not a new chemical. Triclocarban was originally introduced as a surgical scrub, but it has been used in personal care products such as hand soaps, detergents, creams, toothpaste, and detergents since the late 1950s.[16,17] Compared with triclosan, however, triclocarban has received considerably less attention. This reflects the fact that it could not be analyzed by gas chromatography and mass spectroscopy (GC-MS) and had to await the development of liquid chromatography and mass spectroscopy (LC-MS) analytic tools.[39]

The potential endocrine-disrupting abilities of triclocarban have not been studied in detail. Data from in vitro nuclear receptor bioassays, however, suggest that triclocarban may possess unusual endocrine-disrupting ability. Although triclocarban alone exhibits little or no agonist activity, it appears to amplify the response of androgen and estrogen receptors to steroid hormones.[2] Triclocarban also is a potent inhibitor of the human soluble epoxide hydrolase enzyme.[82]

WHERE AND HOW ARE WE EXPOSED?

Like triclosan, human exposure to triclocarban occurs through a wide variety of personal care products and other consumer goods, with oral ingestion and transdermal absorption thought to be the primary routes of exposure. Based on urinary levels, showering with triclocarban-containing soap has been suggested to result in absorption of approximately 0.6% of the triclocarban contained in the product.[81]

Biomonitoring studies have been few and limited in scope. Triclocarban, however, has been detected in human urine[76,97] and cord blood[76] in the United States, with the latest study reporting detectable levels in 87% of urine samples from pregnant women tested at a hospital in Brooklyn, NY.[76] Exposure levels have varied greatly in small biomonitoring studies conducted around the world,[76] likely reflecting in part differences in the analytic methods employed. However, in a biomonitoring study of a Chinese population, the frequency of triclocarban detection exceeded that of triclosan (99% and 69%, respectively) in adult urine samples.[98]

HOW PERSISTENT IS IT IN THE ENVIRONMENT?

Triclocarban is an important environmental contaminant and, together with triclosan, is among the most frequent organic wastewater contaminants.[16]

Triclocarban, however, may be even more environmentally persistent. A study of different environmental compartments calculated half-lives for triclocarban ranging from 0.75 days in air to 540 days in sediment.[38] Triclocarban levels exceeded those of triclosan in an analysis of bioaccumulation in algae in a stream receiving wastewater from a treatment plant in Texas[16] and in samples from urban streams in Baltimore, MD.[38]

Like triclosan, triclocarban is enriched in biosolids and persists under anaerobic conditions. An evaluation of their removal by conventional sludge processing systems reported more rapid removal of triclosan, consistent with the idea that triclocarban is less readily biotransformed.[66] Similarly, in a study using carrot cell cultures, triclocarban proved more resistant to metabolism by plants than triclosan.[95]

WHAT ARE THE CURRENT HEALTH CONCERNS?

As for triclosan, experimental evidence suggests that triclocarban exposure may induce disturbances in thyroid homeostasis. Fewer studies have evaluated the effects of triclocarban, but two in vitro studies using rat cells provide evidence of exposure effects. Altered expression of thyroid hormone responsive genes was observed in pituitary cells exposed to triclocarban,[44] and a slightly stronger inhibition of iodide uptake than triclosan was reported in thyroid cells.[95] The lowest triclocarban concentration eliciting an effect in iodide uptake studies is thought to be within the range of human exposure levels. The limited data available suggest that both broad-spectrum antimicrobials have the potential to disrupt thyroid homeostasis.

TRICLOCARBAN: THE TAKE-HOME MESSAGE

Like triclosan, the use of triclocarban as an antimicrobial is widespread, but its value in personal care products is questionable, especially in light of the high level of environmental contamination caused by this use. Compared with triclosan, triclocarban has been less well studied. Nevertheless, detectable levels in human biospecimens and widespread contamination in wildlife and the environment have been found Evidence that triclosan and triclocarban have endocrine-disrupting properties is accumulating, and the need for studies to assess their biologic activities is urgent.

Quaternary Ammonium Compounds

WHAT ARE THEY AND WHAT ARE THEIR ENDOCRINE-DISRUPTING PROPERTIES?

QACs are cationic disinfectants with antimicrobial, surfactant, and antistatic properties. QACs have been in use for approximately 70 years and serve a variety of applications. In the United States, they are registered as pesticides under the Federal Insecticide, Fungicide, and Rodenticide Act (FIFRA), and many QAC formulations are listed on the federal registry as microbiocides and algaecides.

QACs are effective against most bacteria, fungi, protozoa, and some viruses. The bactericidal effects of QACs are mediated through the adsorption of the cationic molecule to negatively charged proteins on bacterial cell membranes. Their antibacterial value is limited by their lack of sporicidal action and their ineffectiveness against *Clostridium difficile* and some gram-negative bacteria.[92] Nevertheless, QACs have rapidly replaced traditional oxidizing disinfectants such as sodium hypochlorite and hydrogen peroxide because they do not decolorize fabric, are noncorrosive, and leave no odor.[63]

QACs consist of a central nitrogen atom surrounded by four functional groups that influence the antimicrobial, surfactant, and antistatic activity of the molecule. Modifications to QAC functional groups for improved stability, solubility, and product application have generated four chemically diverse groups of QACs. The earliest (i.e., group I QACs) contain long-chain alkyl (C8 to C18) functional groups and have antimicrobial activity. Group II QACs possess nonhalogenated benzyl functional groups and have detergent and biocidal capacity. Group III QACs have dichlorobenzyl and trichlorobenzyl substitutions for enhancement of biocidal activity,[23] and group IV QACs have unusual substituents and are use in textiles, laundry products, and cosmetics.

The most common QACs in commercial cleaning and disinfectant solutions are alkyl dimethyl benzyl ammonium chloride (ADBAC) and didecyl dimethyl ammonium chloride (DDAC). Each compound contains a mix of alkyl chain lengths: C12 to C18 for ADBAC and C8 to C16 for DDAC.

Because oral or inhalation exposure to QACs is considered moderately toxic and dermal exposure slightly irritating, appropriate personal protective equipment is recommended during the application of QACs. Little is known about the endocrine-disrupting potential of QACs. One report suggests that ADBAC (i.e., benzalkonium chloride [BAC]) disrupts cholesterol biosynthesis,[43] and because cholesterol serves as a substrate for all steroid hormones, this raises the possibility that QACs are EDCs. This finding, coupled with the growing evidence of biological effects, indicates that further studies of the mechanisms of action of these compounds are urgently needed.

WHERE AND HOW ARE WE EXPOSED?

Standards set by the U.S. Occupational Safety and Health Administration (OSHA) to mitigate occupational exposure to bloodborne pathogens have resulted in listing by the EPA of several QAC formulations as effective against common clinical pathogens (https://www.osha.gov/pls/oshaweb/owadisp. show_document?p_table=INTERPRETATIONS&p_id=22205). As a result, QACs are common in clinical environments and commercial settings. The efficacy of QACs over a broad range of temperatures and pH levels has led to extensive incorporation of these compounds in consumer applications, including algaecides in swimming pools, antiseptics in candy lozenges, and preservatives in eye drop solutions.

In 2002, QACs were reported to be the most common disinfectant in food production, storage, and preparation facilities in the United Kingdom,[46] and their global use in large-scale agricultural and food processing operations contributes to the prevalence of QACs in commercially prepared food.[88] The extensive use of ADBAC and DDAC QACs in industrial, commercial, and residential settings suggests that humans are chronically exposed. Although little is known about dermal exposure, occupational exposure to ADBAC through inhalation is common among janitorial and health care workers.[10,65,75]

HOW PERSISTENT ARE THEY IN THE ENVIRONMENT?

Because QACs are used as dilute solutions, the contamination potential of these compounds has largely been ignored. ADBAC-containing disinfectant solutions that do not exceed 400 ppm are not considered significant sources of human exposure and are exempt from food residue tolerance requirements in the United States.[30] Extensive commercial use of QACs, however, has led to significant environmental contamination, and there is evidence that these chemicals persist in the environment for many months after their use is discontinued.[61]

In addition to being a wastewater contaminant, QACs are used during municipal wastewater treatment to reduce the coliform load. It is not surprising that analysis of urban sewage runoff suggests that QACs are more prevalent than other aquatic contaminants, including chlorinated pesticides, polychlorinated biphenyls, and polyaromatic hydrocarbons.[56] The propensity for cationic QAC molecules to adsorb sludge and the fact that they undergo little to no biodegradation under anaerobic conditions makes them environmentally persistent.[33] Consequently, QACs have been proposed as useful tools for the evaluation of sewage contamination in aquatic environments.[57] Despite the fact that QAC contamination in aquatic environments is ecologically significant, studies of the toxic effects of these compounds on aquatic organisms are limited.[35]

WHAT ARE THE CURRENT HEALTH CONCERNS?

Experimental studies in rats provide evidence that oral exposure to high concentrations of QACs can be lethal,[28,29] and death after ingestion of a 10% BAC solution has been reported for elderly humans.[45,84] There is some evidence that QACs may be genotoxic, with genetic damage reported in human peripheral lymphocytes from healthy volunteers.[31]

Reports of occupational asthma in health care workers using ADBAC-containing disinfectants suggest that exposure may cause respiratory and mucosal irritation.[75] Sensitization and irritation of skin and mucous membranes have been reported after occupational and residential use of BAC concentrations as low as 0.1% to 0.5%.[91] Experimental studies in mice also provide evidence that QAC inhalation results in pulmonary irritation and inflammation,[55] and in vitro studies of mouse lung fibroblasts implicate DDAC in proinflammatory effects leading to pulmonary fibrosis and disrupted transforming growth factor-β signaling.[67]

ADBAC and DDAC have been identified as reproductive toxicants in the mouse; the chemicals decrease sperm counts in males and ovulation rate and offspring number in females.[61,62] Experimental studies of toxicity in other tissues, however, have been limited to in vitro toxicity studies of ADBAC and DDAC using corneal, epithelial, and pulmonary cell lines. ADBAC is a common preservative in eye drop solutions, and corneal and conjunctival cytotoxicity has been reported at the low concentrations typically present in ophthalmic preparations (0.01% to 0.02%).[37,50,58,79] Spermicidal formulations containing BAC are available outside of the United States, and studies of human vaginal epithelial cell lines suggest that these products may induce mucosal toxicity through the induction of inflammatory interleukin release.[32]

Although relatively few studies of the biological effects of QACs have been undertaken, collective data from in vivo and in vitro studies suggest that ADBAC and DDAC are cytotoxic. In the absence of corroborating data from epidemiologic studies, however, the risk posed to humans (other than for occupational asthma) remains unclear. ADBAC and DDAC are increasingly combined in commercially available products, but few studies have evaluated the toxicity of QAC mixtures.

QACs: THE TAKE HOME MESSAGE

QACs are an important class of disinfectants whose toxicity has been insufficiently evaluated. The prevalence of QACs as disinfectants in occupational settings, as antimicrobials in personal care products, and as common environmental contaminants makes the degree of human exposure significant. Although the lack of research devoted to evaluating the potential health effects of these compounds is surprising, the limited data available data raise serious concerns about the potential adverse effects of exposure on the lung and reproductive health of adults and on the developing fetus.

Because the optimization of QAC moieties for product-specific functions likely influences their ability to exert biologic effects, assessment of different QAC groups is essential. QAC mixtures are commonly used, and because QACs may act synergistically to produce greater toxic effects, assessment of common mixtures is essential to evaluate chemical risk. Given these concerns, identifying the extent of human exposure and understanding the health effects of QACs are critical tasks.

Summary and Future Directions

In this chapter, we have focused on existing evidence of health and ecological effects of four persistent and widespread environmental contaminants. All four have been implicated in reproductive effects, and triclosan and triclocarbon also appear to interfere with thyroid homeostasis. There is concern that the chemicals' antimicrobial properties and widespread use have led to increased bacterial resistance to these biocides. The four chemicals contaminate much of the ecosystem, where they impact many plant and animal species, and the long-term consequences of ecosystem exposures are unknown. Parabens, triclosan, triclocarbon, and QACs represent a tiny subset of the chemicals that enter daily life from the air, food, water, prescription drugs, personal care products, manufactured products, and cleaners used in homes and public spaces, and this select group of biocidal chemicals illustrates several critical concepts.

Chemicals originally designed for clinical and commercial purposes are being used in a wide variety of consumer products. Triclosan and triclocarban proved efficacious in the clinical and industrial realm and were rapidly adapted for use in personal care and other consumer products. The transition occurred in the absence of sufficient safety testing and without sufficient evidence that these chemicals are efficacious in consumer products.

As the number of chemicals in everyday use has expanded, the sense of caution and concern about their use has waned. As illustrated by parabens and QACs, the ability to rapidly engineer man-made compounds to modify or magnify desirable attributes can result in an evolving class of chemicals with different properties. The expanding array of related chemicals impedes efforts to understand biological and environmental effects because each chemical variant has slightly different properties. Because the transition occurs in the absence of sufficient testing, the recognition that a chemical poses a risk to human health or the environment may not occur until exposure or contamination has become widespread.

Our chemical finesse is not without cost. Available evidence suggests that the chemicals reviewed in this chapter have significant potential to harm humans and other species. Their use has become so pervasive that most of the population is exposed. We have allowed inadequately tested chemicals to enter the most intimate aspects of our lives and are conducting population-wide experiments without controls. Elucidating the impacts of chemical exposure on human health means trying to understand the effects of individual chemicals and how their effects are influenced by genetic diversity, lifestyle choices, and other pervasive environmental chemicals.

There are other potentially serious consequences of the extensive and indiscriminant use of biocides, such as possible effects on human immunity and an increased propensity of microbiota to develop resistance. These concerns underscore the urgency of reforms, including testing of chemicals before marketing, devising methods of tracking and controlling applications of approved chemicals, and developing transparency in the use of approved chemicals that provides consumer awareness and facilitates the detection of health or environmental effects.

The role of the clinician is essential. Given the flaws in current chemical safety and risk assessment procedures, the task before us is daunting. Chemical exposures, especially those that occur during development, can affect the incidence of chronic noncommunicable diseases later in life. Ideally, we need a patient *exposome* (i.e., record of in utero and early-life exposure) to understand how specific developmental exposures affect adult health and disease.

In the meantime, clinicians can work with patients to understand how past or current exposures affect their health. By informing patients about growing areas of concern, the medical profession is in a powerful position to affect change. Scientists and clinicians can work with their professional societies to effect change, but a more effective route is through patient education.

Clinicians' most important role is to rationally and responsibly voice their concerns to the general public. Consumers make daily choices, and as a 3-day intervention study involving Latina girls (i.e., HERMOSA study[41]) demonstrated, simple changes in consumer choices can reduce exposure. Citizen concern about the health effects of chemical exposure can drive changes in product formulation and legislation for adequate safety testing of chemicals in consumer products. To feel powerless in the face of information on chemicals such as those reviewed in this chapter is to fail to understand the power of the opinions of scientists and clinicians to influence society.

Addendum

Since this chapter was initially submitted in July 2016, the US Food and Drug Administration (FDA) has banned the use of 19 chemicals used in antibacterial soaps including Triclosan, Triclocarbon and the QAC methylbenzethonium chloride (Hyamine). The FDA stated that the data submitted for these 19 chemicals were insufficient to demonstrate any additional benefit from inclusion in consumer antiseptic wash products. While this decision is a good first step, the reduction in exposure for consumers is likely to be limited. This ruling only applies to consumer products that are intended for use with water and are expected to be rinsed off after use. The ruling does not apply to antiseptic rubs that remain on the skin (hand sanitizers and sanitizing wipes), first aid antiseptics, antiseptic products used in health care settings, nor antiseptic products used in the food industry. In addition, the reason for the ban was not based on safety concerns, but rather lack of increased benefit beyond what is achieved with normal soap and water. The Generally Recognized as Safe (GRAS) designation does evaluate risk vs. benefit. In this case, however, the decision to ban the antiseptics was due to lack of benefit rather than the well documented health and environmental risks associated with use of these chemicals as we outlined in this chapter. It is the opinion of the authors that further restrictions and broader bans need to be placed on these and similar chemicals due to the adverse health effects and environmental concerns following use of these chemicals.

REFERENCES

1. Adolfsson-Erici, M., Pettersson, M., Parkkonen, J., & Sturve, J. 2002. Triclosan, a commonly used bactericide found in human milk and in the aquatic environment in Sweden. *Chemosphere*. 46:1485–1489.

2. Ahn, K.C., Zhao, B., Chen, J., et al. 2008. In vitro biologic activities of the anti-microbials triclocarban, its analogs, and triclosan in bioassay screens: Receptor-based bioassay screens. *Environ Health Perspect.* 116:1203–1210.

3. Alam, M.S., Ohsako, S., Kanai, Y., & Kurohmaru, M. 2014. Single administration of butylparaben induces spermatogenic cell apoptosis in prepubertal rats. *Acta Histochem.* 116:474–480.

4. Allmyr, M., Adolfsson-Erici, M., McLachlan, M.S., & Sandborgh-Englund, G. 2006. Triclosan in plasma and milk from Swedish nursing mothers and their exposure via personal care products. *Sci Total Environ.* 372:87–93.

5. Bester, K. 2005. Fate of triclosan and triclosan-methyl in sewage treatment plants and surface waters. *Arch Environ Contam Toxicol.* 49:9–17.

6. Bledzka, D., Gromadzinska, J., & Wasowicz, W. 2014. Parabens: From environmental studies to human health. *Environ Int.* 67:27–42.

7. Boberg, J., Metzdorff, S., Wortziger, R., et al. 2008. Impact of diisobutyl phthalate and other PPAR agonists on steroidogenesis and plasma insulin and leptin levels in fetal rats. *Toxicology.* 250:75–81.

8. Boberg, J., Taxvig, C., Christiansen, S., & Hass, U. 2010. Possible endocrine disrupting effects of parabens and their metabolites. *Reprod Toxicol.* 30:301–312.

9. Braun, J.M., Just, A.C., Williams, P.L., Smith, K.W., Calafat, A.M., & Hauser, R. 2014. Personal care product use and urinary phthalate metabolite and paraben concentrations during pregnancy among women from a fertility clinic. *J Exposure Sci Environ Epidemiol.* 24:459–466.

10. Burge, P.S., & Richardson, M.N. 1994. Occupational asthma due to indirect exposure to lauryl dimethyl benzyl ammonium chloride used in a floor cleaner. *Thorax.* 49:842–843.

11. Calafat, A.M., Ye, X., Wong, L.Y., Reidy, J.A., & Needham, L.L. 2008. Urinary concentrations of triclosan in the U.S. population: 2003-2004. *Environ Health Perspect.* 116:303–307.

12. Calafat, A.M., Ye, X., Wong, L.Y., Bishop, A.M., & Needham, L.L. 2010. Urinary concentrations of four parabens in the U.S. population: NHANES 2005-2006. *Environ Health Perspect.* 118:679–685.

13. Charles, A.K., & Darbre, P.D. 2013. Combinations of parabens at concentrations measured in human breast tissue can increase proliferation of MCF-7 human breast cancer cells. *J Appl Toxicol.* 33:390–398.

14. Cherednichenko, G., Zhang, R., Bannister, R.A., et al. 2012. Triclosan impairs excitation-contraction coupling and Ca2+ dynamics in striated muscle. *Proc Nat Acad Sci U S A.* 109:14158–14163.

15. Clayton, E.M., Todd, M., Dowd, J.B., & Aiello, A.E. 2011. The impact of bisphenol A and triclosan on immune parameters in the U.S. population, NHANES 2003-2006. *Environ Health Perspect.* 119:390–396.

16. Coogan, M.A., Edziyie, R.E., La Point, T.W., & Venables, B.J. 2007. Algal bioaccumulation of triclocarban, triclosan, and methyl-triclosan in a North Texas wastewater treatment plant receiving stream. *Chemosphere.* 67:1911–1918.

17. Cooney, C.M. 2010. Triclosan comes under scrutiny. Environ Health Perspect. 118:A242.

18. Crofton, K.M., Paul, K.B., Devito, M.J., & Hedge, J.M. 2007. Short-term in vivo exposure to the water contaminant triclosan: Evidence for disruption of thyroxine. *Environ Toxicol Pharmacol*. 24:194–197.

19. Dann, A.B., & Hontela, A. 2011. Triclosan: Environmental exposure, toxicity and mechanisms of action. *J Appl Toxicol*. 31:285–311.

20. Darbre, P.D., Byford, J.R., Shaw, L.E., Horton, R.A., Pope, G.S., & Sauer, M.J. 2002. Oestrogenic activity of isobutylparaben in vitro and in vivo. *J Appl Toxicol*. 22:219–226.

21. Darbre, P.D., & Harvey, P.W. 2008. Paraben esters: Review of recent studies of endocrine toxicity, absorption, esterase and human exposure, and discussion of potential human health risks. *J Appl Toxicol*. 28:561–578.

22. Darbre, P.D., & Harvey, P.W. 2014. Parabens can enable hallmarks and characteristics of cancer in human breast epithelial cells: A review of the literature with reference to new exposure data and regulatory status. *J Appl Toxicol*. 34:925–938.

23. Darragh, J.L., & Ralph, H. 1954. Addition products of halogen and quaternary ammonium germicides and method for making the same. U.S. Patent 2679533A. https://www.google.com/patents/US2679533.

24. Daston, G.P. 2004. Developmental toxicity evaluation of butylparaben in Sprague-Dawley rats. *Birth Defects Res B Dev Reprod Toxicol*. 71:296–302.

25. Dayan, A.D. 2007. Risk assessment of triclosan [Irgasan] in human breast milk. *Food Chem Toxicol*. 45:125–129.

26. Diamanti-Kandarakis, E., Bourguignon, J.P., Giudice, L.C., et al. 2009. Endocrine-disrupting chemicals: An Endocrine Society scientific statement. *Endocr Rev*. 30:293–342.

27. Dodge, L.E., Williams, P.L., Williams, M.A., et al. 2015. Paternal urinary concentrations of parabens and other phenols in relation to reproductive outcomes among couples from a fertility clinic. *Environ Health Perspect*. 123:665–671.

28. Environmental Protection Agency. 2006. Reregistration eligibility decision for aliphatic alkyl quaternaries (DDAC). EPA739-R-06-008. https://archive.epa.gov/pesticides/reregistration/web/pdf/ddac_red.pdf.

29. Environmental Protection Agency. 2006. Reregistration eligibility decision for alkyl dimethyl benzyl ammonium chloride (ADBAC). EPA739-R-06-009. https://nepis.epa.gov/Exe/ZyNET.exe/P1005J4P.TXT?ZyActionD=ZyDocument&Client=EPA&Index=2006+Thru+2010&Docs=&Query=&Time=&EndTime=&SearchMethod=1&TocRestrict=n&Toc=&TocEntry=&QField=&QFieldYear=&QFieldMonth=&QFieldDay=&IntQFieldOp=0&ExtQFieldOp=0&XmlQuery=&File=D%3A%5Czyfiles%5CIndex%20Data%5C06thru10%5CTxt%5C00000011%5CP1005J4P.txt&User=ANONYMOUS&Password=anonymous&SortMethod=h%7C-&MaximumDocuments=1&FuzzyDegree=0&ImageQuality=r75g8/r75g8/x150y150g16/i425&Display=hpfr&DefSeekPage=x&SearchBack=ZyActionL&Back=ZyActionS&BackDesc=Results%20page&MaximumPages=1&ZyEntry=1&SeekPage=x&ZyPURL.

30. Environmental Protection Agency. 2010. Residues of quaternary ammonium compounds, N-Alkyl (C12-14). 40 CFR 180. Final rule 75 FR 40729. https://www.federalregister.gov/documents/2010/07/14/2010-17156/residues-of-quaternary-ammonium-compounds-n-alkyl-c12-14.

31. Ferk, F., Misik, M., Hoelzl, C., et al. 2007. Benzalkonium chloride (BAC) and dimethyldioctadecyl-ammonium bromide (DDAB), two common quaternary ammonium compounds, cause genotoxic effects in mammalian and plant cells at environmentally relevant concentrations. *Mutagenesis.* 22:363–370.

32. Fichorova, R.N., Bajpai, M., Chandra, N., et al. 2004. Interleukin (IL)-1, IL-6, and IL-8 predict mucosal toxicity of vaginal microbicidal contraceptives. *Biol Reprod.* 71:761–769.

33. Flores, G.A., Fotidis, I.A., Karakashev, D.B., Kjellberg, K., & Angelidaki, I. 2015. Effects of Benzalkonium Chloride, Proxel LV, P3 Hypochloran, Triton X-100 and DOWFAX 63N10 on anaerobic digestion processes. *Bioresource Technol.* 193:393–400.

34. Frederiksen, H., Jorgensen, N., & Andersson, A.M. 2011. Parabens in urine, serum and seminal plasma from healthy Danish men determined by liquid chromatography-tandem mass spectrometry (LC-MS/MS). *J Exposure Sci Environ Epidemiol.* 21:262–271.

35. Grillitsch, B., Gans, O., Kreuzinger, N., Scharf, S., Uhl, M., & Fuerhacker, M. 2006. Environmental risk assessment for quaternary ammonium compounds: A case study from Austria. *Water Sci Technol.* 54:111–118.

36. Gritz, E.C., & Bhandari, V. 2015. The human neonatal gut microbiome: A brief review. *Front Pediatr.* 3:17.

37. Guzman-Aranguez, A., Calvo, P., Ropero, I., & Pintor, J. 2014. In vitro effects of preserved and unpreserved anti-allergic drugs on human corneal epithelial cells. *J Ocular Pharmacol Therapeut.* 30:790–798.

38. Halden, R.U., & Paull, D.H. 2005. Co-occurrence of triclocarban and triclosan in U.S. water resources. *Environ Sci Technol.* 39:1420–1426.

39. Halden, R.U. 2014. On the need and speed of regulating triclosan and triclocarban in the United States. *Environ Sci Technol.* 48:3603–3611.

40. Haman, C., Dauchy, X., Rosin, C., & Munoz, J.F. 2015. Occurrence, fate and behavior of parabens in aquatic environments: A review. *Water Res.* 68:1–11.

41. Harley, K.G., Kogut, K., Madrigal, D.S., et al. 2016. Reducing phthalate paraben, and phenol exposure from personal care products in adolescent girls: Findings from the HERMOSA Intervention Study. *Environ Health Perspect.* 124:1600–1607.

42. Heath, R.J., White, S.W., & Rock, C.O. 2002. Inhibitors of fatty acid synthesis as antimicrobial chemotherapeutics. *Appl Microbiol Biotechnol.* 58:695–703.

43. Herron, J., Reese, R.C., Tallman, K.A., Narayanaswamy, R., Porter, N.A., & Xu, L. 2016. Identification of environmental quaternary ammonium compounds as direct inhibitors of cholesterol biosynthesis. *Toxicol Sci.* 151:261–270.

44. Hinther, A., Bromba, C.M., Wulff, J.E., & Helbing, C.C. 2011. Effects of triclocarban, triclosan, and methyl triclosan on thyroid hormone action and stress in frog and mammalian culture systems. *Environ Sci Technol.* 45:5395–5402.

45. Hitosugi, M., Maruyama, K., & Takatsu, A. 1998. A case of fatal benzalkonium chloride poisoning. *Int J Legal Med.* 111:265–266.

46. Holah, J.T., Taylor, J.H., Dawson, D.J., & Hall, K.E. 2002. Biocide use in the food industry and the disinfectant resistance of persistent strains of *Listeria monocytogenes* and *Escherichia coli. J Appl Microbiol.* 92(Suppl):111S–120S.

47. Hoover, R.N., Hyer, M., Pfeiffer, R.M., et al. 2011. Adverse health outcomes in women exposed in utero to diethylstilbestrol. *N Engl J Med.* 365:1304–1314.

48. Jones, R.D., Jampani, H.B., Newman, J.L., & Lee, A.S. 2000. Triclosan: A review of effectiveness and safety in health care settings. *Am J Infect Control.* 28:184–196.

49. Kang, K.S., Che, J.H., Ryu, D.Y., Kim, T.W., Li, G.X., & Lee, Y.S. 2002. Decreased sperm number and motile activity on the F1 offspring maternally exposed to butyl p-hydroxybenzoic acid (butyl paraben). *J Vet Med Sci* 64:227–235.

50. Kim, E.J., Kim, Y.H., Kang, S.H., Lee, K.W., & Park, Y.J. 2013. In vitro effects of preservative-free and preserved prostaglandin analogs on primary cultured human conjunctival fibroblast cells. *Korean J Ophthalmol.* 27:446–453.

51. Kolpin, D.W., Furlong, E.T., Meyer, M.T., et al. 2002. Pharmaceuticals, hormones, and other organic wastewater contaminants in U.S. streams, 1999-2000: A national reconnaissance. *Environ Sci Technol.* 36:1202–1211.

52. Kumar, V., Balomajumder, C., & Roy, P. 2008. Disruption of LH-induced testosterone biosynthesis in testicular Leydig cells by triclosan: Probable mechanism of action. *Toxicology.* 250:124–131.

53. Kumar, V., Chakraborty, A., Kural, M.R., & Roy, P. 2009. Alteration of testicular steroidogenesis and histopathology of reproductive system in male rats treated with triclosan. *Reprod Toxicol.* 27:177–185.

54. Lankester, J., Patel, C., Cullen, M.R., Ley, C., & Parsonnet, J. 2013. Urinary triclosan is associated with elevated body mass index in NHANES. *PloS One.* 8:e80057.

55. Larsen, S.T., Verder, H., & Nielsen, G.D. 2012. Airway effects of inhaled quaternary ammonium compounds in mice. *Basic Clin Pharmacol Toxicol.* 110:537–543.

56. Li, X., & Brownawell, B.J. 2010. Quaternary ammonium compounds in urban estuarine sediment environments: A class of contaminants in need of increased attention? *Environ Sci Technol.* 44:7561–7568.

57. Li, X., Luo, X., Mai, B., Liu, J., Chen, L., & Lin, S. 2014. Occurrence of quaternary ammonium compounds (QACs) and their application as a tracer for sewage derived pollution in urban estuarine sediments. *Environ Pollut.* 185:127–133.

58. Liang, H., Baudouin, C., Daull, P., Garrigue, J.S., Buggage, R., & Brignole-Baudouin, F. 2012. In vitro and in vivo evaluation of a preservative-free cationic emulsion of latanoprost in corneal wound healing models. *Cornea.* 31:1319–1329.

59. MAK. 2012. Chloroform (MAK Value Documentation, 2000). *The MAK Collection for Occupational Health and Safety.* 20–58. http://onlinelibrary.wiley.com/doi/10.1002/3527600418.mb6766e0014/full#leftBorder.

60. Meeker, J.D., Yang, T., Ye, X., Calafat, A.M., & Hauser, R. 2011. Urinary concentrations of parabens and serum hormone levels, semen quality parameters, and sperm DNA damage. *Environ Health Perspect.* 119:252–257.

61. Melin, V.E., Potineni, H., Hunt, P., et al. 2014. Exposure to common quaternary ammonium disinfectants decreases fertility in mice. *Reprod Toxicol.* 50:163–170.

62. Melin, V.E., Melin, T.E., Dessify, B.J., Nguyen, C.T., Shea, C.S., & Hrubec, T.C. 2016. Quaternary ammonium disinfectants cause subfertility in mice by targeting both male and female reproductive processes. *Reprod Toxicol.* 59:159–166.

63. Merianos, J.J. 2001. Surface-active agents. In Block, S.S. (ed.). *Disinfection, Sterilization, and Preservation,* pp 283–316. Philadelphia, PA: Lippincott Williams & Wilkins.

64. Minguez-Alarcon, L., Chiu, Y.H., Messerlian, C., et al. 2016. Urinary paraben concentrations and in vitro fertilization outcomes among women from a fertility clinic. *Fertil Steril.* 105:714–721.

65. Nettis, E., Colanardi, M.C., Soccio, A.L., Ferrannini, A., & Tursi, A. 2002. Occupational irritant and allergic contact dermatitis among healthcare workers. *Contact Dermatitis.* 46:101–107.

66. Ogunyoku, T.A., & Young, T.M. 2014. Removal of triclocarban and triclosan during municipal biosolid production. *Water Environ Res.* 86:197–203.

67. Ohnuma-Koyama, A., Yoshida, T., Tajima-Horiuchi, H., et al. 2013. Didecyldimethylammonium chloride induces pulmonary fibrosis in association with TGF-beta signaling in mice. *Exp Toxicol Pathol.* 65:1003–1009.

68. Oishi, S. 2001. Effects of butylparaben on the male reproductive system in rats. *Toxicol Indus Health* 17:31–39.

69. Oishi, S. 2002. Effects of propyl paraben on the male reproductive system. *Food Chem Toxicol.* 40:1807–1813.

70. Okubo, T., Yokoyama, Y., Kano, K., & Kano, I. 2001. ER-dependent estrogenic activity of parabens assessed by proliferation of human breast cancer MCF-7 cells and expression of ERalpha and PR. *Food Chem Toxicol.* 39:1225–1232.

71. Pan, S., Yuan, C., Tagmount, A., et al. 2016. Parabens and human epidermal growth factor receptor ligands cross-talk in breast cancer cells. *Environ Health Perspect.* 124:563–569.

72. Paul, K.B., Hedge, J.M., DeVito, M.J., & Crofton, K.M. 2010. Short-term exposure to triclosan decreases thyroxine in vivo via upregulation of hepatic catabolism in Young Long-Evans rats. *Toxicol Sci.* 113:367–379.

73. Peretz, J., Vrooman, L., Ricke, W.A., et al. 2014. Bisphenol A and reproductive health: Update of experimental and human evidence, 2007-2013. *Environ Health Perspect.* 122:775–786.

74. Pugazhendhi, D., Sadler, A.J., & Darbre, P.D. 2007. Comparison of the global gene expression profiles produced by methylparaben, n-butylparaben and 17beta-oestradiol in MCF7 human breast cancer cells. *J Appl Toxicol.* 27:67–77.

75. Purohit, A., Kopferschmitt-Kubler, M.C., Moreau, C., Popin, E., Blaumeiser, M., & Pauli, G. 2000. Quaternary ammonium compounds and occupational asthma. *Int Arch Occup Environ Health.* 73:423–427.

76. Pycke, B.F., Geer, L.A., Dalloul, M., Abulafia, O., Jenck, A.M., & Halden, R.U. 2014. Human fetal exposure to triclosan and triclocarban in an urban population from Brooklyn, New York. *Environ Sci Technol.* 48:8831–8838.

77. Rachon, D. 2015. Endocrine disrupting chemicals (EDCs) and female cancer: Informing the patients. *Rev Endocr Metab Disord.* 16:359–364.
78. Reiss, R., Lewis, G., & Griffin, J. 2009. An ecological risk assessment for triclosan in the terrestrial environment. Environ Toxicol Chemistry. 28:1546–1556.
79. Rosin, L.M., & Bell, N.P. 2013. Preservative toxicity in glaucoma medication: Clinical evaluation of benzalkonium chloride-free 0.5% timolol eye drops. *Clin Ophthalmol.* 7:2131–2135.
80. SCCS (Scientific Committee on Consumer Safety). 2010, June 22. Opinion on triclosan (microbial resistance). http://ec.europa.eu/health/scientific_committees/consumer_safety/docs/sccs_o_023.pdf.
81. Schebb, N.H., Inceoglu, B., Ahn, K.C., Morisseau, C., Gee, S.J., & Hammock, B.D. 2011. Investigation of human exposure to triclocarban after showering and preliminary evaluation of its biological effects. *Environ Sci Technol.* 45:3109–3115.
82. Schebb, N.H., Buchholz, B.A., Hammock, B.D., & Rice, R.H. 2012. Metabolism of the antibacterial triclocarban by human epidermal keratinocytes to yield protein adducts. *J Biochem Mol Toxicol.* 26:230–234.
83. Smith, K.W., Souter, I., Dimitriadis, I., Ehrlich, S., Williams, P.L., Calafat, A.M., & Hauser, R. 2013. Urinary paraben concentrations and ovarian aging among women from a fertility center. *Environ Health Perspect.* 121:1299–1305.
84. Spiller, H.A. 2014. A case of fatal ingestion of a 10% benzalkonium chloride solution. *J Forensic Toxicol Pharmacol.* 3:1.
85. Stoker, T.E., Gibson, E.K., & Zorrilla, L.M. 2010. Triclosan exposure modulates estrogen-dependent responses in the female wistar rat. *Toxicol Sci.* 117:45–53.
86. Taxvig, C., Vinggaard, A.M., Hass, U., et al. 2008. Do parabens have the ability to interfere with steroidogenesis? *Toxicol Sci.* 106:206–213.
87. Taxvig, C., Dreisig, K., Boberg, J., et al. 2012. Differential effects of environmental chemicals and food contaminants on adipogenesis, biomarker release and PPARgamma activation. *Mol Cell Endocrinol.* 361:106–115.
88. van Bruijnsvoort, M., Rooselaar, J., Stern, A.G., & Jonker, K.M. 2004. Determination of residues of quaternary ammonium disinfectants in food products by liquid chromatography-tandem mass spectrometry. *J AOAC Int.* 87:1016–1020.
89. Veldhoen, N., Skirrow, R.C., Osachoff, H., et al. 2006. The bactericidal agent triclosan modulates thyroid hormone-associated gene expression and disrupts postembryonic anuran development. *Aquatic Toxicol.* 80:217–227.
90. Vo, T.T., Yoo, Y.M., Choi, K.C., & Jeung, E.B. 2010. Potential estrogenic effect(s) of parabens at the prepubertal stage of a postnatal female rat model. *Reprod Toxicol.* 29:306–316.
91. Wentworth, A.B., Yiannias, J.A., Davis, M.D., & Killian, J.M. 2016. Benzalkonium chloride: A known irritant and novel allergen. *Dermatitis.* 27:14–20.
92. *WHO Guidelines on Hand Hygiene in Health Care: First Global Patient Safety Challenge—Clean Care Is Safer Care.* Geneva, Switzerland: WHO.
93. Witorsch, R.J., & Thomas, J.A. 2010. Personal care products and endocrine disruption: A critical review of the literature. *Crit Rev Toxicol.* 40(Suppl 3):1–30.

94. Wrobel, A., & Gregoraszczuk, E.L. 2013. Effects of single and repeated in vitro exposure of three forms of parabens, methyl-, butyl-and propylparabens on the proliferation and estradiol secretion in MCF-7 and MCF-10A cells. *Pharmacol Rep.* 65:484–493.

95. Wu, X., Fu, Q., & Gan, J. 2016. Metabolism of pharmaceutical and personal care products by carrot cell cultures. *Environ Pollut.* 211:141–147.

96. Xue, J., Sasaki, N., Elangovan, M., Diamond, G., & Kannan, K. 2015. Elevated accumulation of parabens and their metabolites in marine mammals from the United States coastal waters. *Environ Sci Technol.* 49:12071–12079.

97. Ye, X., Bishop, A.M., Needham, L.L., & Calafat, A.M. 2008. Automated on-line column-switching HPLC-MS/MS method with peak focusing for measuring parabens, triclosan, and other environmental phenols in human milk. *Analyt Chim Acta.* 622:150–156.

98. Yin, J., Wei, L., Shi, Y., Zhang, J., Wu, Q., & Shao, B. 2016. Chinese population exposure to triclosan and triclocarban as measured via human urine and nails. *Environ Geochem Health.* 38:1125–1135.

99. Ying, G.G., Yu, X.Y., & Kookana, R.S. 2007. Biological degradation of triclocarban and triclosan in a soil under aerobic and anaerobic conditions and comparison with environmental fate modelling. *Environ Pollut.* 150:300–305.

100. Yueh, M.F., Taniguchi, K., Chen, S., et al. 2014. The commonly used antimicrobial additive triclosan is a liver tumor promoter. *Proc Nat Acad Sci U S A.* 111:17200–17205.

101. Zhang, L., Dong, L., Ding, S., et al. 2014. Effects of n-butylparaben on steroidogenesis and spermatogenesis through changed E(2) levels in male rat offspring. *Environ Toxicol Pharmacol.* 37:705–717.

102. Zorrilla, L.M., Gibson, E.K., Jeffay, S.C., et al. 2009. The effects of triclosan on puberty and thyroid hormones in male Wistar rats. *Toxicol Sci.* 107:56–64.

10

Microwave/Radiofrequency Radiation and Human Health: Clinical Management in the Digital Age

DEVRA DAVIS, MARGARET E. SEARS, ANTHONY B. MILLER, AND RIINA BRAY

Key Concepts

- Increasing numbers of interconnected wireless devices and infrastructure emit nonionizing microwave or radiofrequency radiation (MW/RFR). Higher-frequency, lower-power signals (3G or 4G) may be as harmful as earlier modulations (2G).
- MW/RFR is also applied therapeutically, and exposures substantially below the current regulatory limits affect biochemistry and homeostasis.
- Everyday MW/RFR exposures can impair reproduction, fetal and child development, amplify the effects of other toxicants, and culminate in chronic disease.
- Evidence indicates that the 2011 International Agency for Research on Cancer panel finding that MW/RFR is a *possible* human carcinogen should be upgraded to *probable* or *known*.
- At commonly tolerated MW/RFR exposure levels, some people experience acute and chronic symptoms such as fatigue, headache, tinnitus, and neurologic and cardiac dysfunction.
- The clinical encounter is an important opportunity to educate patients to reduce MW/RFR exposures and to determine relevance to health. Health care professionals can contribute to policies and laws to protect potential parents, the young, and those with chronic conditions.

Introduction

Although emissions from cell phones, cordless phones and other devices are too weak to cause a biologically significant increase in temperature, irregularly pulsed microwave signals, called *radiofrequency radiation* (RFR), can and do exert a broad range of biologic effects.[116] Testing and regulation of permissible radiation has not kept pace with changing technology and applications, or with the medical science indicating that peak exposures may be far more important than averaged exposures in determining impacts.

Although U.S. and many international policies for cell phone and wireless radiation have been set by agencies that are under heavy industry influence and may be subject to regulatory capture (i.e., advancing the commercial or political concerns of the special interest group rather than the public interest),[6] technologically sophisticated nations such as France, Belgium, Israel, and India have taken precautionary steps to reduce exposures. This chapter introduces RFR and the regulation and testing of devices, reviews key research on biologic and health effects, and outlines authoritative practical guidance for clinical management and public policy.

Radiofrequency Radiation Compliance Testing and Bioelectromagnetics

The more than 14 billion wireless transmitting devices globally comply with standards set to prevent heating, which were based on reviews by bodies such as the U.S. Institute of Electrical and Electronic Engineers (IEEE), U.S. National Council on Radiation Protection (NCRP), the European International Commission for Non-Ionizing Radiation Protection (ICNIRP), Health Canada, the Australian Radiation Protection and Nuclear Safety Agency (ARPANSA), and others.[85]

The U.S. Government Accountability Office,[109] U.S. Department of the Interior,[106] American Academy of Pediatrics,[82] Consumer Reports, Environmental Health Trust and others have criticized the 2-decades-old U.S. exposure standard as not protective for children or the natural environment because it fails to take into account chronic health impacts, differential sensitivities of the young, environmental impacts, and simultaneous sources of exposures from combined antennas or multiple devices.

ABSORPTION OF RADIOFREQUENCY RADIATION
BY CHILDREN AND ADULTS

Children are more vulnerable than adults to environmental toxicants,[51,71] including radiation. Sophisticated computer modeling demonstrates higher doses of cell phone radiation to children's bone marrow and critical brain regions such as the cerebellum and hippocampus as a result of differences in geometry (i.e., smaller heads), dielectric constants in thinner skulls with a higher fraction of marrow, and incompletely myelinated brains with higher water content[43,47,87] (Fig. 10.1). An International Agency for Research on Cancer (IARC) working group concluded, "The average RF radiation energy deposition for children exposed to mobile phone RF is two times higher in the brain and 10 times higher in the bone marrow of the skull compared with mobile phone use by adults."[63]

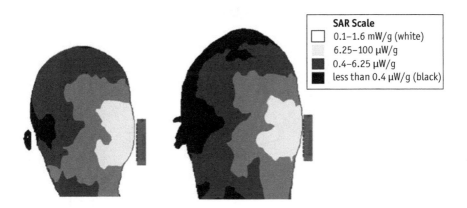

SAR Scale
- 0.1–1.6 mW/g (white)
- 6.25–100 µW/g
- 0.4–6.25 µW/g
- less than 0.4 µW/g (black)

FIGURE 10.1. Radiofrequency radiation doses (i.e., specific absorption rate [SAR]) from a cell phone are absorbed in the head of a 6-year-old child *(left)* and a male adult *(right)*. Finite difference time domain (FDTD) modeling is averaged over 1 g of tissue for a 900-MHz cell phone held to the ear, slice perpendicular to the phone, and through the peak spatial SAR.

Modeling courtesy of C. Fernendez, PhD, Federal Institute of Rio Grande do Sul, Brazil (https://seer.cancer.gov/csr/1975_2013/results_merged/sect_32_aya.pdf#search=glioma+incidence+trend), and Environmental Health Trust, United States (www.EHTrust.org).

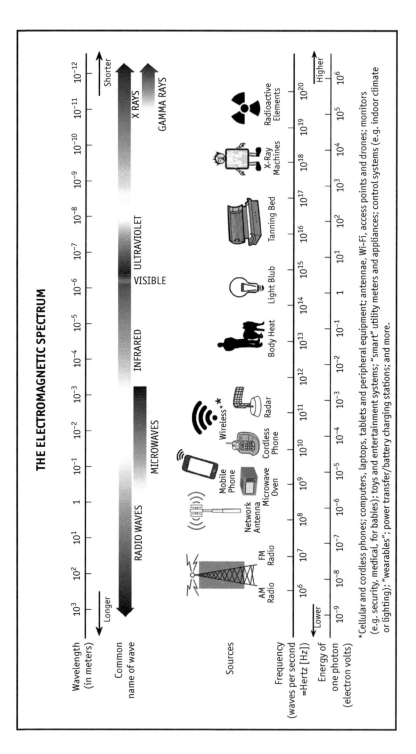

FIGURE 10.2. Electromagnetic spectrum. Wireless devices (*) include cellular and cordless phones; computers, laptops, tablets, and peripheral equipment; antennae, WiFi; access points, and drones; monitors (e.g., security, medical, for babies); toys and entertainment systems; smart utility meters and appliances; control systems (e.g. indoor climate or lighting); "wearables"; and power transfer/battery charging stations.

ELECTROMAGNETICS OVERVIEW

The spectrum of electromagnetic radiation (Fig. 10.2) includes high-energy, ionizing radiation from cosmic rays and x-rays, sunlight (i.e., ultraviolet, visible, and infrared light), longer-wavelength MW/RFR used for wireless two-way communications, and radio and television signals. Household electricity, called *extremely low frequency* (ELF), operates at 50 or 60 cycles per second (Hz), depending on the country. Microwave-emitting devices such as cell phones, tablets, baby monitors, devices for personal fitness, virtual reality systems, and the so-called Internet of things (e.g., smart utility metering, building and appliance monitoring and control) run at between 900 million and 2.4 billion Hz, and newer devices can run at 5 billion Hz (i.e., 900 MHz to 5 GHz).

Whereas a microwave oven and a cell phone rely on similar frequencies, the rates of energy consumption are different. The oven heats with 1000 watts (W) of continuous radiation contained within a metal box, which forms a Faraday cage that contains the radiation. In contrast, a phone works as a two-way microwave radio that communicates with cell towers or routers using on average less than 1 W with an irregular signal. The pulsed nature of the communications signal, with rapid changes in electric and magnetic fields, may be biologically important, including the propensity for cells to undergo carcinogenic transformation.[19]

RADIOFREQUENCY RADIATION EFFECTS IN SIMPLE MIXTURES: CHEMICAL CATALYSIS AND LIPOSOMES

A common misconception is that radiation can result in biologic or chemical changes only by causing atoms to be ionized (i.e., lose electrons), as occurs with ionizing radiation. A peer-reviewed scientific journal, *Current Microwave Chemistry,* is devoted to studies of diverse effects in elementary, nonliving systems.[18] For example, a chemical reaction rate may change with RFR according to the lipid content of mixture examined.[93] Nonthermal, higher-frequency 10.4-GHz exposures can irreversibly inactivate enzymes.[94] In practical applications, however, low-level microwave irradiation greatly reduces the reaction time for a human immunoglobulin G (IgG) enzyme-linked immunosorbent assay (ELISA) test, but heat alone has no effect.[3]

Bioeffects of Radiofrequency Radiation

In living systems, RFR can have beneficial or harmful effects, depending on the frequencies, modulations, and alignments and the underlying conditions of tissues that are being exposed. A recent overview of bioeffects described how nonthermal exposures to RFR can alter the recombination rate of radical pairs (that are tightly controlled in normal metabolism), leading to changes in free radical concentrations.[19] MW/RFR also weakens bonds in biologic membranes, the cellular gatekeepers for essential biochemicals and cellular waste. Structural and functional genetic changes can result from increased free radicals, heat shock proteins, nitric oxide, and other cellular signaling compounds. Nonthermal effects may underlie the adverse impacts on reproduction and development, cardiac and neurologic health, cancer, and other acute and chronic health issues.

Evidence is building that RFR acts synergistically with toxic chemicals and other agents such as drugs. The capacity of RFR to increase the intracellular access of toxicants by activating calcium channels and compromising membranes is being used in several forms of electrochemotherapy.

IN VITRO AND IN VIVO STUDIES

Hundreds of studies over the past 4 decades have reported that nonthermal levels of MW/RFR cause oxidative stress, genetic alterations, and other cellular changes. Many negative studies that purport to be replications have differed from the original studies in important details. Negative results have been more common when research is industry sponsored.[62] Despite the inconsistency of some findings, several authorities, including France's National Health and Safety Agency, have concluded that the biologic impacts of MW/RFR are sufficiently well established that appropriate clinical and public health policies should be mounted and children's exposures should be reduced.

Cellular Responses to Radiofrequency Radiation. Cellular responses are often reported. A 2016 review of 100 peer-reviewed in vitro and in vivo experimental studies at nonthermal RFR exposure levels found that 93 reported significant oxidative biologic activities.[116] RFR increases damaging reactive oxygen species (ROS), including reactive molecules such as hydrogen peroxide (H_2O_2) and free radicals such as nitric oxide (NO) and superoxide (O_2^-), which can interfere with cell signaling and repair.[19]

Of relevance to the changing incidence and types of brain tumor diagnoses,[90] Lu and colleagues[77] found that exposure to 1800 MHz had a significant impact on astrocytes (a cell type present in aggressive brain tumors[105]) compared with microglial cells. The effects included increased production of biomarkers that indicate greater cancer risk, such as changes in interleukin-1b (IL-1b), tumor necrosis factor-α (TNF-α), interleukin-6 (IL-6), prostaglandin

E_2 (PGE2), NO, inducible nitric oxide synthase (iNOS), and cyclooxygenase 2 (COX-2).[77]

Bacterial cells exposed to RFR develop pores that healed when radiation was discontinued.[103] This phenomenon of *reversible electroporation* is being applied clinically in electrochemotherapy,[23] and other electroceutical applications are under development to enhance absorption of therapeutic agents.

Genetic Damage. Several dozen types of in vitro RFR genotoxicity tests have been carried out,[116] with varied responses depending on the cell types and specific RFR signals employed. Stem cells usually exhibit more damage and less adaptive capacity compared with mature lymphocytes, a finding that is relevant for the young and unborn and for cancer treatment.[80] Simulated cell phone signals to human leukemia (HL-60) cells altered 221 genes after 2 hours of exposure and 759 genes after 6 hours.[72]

Animal studies indicate a range of genetic and other types of cellular damage from MW/RFR, including oxidative DNA and lipid membrane damage, single- and double-strand breaks, fragmentation seen in the comet assay (i.e., single-cell gel electrophoresis), and measures of apoptosis such as seen after prenatal and postnatal exposure to simulated cell phone radiation in the brain cells of 1-month-old rabbits.[52] After 2 hours of exposure to cell phone radiation, rats developed dose-dependent inflammation in the liver and pancreas.[83] Exposure altered DNA conformation (but not double-stranded breaks) and altered expression of 11 genes, including encoded proteins affecting neurotransmitter regulation, the blood-brain barrier, and melatonin.[22]

Exposure to very low levels of 1.8-GHz RFR disrupted the circadian rhythm in rats. Compared with those exposed during the day, rats exposed at night had significantly lower levels of melatonin (a sleep-inducing antioxidant) and other detoxifying biochemicals such as glutathione peroxidase and superoxide plasma dismutase.[27]

Voltage-Gated Calcium Channels. Calcium channel–blocking pharmaceuticals can avert some effects of RFR.[91] Although several mechanisms are likely to be involved, voltage-gated calcium channels have been proposed as a major pathway through which RFR operates. RFR triggers polar proteins that regulate ion transport through cellular membrane channels. Resulting spikes in intracellular calcium increase the activity of existing enzymes with calcium cofactors (including nitrite synthases), levels of reactive nitrogen and oxygen species, oxidative damage, changes in cellular signaling, and pathologic manifestations.[10]

Male and Female Reproduction. Reproduction has been shown to be affected by RFR in several in vivo animal studies.[84] One review reported that male effects included decreased testosterone; altered spermatogenesis; increased sperm DNA damage, ROS, lipid peroxidation, and free radicals; and decreased levels of glutathione peroxidase, superoxide dismutase, and fructose. Females had DNA damage in oocytes, decreased numbers of follicles, increased apoptosis and oxidative stress in the endometrium, retarded embryo growth, and increased embryo mortality. The U.S. National Toxicology Program (NTP) found significantly lower average birth weights of rats exposed in utero to simulated common cell phone signals (i.e., Global System for Mobile [GSM] or Code Division Multiple Access [CDMA] modulations) compared with controls.[115]

Developmental and Neurologic Impacts. The effects of RFR exposure on the central nervous system and breaching of the blood-brain barrier have been studied extensively. For example, simulated signals of GSM 900-MHz phones impaired cognition[89] and increased permeability of the blood-brain barrier in rats[88] 7 days after exposure. An Indian research group detailed neurogenotoxicity and cognitive impairment in rats after low-intensity RFR exposures,[36] and a Greek team reported changes in the brain proteome in mice exposed to cell phone or cordless phone (e.g., Digital Enhanced Cordless Telecommunications [DECT]) base station emissions over 8 months.[45]

Cardiovascular Effects. In albino male rabbits, acute exposure to WiFi signals (i.e., 2.45 GHz) significantly increased heart rate, blood pressure, and PR and QT intervals but not maximum amplitude or P waves. RFR also blunted the effects of injected dopamine or epinephrine on heart variability and blood pressure.[97]

Cancer. In May 2016, the U.S. NTP released a partial report of the world's largest and best-designed study of rodents that were exposed to non-thermal microwave radiation pulsed off then on in 20 minute cycles over 18 hours (for a total of 9 hours daily) of whole-body cell phone radiation (GSM or CDMA).[115] NTP scientists confirmed a significantly increased incidence of rare tumors, including gliomas and neoplasias of the brain and schwannomas of the heart in male rats, and found increases in preneoplastic Schwann cell hyperplasia of the heart. In human investigations, gliomas and schwannomas of the auditory nerve (also called vestibular schwannomas or acoustic neuromas) are commonly associated with RFR exposure.[63]

Some have criticized the NTP results because the study controls did not develop any of the rare malignant tumors, whereas control groups used in earlier studies of chemicals had a small numbers of gliomas but none of the malignant schwannomas of the heart. Concurrent controls are always preferred, and in this case it is especially inappropriate to compare results with historical controls because both exposed and control animals in the NTP study were housed in innovative exposure chambers that were also Faraday cages. As a result, the NTP RFR control animals had no confounding exposures to EMF or RFR from laboratory fans, wiring, or use of wireless devices in the laboratory that could have affected the cancer rates observed in the historical controls.

The NTP study is the third positive in vivo study in the past 6 years to find that animals exposed to nonthermal levels of RFR develop some of the same rare cancers as people do. A 2015 study found that levels as low as 0.04 to 0.4 W/kg of Universal Mobile Telecommunications System [UMTS] (i.e., modern signals, similar to a wideband type of CDMA) produced approximately 2-fold higher rates of bronchioalveolar adenomas (i.e., lung tumors) and hepatocellular carcinomas, as well as 2.5-fold higher rates of lymphoma.[73]

RADIOFREQUENCY RADIATION EFFECTS IN HUMANS

Ethical considerations limit human interventional studies when there is no potential benefit, but substantial observational evidence is accruing for the effects of MW/RFR.

Natural Experiments. Despite considerable public concern, few well-designed studies have examined the potential health impacts of exposures to wireless communications infrastructure (e.g., cell towers). In a double-blind study using shielding to control exposure of 57 volunteers to radiation from a 900-MHz mobile phone base station mounted on a kindergarten exterior wall, higher stress markers, saliva cortisol levels, and α-amylase levels were observed with higher unshielded exposures (i.e., low, medium, or high average power fluxes of 5, 150, or 2000 μW/m, respectively).[11]

After installation of a cell phone tower in the center of a Bavarian village, initial significant changes in urine levels of neurotransmitters (i.e., catecholamines) dissipated somewhat over the 1.5-year study duration. In the same group, chronic low levels of the neurotransmitter precursor phenylethylamine were interpreted to indicate physiologic exhaustion (as in Selye's classic general adaptation syndrome). Urine levels reflected a dose-dependent pattern, with exposure estimated from outside the dwelling. All participants were affected. Recovery was delayed for all participants exposed to power density levels greater than 1 μW/cm². Significantly increased sleep and concentration problems, headache, allergy, and dizziness were found. Those using their personal wireless devices tended to be more severely affected, as were children, who exhibited attention deficit disorders.[24]

Reproduction. Reviews of experimental, clinical, and epidemiologic evidence have concluded that cell phone radiation damages male reproductive health, with decreased sperm concentration, motility, and viability occurring at higher exposures to cell phone radiation.[49,70] Oxidative stress leads to membrane lipid and DNA damage in sperm, whereas decreased testosterone production and increased expression of genes for adhesion molecules also potentially contribute significantly.

A 2014 systematic review of in vitro and in vivo studies of human semen confirmed the previous findings along with decreased viability, motility, and concentration of sperm.[1] The use of WiFi-connected laptops on laps also adversely affects sperm quality.[13] Cross-sectional observations by fertility clinic doctors in India, the United States, and Australia have consistently found that men who are the heaviest users of wireless devices have the lowest sperm counts.[2,35,67]

Studies published in 2015 on women in Iran and in China correlated mobile device use with increased abortion risk. Using mobile phones[79] or living close to a mobile communications base station[119] correlated strongly with fetal loss.

Developmental and Neurologic Impacts. In population-based studies, early-life exposure to cell phone radiation was associated with behavioral disturbances,[38,39] asthma[74] (possibly indicating immune disturbance or associated with mucosal membrane damage, as seen in rats[14]), and obesity (i.e., metabolic and endocrine disturbances).[75]

Studies by experts in neuroscience concluded that RFR may be a substantial, multifactorial contributor to autism.[58,59] Myelin, the protective fatty sheath around neurons, which is still developing in the young, may be damaged by repeated exposures to pulsed RFR signals.[95]

An Italian group investigating the effects of cell phone radiation on the human brain found that exposed healthy male volunteers experienced modified brain excitability,[44] decreased cortical activity, and decreased reaction times.[111] Effects were more pronounced in elderly compared with young volunteers.[110] The investigators also found increased coherence of temporal and frontal alpha rhythms measured by electroencephalography (EEG) in epileptic patients, a finding that could be clinically significant in contributing to seizure activity.[112]

Increased frequency of headaches was reported by university students using mobile phones, although not by those using hands-free devices.[31] Greater incidence of headaches in youngsters was also associated with prenatal and postnatal exposures to cell phones.[104] Sleep disturbance and decreased rapid eye movement (REM) sleep has been reported by those using digital devices immediately before bedtime. Many researchers have confirmed previous EEG findings of effects of pulsed 900-MHz GSM cell phone–like emissions, with greater EEG alpha wave activity before and during stage 2 sleep[60,76] and more rapid onset of REM sleep.[76]

Several studies of RFR effects on brain activity have garnered public attention. In randomized, crossover, blinded studies, brain perfusion and metabolic activity were increased after exposure to RFR during a resting state[60,61,113] but decreased after exposures during continuous activities.[69,78] These apparently conflicting significant results initially cast doubt on experimental validity, but the importance of brain activity during exposure is now recognized.[78]

Cardiovascular Effects. The autonomic nervous system is fundamentally electromagnetic and is potentially sensitive to electromagnetic disturbances. Although the subject has not been adequately investigated, some physicians report atrial fibrillation associated with habitual carrying of cell phones in the breast pocket or exposure to MW/RFR, and researchers have reported that cell phone signals can disrupt cardiac signaling and rhythms.[7] In a study of 356 participants, the cell phone signal from the waistline (i.e., clipped to the belt) or midchest (i.e., in a shirt pocket) prolonged the QT interval in males who were healthy or had cardiac conditions not related to ischemia; both signals prolonged QT and changed voltage criteria in male patients with ischemic heart disease.[4] Effects on the autonomic nervous system, including heart rate variability, were demonstrated in a small provocation study using a DECT mobile phone system.[57] Cardiac symptoms are listed by the Austrian Medical Association among possible sequelae of RFR exposure.[12]

Ocular Effects. RFR exposure limits are set to restrict tissue heating, taking into account heat dissipation by blood flow. Eyes are considered sensitive to damage from RFR, in part because transparent structures are not cooled by blood flow,[117] although RFR also causes cataracts by nonthermal mechanisms.[92] Modern devices are being used in manners for which they were never tested. One example is virtual reality devices that work with cell phones in special holders located directly in front of the eyes; this results in much greater exposures of the frontal cortex and the eye (Fig. 10.3) and significant exposure to the young brain compared with standard cell phone use (see Fig. 10.1).

Extended use of digital devices results in high-level exposures to blue and near-ultraviolet light. Blue light decreases melatonin production, which affects sleep, and the light may also damage retinas, particularly of children, potentially predisposing to macular degeneration.[107] (Adults' corneas yellow with age, offering more protection against blue light.) Yellow-tinted glasses are recommended to protect the retina, and they have been reported anecdotally to reduce the symptoms of extended screen time.

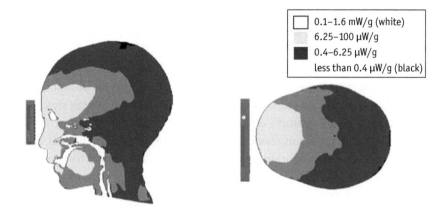

FIGURE 10.3. Modeled exposure of a child's eyes and brain to radiofrequency radiation (RFR) from a cell phone. The absorbed RFR doses (i.e., specific absorption rate [SAR]) using a virtual reality system with a cell phone are shown for the head of a 6-year-old child from two perspectives. The finite difference time domain (FDTD) modeling is averaged over 1 g of tissue for a 900-MHz cell phone used for virtual reality.
Modeling courtesy of C. Fernendez PhD, Federal Institute of Rio Grande do Sul, Brazil and Environmental Health Trust, United States (www.EHTrust.org).

SYNERGISM BETWEEN RADIOFREQUENCY RADIATION AND OTHER TOXICANTS

RFR is a clinical therapeutic tool in addition to being of toxicologic interest. A large 2013 review summarized synergistic effects of RFR and toxicants on carcinogenesis, teratogenesis, mutagenesis, and inflammation; amelioration of RFR effects with agents such as antioxidants (e.g., vitamin C); and use of RFR to enhance therapeutic effectiveness.[68]

Research indicating RFR and chemical synergies includes the following.

- Altered cellular calcium homeostasis with cell phone irradiation (i.e., 800 MHz, 1 hour per week for 4 months) was related to lymphocyte infiltration and tumor induction in a lymphoma-prone mouse model.[10] The same group studied calcium homeostasis related to synergism of RFR with aluminum[9] and with iron,[8] causing increased incidence of cancer in the lymphoma-prone mice.
- Mice prenatally exposed to the carcinogen ethylnitrosourea (ENU) and 2 W/kg of UMTS cell phone signal developed significantly more liver and lung cancers compared with unexposed controls. The lowest-powered (0.04 W/kg) UMTS cell phone signal more than

doubled cancers in the ENU-exposed animals, similar to the number of tumors that developed at the European regulatory exposure limit of 2 W/kg.[73]

Compromise of the blood-brain barrier by RFR may decrease protection of the central nervous system from drugs and toxins and contribute to decreases in important antioxidants and hormones such as melatonin.[65,89] A large study of 2422 children in 27 schools in 10 Korean cities[25] found that among children with higher blood lead levels (i.e., values greater than 2.35 µg/dL, comparable to levels in many developed countries[108]), those making more cell phone voice calls exhibited significantly more attention deficit hyperactivity disorder (ADHD), but no such symptoms were seen in those with lower levels of blood lead or voice calls, or both.

RADIOFREQUENCY RADIATION AND CANCER

In 2011, RFR was classified as a possible carcinogen (i.e., group 2B) by a working group of the IARC.[15] The supporting monograph[63] was a comprehensive, systematic review that included in vitro and in vivo animal studies as well as human epidemiologic studies. The classification applies to RFR from all equipment—baby monitors, WiFi, computers, equipment for the Internet of Things, smart meters, towers, and more—not just cell or cordless phones.[63]

Based on case-control studies, a number of experts have concluded that the evidence is now strong enough for the IARC to designate RFR a *probable* or *known* carcinogen,[54,55,86] a position that was strengthened by the NTP finding of carcinogenicity.[115]

Case-Control Brain Cancer Studies. Studies have evaluated the role of cell phone use and sometimes cordless phone use. As with all studies of environmental exposures, considerable uncertainties exist with respect to estimated histories of exposure and phone use, even when self-report is replaced or supplemented with billing records. A large national case-control study of gliomas in four areas of France conducted between 2004 and 2006[32] found a doubled to tripled risk of glioma among the heaviest users, with a statistically nonsignificant finding of 8-fold increased risk among the heaviest urban users (Fig. 10.4). Those considered to be unexposed in this study had exposures comparable to those of the users in earlier studies.

A 2015 meta-analysis of two brain tumor case-control studies found shorter-term cancer promotion in addition to initiation of gliomas with exposure to cordless phones and cell phones, particularly on the side of the

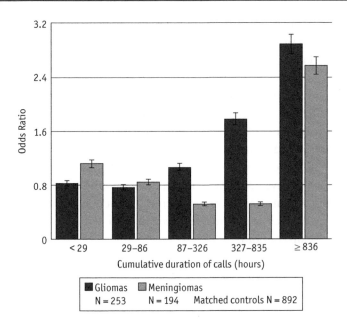

FIGURE 10.4. Association of brain tumors with cell phone use in a French case-control study.

From Coureau, G., Bouvier, G., Lebailly, P., et al. 2014. Mobile phone use and brain tumours in the CERENAT case-control study. *Occup Environ Med.* 2014;71:514–522.

head where phones were habitually used.[55] Patients with an aggressive form of glioma (i.e., astrocytoma grade IV) with heavier and earlier use of mobile and cordless phones had significantly shorter survival times than patients with little exposure.[28]

Prospective Cohort Studies. The prospective cohort study is a strong research design for relatively common end points with short latencies, such as reproductive outcomes or influenza; but for rare occurrences with long latencies (e.g., brain tumors that affect 7 to 12 of 100,000 people), the very large cohort size and extensive, long-term follow-up required to detect significant patterns of disease mean that the prospective cohort study design lacks the power to be useful.

Despite limitations, an often-cited RFR cohort study is that of the Danish Cancer Society.[46] The study began in 1993, when phones cost several thousand dollars to purchase and were expensive to operate. Investigators relied on billing records to identify an exposed group of early cell phone users, but they excluded business users from this group because of the inability to establish users of corporate phones. All subscribers after 1995 were also excluded.[63]

Subsequent updates of this cohort found no difference between the early lim-ited cell phone users and those who were currently using newer phones in many different ways, and the study was assigned zero weight by the IARC working group.

Brain Tumor Registries. The Central Brain Tumor Registry of the United States[29] (CBTRUS) is a large, high-quality brain tumor registry with data on malignant and benign tumors covering more than 10 years and more than 99% of the U.S. population. A 2016 CBTRUS report on adolescents and young adults indicates that brain tumors have become the leading type of cancer among U.S. adolescents, supplanting leukemia and lymphoma as the most common diagnoses among 15- to 19-year-old youth,[90] and that the incidence is rising among adolescents and young adults.[105] The incidence of the most aggressive astrocytomas is rising quickly, whereas that of less aggressive forms of glioma is falling more slowly. Increases in the incidence of astrocytomas are consistent with the proposition that cell phones play a causal role. Another U.S. study of brain tumor location found significantly increasing rates of glioblastoma multiforme in the frontal lobe, temporal lobe, and cerebellum, regions of the brain that receive the highest doses of RFR from phones.[118]

Nonspecific analyses obscure incidence patterns related to phone use. A 2016 Australian registry-based report that brain tumors were increasing only among the oldest citizens claimed to disprove concerns about the role of cell phones.[30] This widely publicized analysis found stable rates for all types of brain cancer but did not examine patterns of those specific brain tumors (i.e., gliomas) associated with cell phone radiation in case-control studies. Among the 7 million people in New South Wales and the Australian Capital Territory, gliomas increased at a rate of 2.5% annually from 2000 through 2008, with an accelerating increase in the final 3 years.[40]

Testicular Cancer. Cell phone radiation is plausibly associated with testicular cancer. Experimental studies of the testicular proteome show that exposures generate precursors to cancer in rodent gonadal tissue.[102] The established genotoxicity of RFR to sperm in extensive experimental and human studies suggests that phones in trouser pockets can contribute to testicular cancer.[56]

Breast Cancers. A case series report by breast cancer surgeons of unusual breast tumors in young women who had no genetic markers for the disease but who kept cell phones in their bras[114] is concerning. The tumors were all located directly under the phone antennae.

Salivary Gland Cancers. The parotid glands receive high levels of RFR from cell phones according to exposure models. The first case-control study (2008) of rare parotid gland malignancy reported significantly higher risk for the heaviest phone users.[96] A 2011 Israeli study of salivary gland tumors reported no change in the number of submandibular tumors but a significant, increasing trend in the incidence of parotid tumors between 1990 and 2006.[33] A 2016 Saudi Arabian case-control study found a 3.5-fold higher risk of parotid tumors among those speaking on a cell phone more than 1 hour daily.[5]

In a Chinese case-control study, parotid gland malignancies were related to cell phone use, with a 10- to 15-fold increased risk of epithelial parotid gland malignancies ($n = 136$) in the longest and heaviest users, and up to a 20- to 30-fold risk of mucoepidermoid carcinoma ($n = 64$).[41] Given that one half of participants reported that they used phones on both sides of the head, there was no correlation with laterality.

Clinical Approaches and Public Policy

For both healthy patients and those with existing chronic conditions such as cancer and neurodegenerative diseases, the clinical encounter provides a teachable moment for guidance about why and how to reduce or avoid critical environmental exposures, including MW/RFR emissions by wireless transmitting devices. Increasingly, physicians are prescribing exercise, meditation, biofeedback, and nutritional changes to promote health. The need to curtail cell phone and other wireless transmitting devices should be added to these important advisories, particularly given the evidence of poorer outcomes with higher exposures.[28]

During these important encounters, exposures contributing to carcinogenesis, adverse reproductive outcomes, and chronic conditions should be identified and discussed. As described elsewhere in this volume, these include exposures to pesticides and chemicals in household cleaning products, plastics, and personal care products.[50]

Public health recommendations regarding wireless transmitting devices and other avoidable environmental health hazards are generally lacking in North America, and there is no accountability for or monitoring of impacts on populations, particularly in residential, daycare, school, and university settings, where developing young people are at greatest risk. For public health, the design and applications of technology should minimize use of and exposure to RFR by substitution with hard (i.e., wire or fiber) connections that do not emit RFR and by innovations to achieve exposures that are as low as reasonably achievable (ALARA)—as is the policy for radiologic procedures.

CLINICAL APPROACHES TO DIAGNOSIS AND MANAGEMENT OF
ELECTROMAGNETICALLY HYPERSENSITIVE INDIVIDUALS

Attitude and Knowledge. Electromagnetic field–related illnesses will never be properly diagnosed, screened, and monitored until physicians routinely collect data on the uses and users of wireless technology, and until health care professionals improve their understanding of the complex concepts of how biologic harm can result from RFR exposure, the constellation of related clinical presentations, and methods to reduce biologic and other resultant harms.

Ignorance due to gaps in university and continuing medical education is preventing management of the growing problem of electromagnetic hypersensitivity (EHS). EHS occurs to some degree in more than 10% of the population according to some estimates,[53] with a fraction of those affected becoming severely disabled. A 2016 international overview of health effects and clinical responses to a range of electromagnetic phenomena provides an extensive overview for clinicians.[21]

With rapidly increasing use of wireless devices, clinicians should screen for device use and degree of exposure to RFR in the everyday lives of all patients (from in utero to old age), including exposures in schools, workplaces and hospitals. In the past 15 years, the number of patients complaining of EHS has risen dramatically in clinics (including practices of our collaborators who specialize in environmental health). This likely reflects a combination of increasing RFR-emitting technology and awareness of the link between exposures and symptoms through self-diagnosis.[17] It is usually after repeated personal experimentation that EHS patients reluctantly conclude that RFR causes symptoms, rather than exhibiting a nocebo response.[37] Physicians who are uneducated about the nature of EHS can mistake patients' symptoms for psychogenic disorders.

Diagnosis. A broad range of symptoms and conditions may be elicited or contributed to by the biochemical effects of RFR,[91,116] such as infertility, developmental and chronic conditions, cancer, and sensitivity responses. Astute questioning about uses of, and second-hand exposures to cell phones and other wireless transmitting devices at home, work, and other routine settings is necessary to understand the etiologic role that wireless devices and infrastructure can play for these and a growing range of otherwise unexplained symptoms. For example, at the Ottawa Environmental Health Clinic, isolated effects have been seen, such as fatigue only in the region of the body or arthritis only in the hip where a cell phone was carried many hours per day. A degree of relief may be achieved with changes in use, distancing from the sources, and other interventions.

At the Environmental Health Clinic at Women's College Hospital, Toronto, Canada, a referral-based, academically affiliated clinic for consultations, patients exhibit a combination of nonspecific neurasthenic, vegetative, and somatic symptoms that manifest or increase during or after exposure to RFR. The most common symptoms include sleep disturbances, headache, difficulty concentrating, fatigue, heart palpitations, dizziness, irritability, nausea, tinnitus, and memory loss.[34] Severity of symptoms ranges from very mild to major impairment. In more severe cases, symptoms can persist with prolonged exposure, can endure even after exposure has ceased, and may interfere with work, family, and social life. Many of these severely affected patients will be disabled by their condition if no accommodation is made. Accommodation includes prudent reduction in the use of wireless technologies, hardwiring of computers (including keyboards, printers, and other peripherals), and remedial action to remove, attenuate, or shield the sources of RFR at home, school, and work, and in health care establishments.

Many factors should be considered in the assessment of possible EHS[12,48,53,66]:

- Assess personal risk factors such as comorbid cardiac, neurologic (e.g., heavy metal overexposure, psychological stress, aging, dementia), dermatologic, and immunologic conditions or multiple chemical sensitivities, which are the most common comorbidity found among EHS patients, although healthy individuals also are affected.
- Assess environmental risk factors, other than heavy use of or exposure to RFR-emitting technology in the home or workplace, such as consuming mercury-contaminated seafood on a weekly basis, eating a very poor diet low in antioxidants or high in oxidative stress foods (e.g., alcohol), having substantial and degrading dental mercury amalgams, and having a high body burden or total load of chemical pollutants.

The limitations in accessibility and cost to carry out biochemical marker screening tests[20] and the resulting nonspecific interpretation mean that the clinician must rely on a thorough history[81] to estimate a patient's exposures and total load of xenobiotics accumulated throughout his or her life span. If feasible, measurement of routine exposure sites (e.g., home, work, school, sleeping quarters) by a building biologist or health care provider with the proper equipment is helpful. The degree of impact correlates with the proximity and power density of the exposure, the duration of exposure, and personal and environmental risk factors. The SF-36 Functional Status questionnaire is useful because the EHS population tends to have lower scores than the normal population in areas of energy, physical functioning, emotional well-being, pain control, and social functioning.

Management. As is standard medical practice for any patient, differential diagnoses are explored and underlying illnesses are treated. Modifiable lifestyle factors are addressed, including limiting exposures to other environmental health risks, avoiding exposures that cause symptoms, and adjusting the diet. The judicious use of indicated supplements (e.g., antioxidants such as vitamin C, melatonin before bedtime, regular consumption of polyphenols) is advised.[48,100] During the environmental history,[81] the clinician can recognize predisposing vulnerabilities such as subnormal abilities to detoxify chemicals (e.g., sensitivity to medications).

Symptoms usually are reduced or eliminated by awareness of RFR sources and avoidance or attenuation of emissions through hardwiring of computers and other devices. If exposures cannot be eliminated or reduced, personal shielding (e.g., use of silver- or copper threaded clothing) and shielding in the workplace or dwelling (e.g., use of paints, foil, metal sheets, and screens or fabrics; reliance on heavy foliage of trees outdoors), distancing from RFR sources, and detoxification of heavy metals (usually mercury)[99,101] can be fairly effective mitigating measures.

Medication and psychotherapy offer little direct help[53] without reduction of exposures. Mindfulness-based stress reduction practices may assist patients in coping with the unseen, ongoing, ubiquitous, and increasingly difficult-to-avoid exposures.

Expert medical groups have addressed RFR-related conditions. The Irish Doctors' Environmental Association has discussed symptoms clearly related to electromagnetic radiation exposure and provided recommendations for patient care and more restrictive regulation of technologies.[64] The Austrian Medical Association has provided guidelines for diagnosis and treatment.[12] The Indian Medical Research Council has also issued guidance to clinicians regarding diagnosis, responses to, and treatment of EHS. Health care providers may support requests from patients with EHS for accommodation in schools, workplaces, hospitals, residential care facilities, and public spaces with letters supporting ALARA approaches such as those outlined here.

PUBLIC POLICY

Several actions and policies[42] that protect public health by reducing expo-sures to RFR are in place in at least one jurisdiction:

- Lowered regulatory limits because the underlying principle that only heating causes harm has been disproved and a greater precautionary margin is chosen
- Requirements and incentives for low-emission equipment, such as wired options or ecologic options (e.g., cordless phones, baby moni-tors) that transmit only when necessary (e.g., voice-activated) and do not maintain continuous contact with a network
- Requiring labeling of devices, packages, and at the point of sale that details the distance the device must be kept from the body to comply with regulatory requirements (i.e., "tested at" distances)
- Providing headsets with all phones as is required by law in Israel and other countries
- Discouraging the use of wireless devices by children
- Education of medical professionals in bioelectromagnetics and diag-nosis and management of related conditions
- Requiring accommodation of environmental sensitivities, including EHS in clinics, hospitals, schools, and workplaces, as is required by the Canadian Human Rights Commission[26,98]
- Banning sales and advertising of RFR-emitting toys and devices for children, especially for infants and toddlers, such as teething rattle cases for phones and tablets
- Banning use by youngsters of devices when they are connected to wireless networks (i.e., devices must be on airplane mode with all wireless features turned off)
- Banning wireless equipment from daycare centers and schools (at least for lower grades)

There are ways to reduce risks while using wireless devices:

- Keeping devices away from the body, particularly the head, repro-ductive organs, heart, and pregnant abdomen (recommended by the Baby-Safe Project, a group of more than 150 physicians and experts advising practical means to protect pregnancy[16])
- Texting rather than talking
- Using the speaker phone or a headset and keeping calls short

- Turning the device to airplane mode or off when carrying it next to the body
- Keeping phones at a distance (i.e., not in the pocket) or on airplane mode at night
- Avoiding use of phones when signals are weak because the phone emits at maximum power (i.e., signaled by rapid discharge of batteries)
- Using a phone in the car through the radio or bluetooth system because maximum power is emitted when the vehicle moves from one cell tower area to another, and the metal vehicle contains the RFR and further increases occupants' exposure

Laws, regulations, and policies regarding RFR are changing, but they are not keeping up with the rapidly evolving science. Clinicians and patients who may have some symptoms associated with RFR exposures do not have the luxury of waiting to address ill health years after the research has been completed. Efforts to reduce RFR exposures, especially in the environments of infants, toddlers, young children, and men and women who wish to produce healthy children should be promoted during the clinical encounter. Advances in hardware and software are also likely to result in lower exposures overall. As questions about regular uses and exposures to RFR are incorporated into medical practice and awareness grows about adverse health impacts, clinicians will play an important role in advancing medical understanding and in alleviating a host of conditions that may be associated with important, avoidable environmental exposures.

Current details about existing laws and policies, along with resources for public health and medical professionals, politicians, educators, and citizens, are maintained by the Environmental Health Trust (www.EHTrust.org) and Canadians for Safe Technology (www.C4ST.org).

Acknowledgments

We thank Lucy R. Wiletzky, who generously sponsored the work of the Environmental Health Trust and Prevent Cancer Now for this project. Clinicians at the cutting-edge of diagnosing and treating conditions affected by EMF provided invaluable constructive clinical advice: Dana F. Flavin, PhD, Dr med Pharmacology, DeMontfort University, Leicester, UK; Jennifer Armstrong, BSc, MD, DIBEM, Medical Director, Ottawa Environmental Health Clinic, Canada; and Alison C. Bested, MD, FRCPC, Clinical Associate

Professor, Faculty of Medicine, University of British Columbia, Vancouver, BC, Canada. Claudio Fernández, PhD, Federal Institute of Rio Grande do Sul, Canoas, Brazil, generously provided gray-scale images of RFR absorption in the brain. Frank Barnes, PhD, Distinguished Emeritus Professor University of Colorado, Boulder, CO, and member of the National Academy of Engineering, generously provided technical review. We also thank Barb Payne for editorial review.

REFERENCES

1. Adams, J.A., Galloway. T.S., Mondal, D., Esteves, S.C., & Mathews, F. 2014. Effect of mobile telephones on sperm quality: A systematic review and meta-analysis. *Environ Int.* 70:106–112.

2. Agarwal, A., Singh, A., Hamada, A., & Kesari, K. 2011. Cell phones and male infertility: A review of recent innovations in technology and consequences. *Int Braz J Urol Off J Braz Soc Urol.* 37:432–454.

3. Ahirwar, R., Tanwar, S., Bora, U., & Naharm P. 2016. Microwave non-thermal effect reduces ELISA timing to less than 5 minutes. *RSC Adv.* 6:20850–20857.

4. Alhusseiny, A., Al-Nimer, M., & Majeed, A. 2012. Electromagnetic energy radiated from mobile phone alters electrocardiographic records of patients with ischemic heart disease. *Ann Med Health Sci Res.* 2:146–151.

5. Al-Qahtani, K. 2016. Mobile phone use and the risk of parotid gland tumors: A retrospective case-control study. *Gulf J Oncol.* 1:71–78.

6. Alster, N. 2015. Captured agency: How the Federal Communications Commission is dominated by the industries it presumably regulates. http://ethics.harvard. edu/files/center-for-ethics/files/capturedagency_alster.pdf.

7. Andrzejak, R., Poreba, R., Poreba, M., et al. 2008. The influence of the call with a mobile phone on heart rate variability parameters in healthy volunteers. *Ind Health.* 46:409–417.

8. Anghileri, L., Mayayo, E., & Domingo, J. 2006. Iron-radiofrequency synergism in lymphomagenesis. *Immunopharmacol Immunotoxicol.* 28:175–183.

9. Anghileri, L., Mayayo, E., & Domingo, J. 2009. Aluminum, calcium ion and radiofrequency synergism in acceleration of lymphomagenesis. *Immunopharmacol Immunotoxicol.* 31:358–362.

10. Anghileri, L., Mayayo, E., Domingo, J., & Thouvenot, P. 2005. Radiofrequency-induced carcinogenesis: Cellular calcium homeostasis changes as a triggering factor. *Int J Radiat Biol.* 81:205–209.

11. Augner, C., Hacker, G.W., Oberfeld, G., et al. 2010. Effects of exposure to GSM mobile phone base station signals on salivary cortisol, alpha-amylase, and immunoglobulin A. *Biomed Environ Sci.* 23:199–207.

12. Austrian Medical Association. 2012. Guideline of the Austrian Medical Association for the diagnosis and treatment of EMF-related health problems and illnesses (EMF syndrome). Consensus paper of the Austrian Medical

Association's EMF Working Group. http://www.ehsf.dk/dokumenter/7810-Austrian-EMF-Guidelines-2012.pdf.

13. Avendaño, C., Mata, A., Sanchez Sarmiento, C.A., & Doncel, G.F. 2012. Use of laptop computers connected to internet through Wi-Fi decreases human sperm motility and increases sperm DNA fragmentation. *Fertil Steril.* 97:39–45.e2.

14. Aydoğan, F., Aydın, E., Koca, G., et al. 2015. The effects of 2100-MHz radiofrequency radiation on nasal mucosa and mucociliary clearance in rats. *Int Forum Allergy Rhinol.* 5:626–632.

15. Baan, R., Grosse, Y., Lauby-Secretan, B., et al. 2011. Carcinogenicity of radiofrequency electromagnetic fields. *Lancet Oncol.* 12:624–626.

16. The BabySafe Project: Know your exposure. http://www.babysafeproject.org/.

17. Baliatsas, C., Kamp, I.V., Lebret, E., & Rubin, G.J. 2012. Idiopathic environmental intolerance attributed to electromagnetic fields (IEI-EMF): A systematic review of identifying criteria. *BMC Public Health.* 12(1):643.

18. Banik, B.K. (ed.) *Current Microwave Chemistry.* Sharjah, UAE: Bentham Science Publishers. http://benthamsciencepublisher.org/journals/current-microwave-chemistry/aims-scope/#top.

19. Barnes, F., & Greenenbaum, B. 2016. Some effects of weak magnetic fields on biological systems: RF fields can change radical concentrations and cancer cell growth rates. *IEEE Power Electron Mag.* 3:60–68.

20. Belpomme, D., Campagnac, C., & Irigaray, P. 2015. Reliable disease biomarkers characterizing and identifying electrohypersensitivity and multiple chemical sensitivity as two etiopathogenic aspects of a unique pathological disorder. *Rev Environ Health.* 30:251–271.

21. Belyaev, I., Dean, A., Eger, H., et al. 2016. EUROPAEM EMF Guideline 2016 for the prevention, diagnosis and treatment of EMF-related health problems and illnesses. *Rev Environ Health.* 31:363–397.

22. Belyaev, I.Y., Koch, C.B., Terenius, O., et al. 2006. Exposure of rat brain to 915 MHz GSM microwaves induces changes in gene expression but not double stranded DNA breaks or effects on chromatin conformation. *Bioelectromagnetics.* 27:295–306.

23. Bimonte, S., Leongito, M., Granata, V., et al. 2016. Electrochemotherapy in pancreatic adenocarcinoma treatment: Pre-clinical and clinical studies. *Radiol Oncol.* 50:14–20.

24. Buchner, K., & Eger, H. 2011. Changes of clinically important neurotransmitters under the influence of modulated RF fields: A long-term study under real-life conditions. *Umwelt-Medizin-Gesellschaft.* 24:44–57.

25. Byun, Y-H., Ha, M., Kwon, H-J., et al. 2013. Mobile phone use, blood lead levels, and attention deficit hyperactivity symptoms in children: A longitudinal study. *PLoS One.* 8:e59742.

26. Canadian Human Rights Commission. 2007. Policy on Environmental Sensitivities. http://www.chrc-ccdp.ca/eng/content/policy-environmental-sensitivities.

27. Cao, H., Qin, F., Liu, X., et al. 2015. Circadian rhythmicity of antioxidant markers in rats exposed to 1.8 GHz radiofrequency fields. *Int J Environ Res Public Health.* 12:2071–2087.

28. Carlberg, M., & Hardell, L. 2014. Decreased survival of glioma patients with astrocytoma grade IV (glioblastoma multiforme) associated with long-term use of mobile and cordless phones. *Int J Environ Res Public Health.* 11:10790–10805.

29. Central Brain Tumor Registry of the United States. http://www.cbtrus.org/aboutus/aboutus.html.

30. Chapman, S., Azizi, L., Luo, Q., & Sitas, F. Has the incidence of brain cancer risen in Australia since the introduction of mobile phones 29 years ago? *Cancer Epidemiol.* 42:199–205.

31. Chu, M.K., Song, H.G., Kim, C., & Lee, B.C. 2011. Clinical features of headache associated with mobile phone use: A cross-sectional study in university students. *BMC Neurol.* 11:115.

32. Coureau, G., Bouvier, G., Lebailly, P., et al. 2014. Mobile phone use and brain tumours in the CERENAT case-control study. *Occup Environ Med.* 71:514–522.

33. Czerninski, R., Zini, A., & Sgan-Cohen, H.D. 2011. Risk of parotid malignant tumors in Israel (1970–2006). *Epidemiology.* 22:130–131.

34. de Graaff, M., & Bröer, C. 2012. "We are the canary in a coal mine": Establishing a disease category and a new health risk. *Health Risk Soc.* 14:129–147.

35. De Iuliis, G.N. King, B.V., & Aitken, R.J. 2012. Electromagnetic radiation and oxidative stress in the male germ line. In: Agarwal, A., Aitken, R.J., & Alvarez, J.G. (eds.). *Studies on Men's Health and Fertility,* pp 3–20.

36. Deshmukh, P.S., Nasare, N., Megha, K., et al. 2015. Cognitive impairment and neurogenotoxic effects in rats exposed to low-intensity microwave radiation. *Int J Toxicol.* 34:284–290.

37. Dieudonné, M. 2016. Does electromagnetic hypersensitivity originate from nocebo responses? Indications from a qualitative study. *Bioelectromagnetics.* 37:14–24.

38. Divan, H.A., Kheifets, L., Obel, C., & Olsen, J. 2008. Prenatal and postnatal exposure to cell phone use and behavioral problems in children. *Epidemiology.* 19:523–529.

39. Divan, H.A., Kheifets, L., Obel, C., & Olsen, J. 2010. Cell phone use and behavioural problems in young children. *J Epidemiol Commun Health.* 66:524–529.

40. Dobes, M., Khurana, V.G., Shadbolt, B., et al. 2011. Increasing incidence of glioblastoma multiforme and meningioma, and decreasing incidence of Schwannoma (2000–2008): Findings of a multicenter Australian study. *Surg Neurol Int.* 2:176.

41. Duan, Y., Zhang, H.Z., & Bu, R.F. 2011. Correlation between cellular phone use and epithelial parotid gland malignancies. *Int J Oral Maxillofac Surg.* 40:966–972.

42. Environmental Health Trust. 2016. Policy. http://ehtrust.org/policy/.

43. Fernandez-Rodriguez, C.E., De Salles, A.A., & Davis, D.L. 2015. Dosimetric simulations of brain absorption of mobile phone radiation: The relationship between psSAR and age. *IEEE Access.* 3:2425–2430.

44. Ferreri, F., Curcio, G., Pasqualetti, P., et al. 2006. Mobile phone emissions and human brain excitability. *Ann Neurol.* 60:188–196.

45. Fragopoulou, A.F., Samara, A., Antonelou, M.H., et al. 2012. Brain proteome response following whole body exposure of mice to mobile phone or wireless DECT base radiation. *Electromagn Biol Med.* 31:250–274.

46. Frei, P., Poulsen, A.H., Johansen, C., et al. 2011. Use of mobile phones and risk of brain tumours: Update of Danish cohort study. *BMJ.* 343:d6387–d6387.

47. Gandhi, O.P., Morgan, L.L., de Salles, AA, et al. 2012. Exposure limits: The underestimation of absorbed cell phone radiation, especially in children. *Electromagn Biol Med.* 31:34–51.

48. Genuis, S.J. 2008. Fielding a current idea: Exploring the public health impact of electromagnetic radiation. *Public Health.* 122:113–124.

49. Glantz, S. 2011. *Primer of Biostatistics,* 7th ed. New York, NY: McGraw Hill Professional.

50. Goodson, W.H., Lowe, L., Carpenter, D.O., et al. 2015. Assessing the carcinogenic potential of low-dose exposures to chemical mixtures in the environment: The challenge ahead. *Carcinogenesis.* 36(Suppl 1):S254–S296.

51. Gosselin. M-C., Neufeld. E., Moser. H., et al. 2014. Development of a new generation of high-resolution anatomical models for medical device evaluation: The Virtual Population 3.0. *Phys Med Biol.* 59:5287.

52. Güler, G., Ozgur, E., Keles, H., et al. 2015. Neurodegenerative changes and apoptosis induced by intrauterine and extrauterine exposure of radiofrequency radiation. *J Chem Neuroanat.* 75(Pt B):128–133.

53. Hagström, M., Auranen, J., & Ekman, R. 2013. Electromagnetic hypersensitive Finns: Symptoms, perceived sources and treatments; a questionnaire study. *Pathophysiol Off J Int Soc Pathophysiol ISP.* 20:117–122.

54. Hardell, L., & Carlberg, M. 2013. Using the Hill viewpoints from 1965 for evaluating strengths of evidence of the risk for brain tumors associated with use of mobile and cordless phones. *Rev Environ Health.* 28:97–106.

55. Hardell, L., & Carlberg, M. 2015. Mobile phone and cordless phone use and the risk for glioma: Analysis of pooled case-control studies in Sweden, 1997–2003 and 2007–2009. *Pathophysiology.* 22:1–13.

56. Hardell, L., Carlberg, M., Ohlson, C-G., et al. 2007. Use of cellular and cordless telephones and risk of testicular cancer. *Int J Androl.* 30:115–122.

57. Havas, M., Marrongelle, J., Pollner, B., et al. 2010. Provocation study using heart rate variability shows microwave radiation from 2.4 GHz cordless phone affects autonomic nervous system. *Eur J Oncol.* 5:273–300.

58. Herbert, M.R., & Sage, C. 2013. Autism and EMF? Plausibility of a pathophysiological link—Part I. *Pathophysiology.* 20:191–209.

59. Herbert, M.R., & Sage, C. 2013. Autism and EMF? Plausibility of a pathophysiological link—Part II. *Pathophysiology.* 20:211–234.

60. Huber, R., Treyer, V., Borbély, A.A., et al. 2002. Electromagnetic fields, such as those from mobile phones, alter regional cerebral blood flow and sleep and waking EEG. *J Sleep Res.* 11:289–295.

61. Huber, R., Treyer, V., Schuderer, J., et al. 2005. Exposure to pulse-modulated radio frequency electromagnetic fields affects regional cerebral blood flow. *Eur J Neurosci.* 21:1000–1006.

62. Huss, A., Egger, M., Hug, K., Huwiler-Müntener, K., & Röösli, M. 2007. Source of funding and results of studies of health effects of mobile phone use: Systematic review of experimental studies. *Environ Health Perspect.* 115:1–4.

63. International Agency for Research on Cancer. 2013. *Non-ionizing Radiation, Part 2: Radiofrequency Electromagnetic Fields.* IARC Monographs on the Evaluation of Carcinogenic Risks to Humans, vol 102. http://monographs.iarc.fr/ENG/Monographs/vol102/index.php.

64. Irish Doctors' Environmental Association. 2004. IDEA Position on Electro-Magnetic Radiation. http://emrpolicy.org/regulation/international/docs/idea_emr.pdf.

65. Johansson, O. 2006. Electrohypersensitivity: State-of-the-art of a functional impairment. *Electromagn Biol Med.* 25:245–258.

66. Kato, Y., & Johansson, O. 2012. Reported functional impairments of electro-hypersensitive Japanese: A questionnaire survey. *Pathophysiol Off J Int Soc Pathophysiol ISP.* 19:95–100.

67. Kesari, K.K., Kumar, S., Nirala, J., Siddiqui, M.H., & Behari, J. 2013. Biophysical evaluation of radiofrequency electromagnetic field effects on male reproductive pattern. *Cell Biochem. Biophys.* 65:85–96.

68. Kostoff, R.N., & Lau, C.G.Y. 2013. Combined biological and health effects of electromagnetic fields and other agents in the published literature. *Technol Forecast Soc Change.* 80:1331–1349.

69. Kwon, M.S., Vorobyev, V., Kännälä, S., et al. 2011. GSM mobile phone radiation suppresses brain glucose metabolism. *J Cereb Blood Flow Metab* 31:2293–2301.

70. La Vignera, S., Condorelli, R.A., Vicari, E., D'Agata, R., & Calogero, A.E. 2012. Effects of the exposure to mobile phones on male reproduction: A review of the literature. *J Androl.* 33:350–356.

71. Landrigan, P.J., & Goldman, L.R. Children's vulnerability to toxic chemicals: A challenge and opportunity to strengthen health and environmental policy. 2011. *Health Aff. (Millwood).* 30:842–850.

72. Lee, S., Johnson, D., Dunbar, K., et al. 2005. 2.45 GHz radiofrequency fields alter gene expression in cultured human cells. *FEBS Lett.* 579:4829–4836.

73. Lerchl, A., Klose, M., Grote, K., et al. 2015. Tumor promotion by exposure to radiofrequency electromagnetic fields below exposure limits for humans. *Biochem Biophys Res Commun.* 459:585–590.

74. Li, D-K., Chen, H., & Odouli, R. 2011. Maternal exposure to magnetic fields during pregnancy in relation to the risk of asthma in offspring. *Arch Pediatr Adolesc Med.* 165:945–950.

75. Li, D-K., Ferber, J.R., Odouli, R., & Quesenberry, C.P. Jr. 2012. A prospective study of in-utero exposure to magnetic fields and the risk of childhood obesity. *Sci Rep.* 2:540.

76. Loughran, S.P., Wood, A.W., Barton, J.M., et al. 2005. The effect of electromagnetic fields emitted by mobile phones on human sleep. *Neuroreport.* 16:1973–1976.

77. Lu, Y., He, M., Zhang, Y., et al. 2014. Differential pro-inflammatory responses of astrocytes and microglia involve STAT3 activation in response to 1800 MHz radiofrequency fields. *PLoS One.* 9:e108318.

78. Lv, B., Chen, Z., Wu, T., et al. 2014. The alteration of spontaneous low frequency oscillations caused by acute electromagnetic fields exposure. *Clin Neurophysiol.* 125:277–286.

79. Mahmoudabadi, F.S., Ziaei, S., Firoozabadi, M., & Kazemnejad, A. 2015. Use of mobile phone during pregnancy and the risk of spontaneous abortion. *J Environ Health Sci Eng.* 13:34.

80. Markovà, E., Malmgren, L.O.G., & Belyaev, I.Y. 2010. Microwaves from mobile phones inhibit 53BP1 focus formation in human stem cells more strongly than in differentiated cells: Possible mechanistic link to cancer risk. *Environ Health Perspect.* 118:394–399.

81. Marshall, L. 2004. Taking An Exposure History. http://www.ocfp.on.ca/docs/public-policy-documents/taking-an-exposure-history.pdf.

82. McInerny, T. 2013. Letter from the American Academy of Pediatrics to Commissioners of the U.S. Federal Communications Commission regarding regulation of wireless technology. http://apps.fcc.gov/ecfs/document/view?id=7520941318.

83. Meo, S.A., Arif, M., Rashied, S., et al. 2013. Morphological changes induced by mobile phone radiation in liver and pancreas in Wistar albino rats. *Eur J Anat.* 14:105–109.

84. Merhi, Z.O. 2012. Challenging cell phone impact on reproduction: A review. *J Assist Reprod Genet.* 29:293–297.

85. Morgan, L.L., Kesari, S., & Davis, D,L. 2014. Why children absorb more microwave radiation than adults: The consequences. *J Microsc Ultrastruct.* 2:197–204.

86. Morgan, L.L., Miller, A.B., Sasco, A., & Davis, D.L. 2015. Mobile phone radiation causes brain tumors and should be classified as a probable human carcinogen (2A). Review. *Int J Oncol.* 46:1865–1871.

87. Morris, R.D., Morgan, L.L., & Davis, D. 2015. Children absorb higher doses of radio frequency electromagnetic radiation from mobile phones than adults. *IEEE Access.* 3:2379–2387.

88. Nittby, H., Brun, A., Eberhardt, J., et al. 2009. Increased blood–brain barrier permeability in mammalian brain 7 days after exposure to the radiation from a GSM-900 mobile phone. *Pathophysiology.* 16:103–112.

89. Nittby, H., Grafström, G., Eberhardt, J.L., et al. 2008. Radiofrequency and extremely low-frequency electromagnetic field effects on the blood-brain barrier. *Electromagn Biol Med.* 27:103–126.

90. Ostrom, Q.T., Gittleman, H., de Blank, P.M., et al. 2016. American Brain Tumor Association adolescent and young adult primary brain and central nervous system tumors diagnosed in the United States in 2008-2012. *Neuro-oncology.* 18(Suppl 1):i1–i50.

91. Pall, M. 2013. Electromagnetic fields act via activation of voltage-gated calcium channels to produce beneficial or adverse effects. *J Cell Mol Med.* 17:958–965.

92. Pall, M.L. 2015. Scientific evidence contradicts findings and assumptions of Canadian Safety Panel 6: Microwaves act through voltage-gated calcium channel activation to induce biological impacts at non-thermal levels, supporting a

paradigm shift for microwave/lower frequency electromagnetic field action. *Rev Environ Health*. 30:99–116.

93. Parker, M-C., Besson, T., Lamare, S., & Legoy, M-D. 1996. Microwave radiation can increase the rate of enzyme-catalysed reactions in organic media. *Tetrahedron Lett*. 37:8383–8386.

94. Porcelli, M., Cacciapuoti, G., Fusco, S., et al. 1997. Non-thermal effects of microwaves on proteins: Thermophilic enzymes as model system. *FEBS Lett*. 402:102–106.

95. Redmayne, M., & Johansson, O. 2015. Radiofrequency exposure in young and old: Different sensitivities in light of age-relevant natural differences. *Rev Environ Health*. 30:323–335.

96. Sadetzki, S., Chetrit, A., Jarus-Hakak, A., et al. 2008. Cellular phone use and risk of benign and malignant parotid gland tumors: A nationwide case-control study. *Am J Epidemiol*. 167:457–467.

97. Saili, L., Hanini, A., Smirani, C., et al. 2015. Effects of acute exposure to WIFI signals (2.45 GHz) on heart variability and blood pressure in Albinos rabbit. *Environ Toxicol Pharmacol*. 40:600–605.

98. Sears, M. 2007. *The Medical Perspective on Environmental Sensitivities*. Canadian Human Rights Commission. http://www.chrc-ccdp.gc.ca/sites/default/files/envsensitivity_en_1.pdf.

99. Sears, M.E. 2013. Chelation: Harnessing and enhancing heavy metal detoxification—A review. *Sci World J*. (2013):219840.

100. Sears, M.E., & Genuis, S.J. 2012. Environmental determinants of chronic disease and medical approaches: Recognition, avoidance, supportive therapy, and detoxification. *J Environ Public Health*. (2012):356798.

101. Sears, M.E., Kerr, K.J., & Bray, R.I. 2012. Arsenic, cadmium, lead, and mercury in sweat: A systematic review. *J Environ Public Health*. (2012):184745.

102. Sepehrimanesh, M., Kazemipour, N., Saeb, M., & Nazifi, S. 2014. Analysis of rat testicular proteome following 30-day exposure to 900 MHz electromagnetic field radiation. *Electrophoresis*. 35:3331–3338.

103. Shamis, Y., Croft, R., Taube, A., Crawford, R.J., & Ivanova, E.P. 2012. Review of the specific effects of microwave radiation on bacterial cells. *Appl Microbiol Biotechnol*. 96:319–325.

104. Sudan, M., Kheifets, L., Arah, O., Olsen, J., & Zeltzer, L. 2012. Prenatal and postnatal cell phone exposures and headaches in children. *Open Pediatr Med J*. 6:46–52.

105. Surveillance, Epidemiology, and End Results Program. 2013. *SEER Cancer Statistics Review, 1975–2010*. http://seer.cancer.gov/csr/1975_2010/.

106. Taylor, W. 2014. Letter from the U.S. Department of the Interior to Mr. Eli Veenendaal, U.S. National Telecommunications and Information Administration, regarding ER 14/0001, 14/0004. https://skyvisionsolutions.files.wordpress.com/2014/03/us-dept-of-interior-letter-2014.pdf.

107. Tosini, G., Ferguson, I., & Tsubota, K. 2016. Effects of blue light on the circadian system and eye physiology. *Mol Vis*. 22:61–72.

108. U.S. Centers for Disease Control and Prevention. 2015. *Fourth National Report on Human Exposure to Environmental Chemicals.* http://www.cdc.gov/biomonitoring/pdf/FourthReport_UpdatedTables_Feb2015.pdf.

109. U.S. Government Accountability Office. 2012. *Telecommunications: Exposure and Testing Requirements for Mobile Phones Should Be Reassessed.* GAO-12-771. http://www.gao.gov/products/GAO-12-771.

110. Vecchio, F., Babiloni, C., Ferreri, F., et al. 2010. Mobile phone emission modulates inter-hemispheric functional coupling of EEG alpha rhythms in elderly compared to young subjects. *Clin Neurophysiol.* 121:163–171.

111. Vecchio, F., Buffo, P., Sergio, S., et al. 2012. Mobile phone emission modulates event-related desynchronization of alpha rhythms and cognitive–motor performance in healthy humans. *Clin Neurophysiol.* 123:121–128.

112. Vecchio, F., Tombini, M., Buffo, P., et al. 2012. Mobile phone emission increases inter-hemispheric functional coupling of electroencephalographic alpha rhythms in epileptic patients. *Int J Psychophysiol.* 84:164–171.

113. Volkow, N.D., Tomasi, D., Wang, G-J., et al. 2011. Effects of cell phone radiofrequency signal exposure on brain glucose metabolism. *JAMA.* 305:808–813.

114. West, J.G., Kapoor, N.S., Liao, S-Y., et al. 2013. Multifocal breast cancer in young women with prolonged contact between their breasts and their cellular phones. *Case Rep Med.* (2013):354682.

115. Wyde, M., Cesta, M., Blystone, C., et al. 2016, June 23. Report of partial findings from the National Toxicology Program carcinogenesis studies of cell phone radiofrequency radiation in Hsd: Sprague Dawley SD rats (whole body exposure). *bioRxiv* 2016:55699.

116. Yakymenko, I., Tsybulin, O., Sidorik, E., et al. 2016. Oxidative mechanisms of biological activity of low-intensity radiofrequency radiation. *Electromagn Biol Med.* 35:186–202.

117. Yu, Y., & Yao, K. 2010. Non-thermal cellular effects of lowpower microwave radiation on the lens and lens epithelial cells. *J Int Med Res.* 38:729–736.

118. Zadac G., Bond, A.E., Wang, Y-P., Giannotta, S.L., & Deapen, D. 2012. Incidence trends in the anatomic location of primary malignant brain tumors in the United States: 1992–2006. *World Neurosurg.* 77:518–524.

119. Zhou, L-Y., Zhang, H-X., Lan, Y-L., et al. 2015, April 14. Epidemiological investigation of risk factors of the pregnant women with early spontaneous abortion in Beijing. *Chin J Integr Med.* doi:10.1007/s11655-015-2144-z.

Regulatory Issues, Exposure Mitigation, and Resources for Clinicians and Patients

11

Food Additives: Health Consequences of Regulatory Oversight Failure

MARICEL V. MAFFINI AND SARAH VOGEL

Key Concepts

- The Food Additive Amendment of 1958 was intended to protect the public from harmful chemicals by requiring an affirmation of safety by the Food and Drug Administration (FDA) and testing before they are used in or on foods.
- There is far less safety information today than in 1958, whereas the estimated number of additives allowed in food has increased more than 1000%.
- Ongoing exposures to small amounts of chemicals in the diet during susceptible life stages may contribute to increased risk of chronic diseases.
- An exemption in the law for vinegar, oil, and the like, has been abused by industry to bring at least 1000 chemicals to market without safety review by the FDA.
- Ingredients listed on packages are just a few of the chemicals we eat. Labeling exemptions leave out classes of chemicals that are part of our diet.

Introduction

Most of the food we eat is processed in some way, such as freezing, curing, coloring, and flavoring. Humans have been processing food for several thousand years.[26] Noodles were created around 2000 BC, bacon around 1500 BC, and tofu around 965 AD. It was not until the early 1900s, thanks to new methods and technologies, that more ready-to-eat foods with longer shelf lives became available, including canned pork and beans, jelly, cereal, and peanut butter. In the second half of the 20th century, spurred by the commercialization of new technologies and innovations from World War II, the mass distribution of processed and packaged foods became increasingly available to every household. From Saran Wrap and Teflon pans to food dyes and artificial preservatives, chemicals used to prevent spoiling, add flavor, and restore color lost during manufacturing and to improve packaging, handling, and holding of food transformed how Americans consumed food and what they consumed. These chemicals, referred to as *food additives*, became essential to produce stable, practical, tasty, and appealing foods, but were they safe for human consumption?

In the early 1950s, Congress investigated the impact of the rapid growth in the use of chemical additives in manufacturing, processing, handling, and packaging of food. What became evident through the investigation and many Congressional hearings was that the food law, the 1938 Federal Food, Drug and Cosmetics Act, inadequately protected the public from the new and expanding uses of chemicals.[62] Among the major concerns at the time were that chemicals were being added to conceal the inferior quality of food, that use of unnecessary chemicals could diminish nutritional value or replace nutrients, and that the safety of many of these chemicals was unknown.

Congressional hearing records revealed that the U.S. Food and Drug Administration (FDA), the regulatory agency responsible for food safety, and the scientific community feared that many of the chemicals being added to food had not been adequately tested to establish their safe use in food.[25] The main concern was with chemicals that might cause harmful effects after being consumed for months or years. After years of debate, in 1958, Congress passed the Food Additive Amendment to the Federal Food, Drug, and Cosmetics Act,[43] which gave the FDA new authority to regulate food additives.

The following sections explore the current universe of food chemicals, how their safety is determined, and by whom, with a focus on the role of the FDA. We describe specific examples of food chemicals associated with adverse human health outcomes and detail some of the limitations and flaws in the food additives law. We also discuss why reading labels may not be as helpful as you think.

What are Food Additives?

The purpose of the 1958 Food Additives Amendment was twofold: (1) to protect the health of consumers by requiring manufacturers of food additives and food processors to pretest any potentially unsafe substances that will be added to food and (2) to advance food technology by permitting the use of food additives at safe levels. The law defines a food additive as "any substance the intended use of which results or may reasonably be expected to result, directly or indirectly, in its becoming a component or otherwise affecting the characteristics of any food."[10] This includes chemical ingredients intentionally added to foods, or *direct additives*, such as preservatives, flavors, sweeteners, and emulsifiers. It also includes chemicals unintentionally added to foods such as chemicals used in production, packaging, preparing, or transporting foods that may enter the food supply through migration or leaching. Examples of these *indirect additives* are bisphenol A (BPA), ortho-phthalates, perchlorate, and tetrafluoroethylene-hexafluoropropylene-vinylidene fluoride copolymers.

Excluded from the legal definition of food additive are *generally recognized as safe* (GRAS) substances. These are substances "generally recognized, among experts qualified by scientific training and experience to evaluate its safety, as having been adequately shown through scientific procedures (or, in the case of a substance used in food before January 1, 1958, through scientific procedures or experience based on common use in food) to be safe under the conditions of its intended use."[10] According to Congressional intent and the FDA's regulations, the amount and type of toxicity and exposure data needed to make a safety determination for a GRAS substance are comparable to that for a food additive. Unlike food additives whose safety data could be unpublished, for a chemical use to be considered GRAS, its safety assessment must be published so that the scientific community can assert its general recognition. Unfortunately, as discussed later, this is not always the case. The GRAS exemption has become the rule that has left the FDA and the public in the dark.

The GRAS exemption was intended for common food ingredients such as vinegar, oil, salt, and sugar; Congress interpreted that the use of those substances did not necessitate FDA review of their safety.[40] However, it has become increasingly evident that the FDA and industry have a different interpretation of GRAS[41]: as long as the use of a substance is determined to be GRAS by somebody, there is no requirement to inform the FDA of its identity, safety assessment, and uses. This appears to hold even if the determination is made in secret with no review by or reporting to the FDA. In other words, according to the FDA it is legal for a company to make its own decision that a chemical is GRAS, market it as GRAS, and completely bypass the agency in charge of ensuring food safety and public health. This is exemplified on the left side of Figure 11.1.

Alternatively, some companies may seek FDA review of their safety assessment by voluntarily submitting data to the agency, but this has not been required. In cases of voluntary submission, the FDA acts more as an auditor or a peer reviewer than as a regulator; although it offers an opinion about

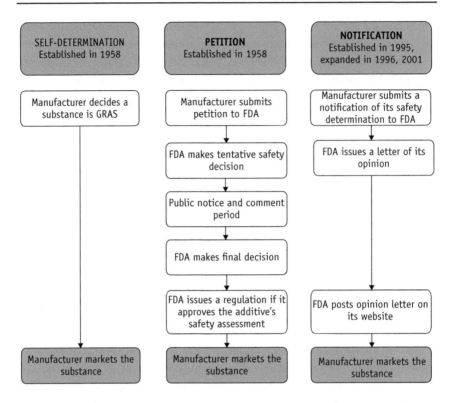

FIGURE 11.1. Schematic representation of the decision-making process for chemicals allowed to be used in food. FDA = Food and Drug Administration; GRAS = generally recognized as safe.

whether it agrees or disagrees with the industry assessment, the agency's last word is not binding. If the company perceives that the FDA may disagree with the GRAS determination, it can withdraw the notification at any time, asking the FDA to stop its review.

Regardless of potential concerns expressed by the FDA about the safe use of a voluntarily submitted chemical, companies are still allowed to market and sell the substance as GRAS. Although the FDA indicates in its website that a GRAS notification has been withdrawn, it does not publish the reasons. If the FDA does not have any concerns and agrees with the company's GRAS determination, it expresses that opinion in a letter (see Fig. 11.1, right side). Because it is only an opinion, it cannot be challenged in court. The following sections discuss how this flawed system works against protecting food safety and human health.

There are also 120 chemicals used in food that were grandfathered in through a "prior sanctioned"[2] process after the Food Additives Amendment was passed. The use of these chemicals was explicitly approved by the FDA or by the U.S. Department of Agriculture before September 6, 1958.[4] The prior sanctioned uses are exempted from the food additive regulations.

Today, other chemicals that may be present in the diet (e.g., color additives, pesticide chemicals or pesticide residues, animal drugs, dietary supplements) are regulated under different laws. Unless otherwise specified, the terms *additives* and *food chemicals* are used as synonyms throughout this chapter.

When the Food Additives Amendment was signed into law in 1958, according to the FDA, "approximately 842 chemicals are used, have been used, or have been suggested for use in foods. Of this total, it was estimated that 704 are employed today."[25] Today, the universe of food chemicals is roughly 10,000,[40] with an approximately even split between direct and indirect additives. It is unknown how many of these additives are in use currently or have been used in the past and at what volume. An estimated 10% of the 10,000 chemicals have been declared GRAS by manufacturers with no review or disclosure to the FDA.[40] This absence of information results from the lack of requirements in the law for chemical manufacturers to report uses to the FDA.

The substantial increase in the number of food additives over the past 60 years reflects the continued transformation of food. Many of the foods and beverages found in a mainstream grocery store are highly engineered products in terms of the food itself and its packaging. According to the most recent data, almost 60% of the American diet is composed of ultra-processed foods.[31] A new food classification system based on the extent and purpose of industrial food processing[34] defines ultra-processed foods as "formulation of several ingredients, which, besides salt, sugar, oils and fats, include food substances not used in culinary preparations, in particular, flavors, colors, sweeteners, emulsifiers, and other additives used to imitate sensorial qualities of unprocessed or minimally processed foods and their culinary preparations or to disguise undesirable qualities of the final product."[31]

The proliferation of food chemicals and the incredible variety of foods in the marketplace suggest that the law has allowed food technology to advance at a rapid pace. However, in the face of rapid innovation and change, has the law adequately protected consumer health?

Safety of Food Chemicals

The Food Additive Amendment of 1958 fundamentally changed the way chemicals were supposed to come into use in or on food. Under the Federal Food, Drug, and Cosmetics Act of 1938, no testing of chemicals was required. In 1952, the FDA described to members of Congress that it knew that roughly one half of the chemicals in use (428 of the 842) were "known to be safe." The Food Additives Amendment mandated that industry test "any potentially unsafe substances that are to be added to food,"[22] in order to provide the FDA with the information needed to make safety decisions.

Although the law did not define *safe* or *safety*, the FDA has used language from the legislative history to define safe or safety to mean "a reasonable certainty in the minds of competent scientists that the substance is not harmful under the intended conditions of use."[1] This definition applies to all food additives and GRAS substances. In other words, a chemical is considered unsafe until proved safe.

Another important term that was not defined in the law or by the FDA is *harm*[28]; this lack of clarity has been the source of many controversies about the safety of chemicals, including debates about the safety of chemicals that have been shown to have hormonal activity and may cause chronic health effects.

The concern about chronic health effects of exposure to food chemicals was foremost in the Congressional investigation in the early 1950s. The Surgeon General pointed out that "the lack of adequate information on the chronic health effects" of chemicals precluded understanding the extent of the public health impact. Similar statements about the unknown impact of chemicals used in production and processing of foods on chronic health effects were made by the American Public Health Association and the American Medical Association.[25]

Despite the law's original intent to promote safety testing for food additives, there are significant information gaps, and the FDA has made minimal effort to conduct another review the additive safety, even in the face of new scientific evidence. The percentage of chemicals tested has decreased since the 1950s. A 2013 report by The Pew Charitable Trusts on toxicity testing of chemicals allowed in foods showed that information sufficient to estimate a safe level of exposure is available for a mere 21% of direct additives.[38] An even more disturbing fact is that fewer than 7% of those additives have been tested for developmental or reproductive toxicity. If in vitro and computer-based (e.g. in silico) studies are taken into account, more than 50% of direct additives still lack information. Overall, the 2013 report found that fewer than 38% of FDA-regulated additives (i.e., direct and indirect additives and GRAS substances) have been investigated in studies that included feeding the chemical to laboratory animals and evaluating for health effects.

There are several explanations for the lack of safety data based on laboratory animal feeding studies.[38] First, the GRAS exemption allows food manufacturers to determine that a chemical use is GRAS based on common uses before 1958 or on scientific procedures (e.g., toxicity testing, exposure estimates). A claim of common uses releases the manufacturer from performing a safety assessment. Second, the FDA approved thousands of chemicals before it defined safety or established how a safety determination should be conducted. An example is BPA, which was approved in 1963 together with hundreds of other can-coating chemicals with few or no data.[14] Third, the industry and FDA rely heavily on estimated (not experimentally determined) thresholds of exposure below which few (mostly in vitro) or no data are generated. The assumption is that at very low exposures, chemicals cannot present a risk.[9,29]

This is a very common practice for indirect additives[53] and flavors.[24] For example, in 2005, the FDA approved the chemical perchlorate, a well-known thyroid disruptor, as a component of plastics designed to hold dry food without any toxicity testing. The manufacturer claimed that the dietary exposure would be below the threshold of 0.5 parts per billion (ppb) and therefore would be considered toxicologically insignificant.[29] The manufacturer invoked a 1995 regulation that exempts chemicals from regulation as food additives if they are in the diet at levels below 0.5 ppb and the chemical has not been shown to be a carcinogen.[54]

The fourth explanation for the lack of safety studies is that academic researchers are unlikely to conduct research aimed at filling data gaps, particularly in the absence of existing data indicating that there may be hazardous characteristics to explore, and there is no significant available funding for such work. Finally, industry has little or no incentive to generate additional information, particularly given that the FDA does not systematically review additive safety.[29]

The lack of review by the FDA of previous decisions about additive safety, even in the presence of new data indicating the existence of new hazards or exposures exceeding safe amounts, is particularly troubling. For instance, diethylhexyl phthalate (DEHP) is an industrial chemical commonly used to make plastics flexible. DEHP has been used as an indirect food additive since before 1958, and when the law was passed, it was grandfathered in as a "prior sanctioned" chemical for use as a plasticizer in food packaging for foods of high water content only.[3] It is unclear what type, if any, of safety data was available at that time. However, over the past 15 years, DEHP has been well characterized as an endocrine disruptor with antiandrogenic properties,[35] and its use has been effectively banned in children's toys and care articles[18] due to adverse health effects associated with exposure.[48,49] Despite the FDA's knowledge of its toxic effects in 1973[47] and the additional evidence concerning human and animal health effects,[17] DEHP is still allowed to be used in the manufacture of materials in contact with food without any limitation on the quantities that could migrate into food.

There are a few notable examples of FDA reassessment of the safety of food chemicals. In 1969, President Richard Nixon issued a directive[42] that ordered the agency to perform a full review of food additives, with a focus on the safety of chemicals that the FDA had designated as GRAS. Specifically, the FDA was directed to reexamine the structure and procedures used by the agency to approve chemical additives to ensure they were "fully adequate."[42] In response, the FDA established the Select Committee on GRAS Substances (SCOGS)[51] and charged it with the task of "evaluating the safety" of 468 substances (i.e., 422 for direct addition to food and 46 as components of packaging materials).[46] The committee, made up of experts in biochemistry, pharmacology, and medicine, conducted its analysis from 1972 to 1982 and published its decisions in 115 reports.[61] It agreed that 92% of the chemicals were safe for direct use in foods. However, it stated that 35 chemicals required either "that safe conditions of use be established" or that, in the absence of relevant data submission, the FDA should move to "rescind GRAS status."[46] To our knowledge, the GRAS status of those substances has not been revoked.[29]

In 2009, a University of Illinois professor sued the FDA after its failure to respond to his citizen petition requesting a ban on the use of partially hydrogenated oils (the main source of artificial *trans* fats) due to their association with heart disease.[63] In 2015, after reviewing the evidence, the FDA determined that partially hydrogenated oils were not "generally recognized as safe for use in human food."[55]

The FDA took its most recent action in January of 2016, banning the use of long-chain perfluorinated compounds (PFCs) as indirect food additives because the chemicals are unsafe (i.e., they bioaccumulate and cause developmental and reproductive toxicity).[19] The decision was made in response to a food additive petition submitted by a group of public interest organizations.[36] These recent efforts to direct the agency to again review the safety of food additives suggest that the agency has the authority and the capacity to better manage these chemicals.

Who Determines the Safety of Food Chemicals, and Why is it Important?

According to the law, a chemical must be shown to be safe before is used in or on food. The FDA states that it is the manufacturer's responsibility to demonstrate the safe use of its chemical. After a safety assessment is conducted, the manufacturer has three options to get its additive approved or cleared for use in food (see Fig. 11.1). First, it can submit a food additive petition to the FDA. The agency reviews the safety assessment and publishes its decision; the public submits comments; and the FDA eventually approves the chemical's safe uses. In the process Congress intended, the FDA reviews and approves the safety of chemicals and codifies its decision in the Code of Federal Regulations (CFR).

Second, a manufacturer can submit a notification informing the agency of its safety determination and asking for its review. If the FDA agrees with the manufacturer, the agency publishes its decision on its website. This is not an approval but rather an opinion, and as such, it lacks the same legal weight. Figure 11.2 shows changes in the FDA's role over time.

Third, a manufacturer can make a GRAS determination and immediately market the chemical. The FDA is completely bypassed and therefore remains unaware of the chemical's identity and presence in the food supply. There are an estimated 1000 substances that have been determined by their manufacturers to be GRAS without notification to the FDA (Fig. 11.3).

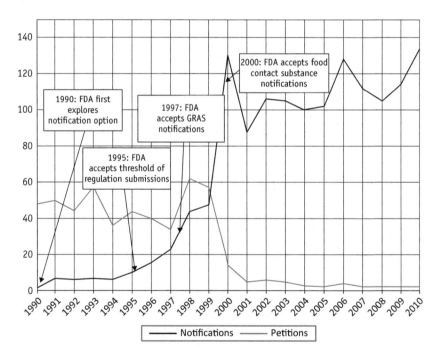

FIGURE 11.2. Trends in filings of petitions and notifications for food additives and GRAS substances directly added to human food submitted to the FDA from 1990 to 2010. Most decisions are made by companies, whereas the role of FDA as decision-maker has plummeted. FDA = Food and Drug Administration; GRAS = generally recognized as safe.

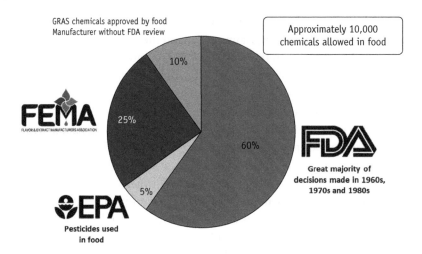

FIGURE 11.3. Relative contributions to the total estimated number of substances allowed in human food grouped by organization making the final decision. Most of the FDA's decisions were made decades ago. The EPA makes safety decisions about pesticides used in food. The safety of at least 10% of the more than 10,000 chemicals allowed in food has not been reviewed by the FDA. FDA = Food and Drug Administration; FEMA = Flavor and Extract Manufacturers Association; GRAS = generally recognized as safe.

These GRAS self-determinations are riddled with conflicts of interest. When researchers analyzed more than 450 GRAS determinations voluntarily submitted to the FDA, they found that 22% of the safety assessments were made by an employee of the chemical manufacturer, 13% by an employee of a consulting firm hired by the company, and 65% by an expert panel selected by the manufacturer or its consulting firm.[39] The lack of independent review in GRAS determinations raises concerns about the integrity of the process and the safety of the chemicals, especially when the manufacturers do not notify the FDA. In the past 2 decades, the private sector has made more safety decisions than the FDA (see Fig. 11.2).

A 2014 report by the Natural Resources Defense Council (NRDC)[41] identified 275 chemicals from 56 companies that were marketed for use in food based on undisclosed GRAS safety determinations. In other words, the investigators found no evidence that the FDA had reviewed and cleared their use in food. Most of the GRAS chemicals the NRDC examined were primarily marketed as active ingredients in dietary supplements, suggesting that the market for such substances has expanded into conventional foods with claims that they make food "better for you." Many of the chemicals were extracts of plants or highly purified or synthetic versions of biologically active chemicals in plants, such as antioxidants, that are purported to have health benefits.[41]

It is fair to assume that it is not in a company's best interest to commercialize an unsafe or questionable GRAS substance. However, there are examples of GRAS substances that raise considerable concerns about the effectiveness of this kind of self-policing. The following are examples of self-determined GRAS substances submitted to the FDA for review that were found to have serious safety issues but are nevertheless used in and on food.

- *Epigallocatechin-3-gallate (EGCG):* EGCG is a highly purified chemical from green tea extract; it can be labeled as EGCG or with the more appealing name of green tea extract. The FDA had serious concerns[59] about its safety due to evidence that it might cause fetal leukemia based on in vitro studies using newborn and adult human cells. The FDA pointed out the lack of explanation for potentially dangerous interactions with sodium nitrite, a common preservative, or with acetaminophen (see Chapter 7), the active ingredient in Tylenol and many other over-the-counter pain killers. EGCG was declared to be GRAS for use in beverages, including teas, sport drinks, and juices.
- *Sweet lupin protein, fiber, and flour:* Lupin is a legume belonging to the same plant family as peanuts. Lupin has been shown to cause allergic reactions[12] similar to those from peanuts. In its review, the FDA raised concerns that people with peanut allergies[11] would be exposed to a similar allergen without any warning labels on the products. Lupin products are commonly used in gluten-free baked goods. They were declared GRAS also for use in dairy products, gelatin, meats, and candy.[52]
- *γ-Amino butyric acid (GABA):* GABA is a neurotransmitter that is naturally present in the central nervous system and inhibits brain signals. The FDA's chief concern[37] was that the company's estimated exposure, based on its intended uses, was well in excess of what it had considered safe. If estimated exposure levels exceed the estimated safe level, the chemical cannot be used safely. The company also failed to consider the contribution from natural sources of GABA (e.g., meats), which could increase exposure levels even further beyond a safe amount. The company also relied on unpublished data. Nevertheless, GABA was declared GRAS for use in beverages, chewing gum, coffee, tea, and candy.[60]

Although it is fairly certain that there is high degree of confidence that all ingredients listed on a label are legal for use in food under the current laws,[41] the safety in many cases appears uncertain. For many food chemicals, safety largely boils down to blind trust in the manufacturer. Given the chronic, long-term exposures to chemicals in the diet, determinations of safety demand rigorous, independent review of scientific evidence.

Cumulative Effects of Chemicals and Human Health

In its *Global Status Report on Noncommunicable Diseases* (NCDs), the World Health Organization (WHO) recognized that chronic diseases have become one of the "major health and developmental challenges of the 21st century in terms of the human suffering they cause and the harm they inflict on the socioeconomic fabric of countries."[65] NCDs are the leading cause of death globally. *Noncommunicable* means that the disease, usually chronic and with slow progression, is not transmittable from person to person. Examples are diabetes, cancer, obesity, and cardiovascular and chronic respiratory diseases.

The incidence of NCDs has increased in the past 40 years due to environmental changes—not only lifestyle, diet, and behavioral changes but also environmental chemical exposures, and in particular, exposures that occur during fetal development.[13] Food is a constant source of environmental exposures ranging from fats, salts, and sugar to DEHP and other endocrine disrupting compounds present in the diet. Exposure to chemicals in food is ongoing and occurs throughout all life stages, including the highly susceptible period of prenatal development.

When Congress passed the food additives law in 1958, it intended that the FDA determine the safety of chemicals in food. Discussions of lawmakers at the time reflect an understanding that some chemicals could pose potential health hazards and that co-exposure to chemicals is the norm because many additives are present in the diet. The law therefore mandates that the FDA require three factors in determining the safety of a food chemical.[1]

The first factor is the probable consumption of the substance and of any substance formed in or on food because of its use. To determine the risk of the chemical, there needs to be evidence of exposure (risk = exposure × health hazard). The second factor deals with the uncertainty of data and requires the use of safety factors that in the opinion of experts are appropriate. A 10-, 100-, or 1000-fold safety factor is applied to the exposure level that does not cause harm, with the goal of lowering the risk. The third factor in a safety assessment states that the "cumulative effect of the substance in the diet, taking into account any chemically or pharmacologically related substance or substances in such diet" must be considered. In other words, chemicals that are structurally similar, such as ortho-phthalates (e.g., DEHP, benzyl butyl phthalate [BBP], di-isononyl phthalate [DINP]) should be assessed for safety together as a class.[35] The reasoning behind this approach is that structurally similar substances may have similar toxic effects. By assessing them cumulatively, the logic follows, a more accurate safe level for the class can be determined and the public can be better protected. The FDA did not define *pharmacologically related* substances, but in a decision on the unsafe use as indirect additives of long-chain PFCs,[57] it implied that such substances are those that have similar toxicity effects.[56]

The implications for considering the cumulative effects of pharmacologically related substances are significant. If this is how the agency should be interpreting the safety of food additives, it could be argued that even structurally unrelated chemicals such as perchlorate (used in plastic packaging), nitrate (used in processed meats), and thiocyanate (food contaminant) should be assessed together. All three of these chemicals found in the diet share a common toxic effect on the thyroid gland: inhibition of iodine uptake, which leads to decreased levels of thyroid hormone.[30]

Decreased levels of thyroid hormone can present harm, and pregnant women are particularly vulnerable due to the permanent effects of low thyroid hormone levels on fetal brain development. One half of pregnant women in the United States[16] already have inadequate iodine intake according to the WHO,[64] and almost 16% are clinically deficient in iodine. The risk of perchlorate, nitrate, and thiocyanate exposure is particularly high for these women and their fetuses. Thyroid hormone is fundamental for normal brain development, and long-term hormone deficiency, either maternal or after birth due to low iodine intake, is known to cause neurologic impairment.[44] Additional additives with thyroid-adverse effects in the FDA's toxicology database include flavors (e.g., brominated vegetable oil, butyl alcohol, ethyl isovalerate), synthetic colors (e.g., FD&C Red No. 3), preservatives (e.g., heptyl paraben, sodium nitrite), nutrients (e.g., tocopherols, vitamin D_3), and dough conditioners (e.g., potassium bromate).

Direct adverse effects on the brain or hypothalamus in animal studies are also documented for many food chemicals in the FDA's toxicology database. They include preservatives (e.g., butylated hydroxyanisole [BHA]), artificial sweeteners (e.g., aspartame, neotame), flavors (e.g., taurine [a common ingredient of energy drinks], theobromine, styrene, pulegone, peppermint oil), and the widespread ingredients monosodium glutamate (MSG) and caffeine.[27] Contemporary data indicate that BPA[45] and some ortho-phthalates[33] also adversely affect the developing brain.

There are more examples of additives adversely affecting the same organs or systems. However, it is unclear whether the cumulative effect of pharmacologically related substances in the diet was ever considered when any of the chemicals mentioned previously were approved for uses in or in contact with food. It appears that this fundamental requirement has been ignored. The current safety or risk assessment approach is chemical-centric: the agency evaluates a single chemical and how it affects many organs.[27] Although this is an important step in understanding how the body reacts to a particular chemical in isolation and the potential health effects resulting from such exposure, it is not equivalent to the safety assessment requirements mandated by Congress.

In the safety assessment process, a chemical's contribution to the health outcome of concern should take into account the cumulative biologic effects of multiple chemicals on the same organ or system. This health outcome–centric approach to assessing chemical safety was proposed by the National Research Council in its report on phthalates. Its Committee on Health Risks of Phthalates stated that "[m]ultiple pathways can lead to a common outcome" and that "the chemicals that should be considered for cumulative risk assessment should be ones that cause the same health outcomes or the same type of health outcomes."[35]

Consideration of the cumulative effects of pharmacologically related substances can better inform the social and financial costs of exposure. For example, Bellinger estimated that exposures to neurotoxic chemicals (e.g., methylmercury, organophosphate pesticides, lead) alone accounted for more than 40 million lost full-scale IQ points in a population of 25.5 million American children 0 to 5 years of age.[15] Other researchers have estimated the cost of disease and dysfunction (e.g., intellectual disability, autism, attention deficit hyperactivity disorder, childhood and adult obesity, endometriosis, male infertility, adult diabetes) associated with endocrine-disrupting chemicals at €163 billion per year.[50]

A better understanding of the contribution of chemical exposures to the rising incidence of chronic diseases demands moving beyond a chemical-centric focus to consider the cumulative biologic effects on organs and their role in the onset of chronic diseases. For chemicals in food, this was the approach Congress intended in 1958.

Can We Buy Our Way Out of Hazardous Additives?

Foods, unlike many other consumer products, must carry a label listing their ingredients to allow people to make informed choices and avoid substances that may compromise their health (e.g., allergens, artificial colors, *trans* fats). The Nutrition Labeling and Education Act of 1990 requires that most foods

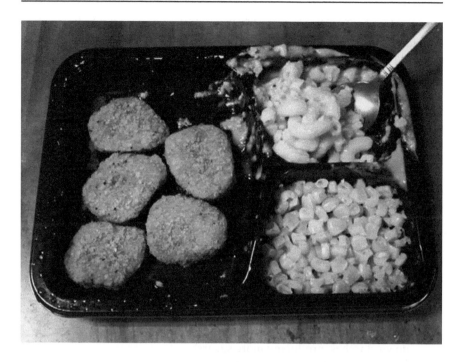

FIGURE 11.4. Picture of a microwave-ready frozen children's meal. Its ingredients list identifies 68 items, which range from whole-grain flour to microcrystalline and carboxymethyl cellulose. However, the meal contains many additional substances not listed, such as chemicals used in packaging or during the manufacturing process and processing aids.

bear nutrition labeling. There are specific requirements for the type of information that may be placed on a product, where the label may be placed on the package, and the size of typeface on the printed information.[58] In one survey, 68% of respondents said they looked at the nutrition facts panel when deciding what foods to purchase, 63% looked at the expiration date, 50% looked at the brand name, and 49% looked at the ingredients list.[32]

The ingredients list on a food label cites each of the ingredients in descending order of predominance in the food by weight.[8] The common or usual name should be used rather than the ingredient's scientific designation (e.g., *sugar* rather than *sucrose*). Although a considerable amount of information can be obtained from the ingredients list, when it comes to all food additives, what is listed is less than what is contained in the food (Fig. 11.4).

There are several labeling exceptions made for additives. One example is the so-called *incidental additives*. The FDA defines them as additives that are "present in a food at insignificant levels and do not have any technical or functional effect in that food."[5] For sulfiting agents (including sulfur dioxide, sodium or potassium sulfite, bisulfite, and metabisulfite), which are used to prevent spoilage and discoloration, the detectable amount was set at 10 parts per million (ppm). For all other incidental additives, the term "insignificant level" is unspecified by the FDA; that is, it is defined by the manufacturer.

There are three types of incidental additives. The first are processing aids, which are chemicals used during the manufacturing process to perform specific functions, including reducing potential bacterial contamination, facilitating removal of impurities, controlling pH, bringing clarity, or preventing crystallization or clumping. The FDA defines processing aids as follows:[21]

- Substances that are added during the processing of a food but are removed in some manner before the food is packaged in final form (e.g., methylene chloride used to decaffeinate coffee)
- Substances that when added to a food are converted into other substances already present in the food and do not significantly increase the amount naturally found in the food (e.g., enzymes that break down starches, producing more sugars)
- Substances that are added to a food for their technical or functional effect in the processing but are present in the finished food at insignificant levels and do not have any technical or functional effect in that food (e.g., rennet that coagulates milk to form cheese curds)

The second category of incidental additives comprises substances that migrate into food from equipment or packaging (final or raw materials). They are indirect food additives and are referred to as *food-contact chemicals*. Examples are fluorinated compounds, perchlorate, ortho-phthalates (e.g., DEHP, DINP, DIDP), and BPA. There are almost 4000 food-contact chemicals, all of which are exempted from ingredient listing.[40]

The third category of incidental additives includes substances that have no technical or functional effect in food but are incorporated into the food as an ingredient of another food in which the substance did have a functional or technical effect. An example is dimethylamine epichlorohydrin copolymer, which is used as a decoloring agent in the refinement of sugar, a common ingredient in many foods.

Another large group of additives exempted from being included by name on the label are flavors or flavoring agents. In 1981, Hall and Merwin defined a flavor as "a substance that may be a single chemical entity or a blend of chemicals of natural or synthetic origin whose primary purpose is to provide all or part of the particular flavor effect to any food or other product taken in the mouth."[23,24] More than 2700 flavors are authorized for use in food, most of which are GRAS substances.

The FDA defines distinguishes between natural and artificial flavors. *Natural flavors* means "the essential oil, oleoresin, essence or extractive, protein hydrolysate, distillate, or any product of roasting, heating, or enzymolysis, which contains the flavoring constituents derived from a spice, fruit or its juice, vegetable or its juice, edible yeast, herb, bark, bud, root, leaf or similar plant material, meat, seafood, poultry, eggs, dairy products, or fermentation products thereof whose significant function in food is flavoring rather than nutritional."[7] *Artificial flavors* are defined as "any substance, the function of which is to impart flavor, which is not derived from a spice, fruit or fruit juice, vegetable or vegetable juice, edible yeast, herb, bark, bud, root, leaf or similar plant material, meat, fish, poultry, eggs, dairy products, or fermentation products thereof."[6] In short, artificial flavors are usually created in a laboratory.

Although they are derived from different sources, natural and artificial flavors are both labeled in a generic manner (i.e., as simply "artificial flavor" or "natural flavor") without specification of their composition. However, both can be complex substances. It is fair to assume that flavors such as hot wings, zesty taco, chile limon, and guacamole are more than just a single chemical.

Like flavors, spices are not required to be identified and are labeled as "spice." The FDA defines them as any vegetable used to add flavor, with the exception of onions, garlic and celery, which are considered foods.

Although most flavors have been designated as GRAS substances, there is no published information about their safety assessment, including hazard and exposure data. In 1959, the Flavor and Extract Manufacturers Association (FEMA), the industry trade association, began a program to assess the safety and GRAS status of flavors. Its panel of experts determined that more than 2000 flavors are GRAS, but there are no public records of their safety assessments. Only flavor names, Chemical Abstracts Service (CAS) Registry Numbers, and flavor profiles (e.g., butter, creamy, green pepper, fruit, flower, wax, banana, green, rubber) are available to the public.[21] The identity of specific flavors (i.e., their chemical ingredients), like fragrances is secret. According to FEMA, "[t]he recipes used to create the flavors we recognize are protected as intellectual property by flavor manufacturers. The most important thing to remember is that the individual ingredients used to create these flavors have all been determined to be safe."[20] This suggests that the safety of flavors, like that of many GRAS substances, depends solely on blind trust in the manufacturer.

Given the wide range of exemptions for labeling requirements, it is clear that no individual can know the full scope of chemicals consumed in a meal.

It would be daunting for the consumer to read and understand labels that did list every chemical. For many, the assumption may follow that the chemicals in food that do not appear on the label, such as those from packaging and in flavors, have been rigorously and independently evaluated for their safety. However, that is far from reality despite the original intent of the 1958 food additives law.

Conclusions

The American diet is dramatically different today than in 1958, when Congress passed the Food Additives Amendment. Our food supply is more diverse and more processed. Food tends to be produced farther from where it is consumed. Innovations in processing, preserving, and packaging have made food more affordable, convenient, and available to all, but this transformation has brought with it thousands of new chemicals that have become an integral part of our daily diet. The unsettling aspect of this change is that the long-term, chronic effects of the use of these chemicals have rarely been studied or considered in the assessment of their safe use in food.

Today there are more than 10,000 additives allowed in food. The regulatory system designed to evaluate these additives for safety is plagued with problems. As a result, if a food additive is causing serious chronic health problems short of immediate serious injury, it is unlikely that the FDA would detect the problem unless the food industry alerted the agency.

Absent a robust regulatory review process for food additive safety, there are a few options available to individuals for limiting exposure. Eating more fresh, frozen, or minimally processed foods may reduce exposures. However, GRAS exemptions, lack of safety assessments that consider cumulative effects of chemically and pharmacologically related substances, and industry-determined safety assessments have created considerable uncertainty about the safety of food additives. When Congress passed the Food Additive Amendment in 1958, it was in response to a rapidly changing food system and rising public and scientific concerns about the potential health risks of the use of new chemicals.[62] In the almost 60 years since that time, the number of chemicals used in food processing, packaging, transport, and handling has risen dramatically. During this same period, chronic diseases have become the leading cause of mortality and morbidity globally. Scientific knowledge about the impacts of chemical exposures—even very low-level exposures considered to be inconsequential by corporations and the FDA—on normal development and disease processes have raised new questions and concerns about chronic exposures to chemicals (see Chapter 12).

We are faced with a regulatory system that has fallen short of being fully implemented and is weakened by decades of limited resources. The GRAS exemption has been exploited to the point that it is almost swallowing the law. The result is that consumers bear the burden of deciding what is safe to eat but have very limited information on which to base such decisions. Without adequate, robust review of the safety of chemicals in foods, we have little insight into the extent to which they may be contributing to chronic diseases or how we can safely use them in our food supply.

Actionable Recommendations

A balanced diet is important for the well-being of an individual. The idea of preparing homemade whole foods usually collides with a reality of conflicting priorities and demanding schedules, resources, or training. Ready-to-eat foods continue to be a staple in American kitchens. Here are some tips to reduce exposure to food additives:

1. Reduce consumption of processed foods in general. In addition to being high in sodium, these foods are low in iodine, a very important element needed to produce thyroid hormone, which is fundamental for fetal brain development. Normal levels of iodine can reduce the effect of perchlorate, a known thyroid endocrine disruptor.
2. It is important to limit intake of sodium, but if one is using salt at home, iodized salt rather than sea salt or regular salt can protect against the effects of perchlorate.
3. Limit consumption of canned foods to minimize exposure to BPA. If possible, choose fresh or frozen foods and glass- or carton-based packages.
4. Limit foods with synthetic colors; they appear on package labels with the letters FD&C preceding the color additive name.
5. Reduce consumption of fast foods; they are nutritionally poor and contain ortho-phthalates, which are known endocrine disruptors.
6. Avoid heating breast milk or formula in plastic containers or plastic baby bottles.
7. Avoid heating foods in plastic containers, and discard containers when they change color or are scratched. Components of the plastic can migrate into the food.
8. If bleach is used to clean kitchen surfaces, make sure it is less than 6 months old. Bleach or sodium hypochlorite degrades to perchlorate with time. Perchlorate remains on surfaces that touch foods.

REFERENCES

1. 21 CFR §170.3(i).
2. 21 CFR §181.
3. 21 CFR §181.27. Plasticizers.
4. 21 CFR §181.5.
5. 21 CFR 101.100(a)(3).
6. 21 CFR 101.22(a)(1).
7. 21 CFR 101.22(a)(3).
8. 21 CFR 101.4(a).
9. 21 CFR 170.39. Threshold of regulation for substances used in food-contact articles.
10. 21 USC §321(s).
11. Ballabio, C., Peñas, E., Uberti, F., et al. 2013. Characterization of the sensitization profile to lupin in peanut-allergic children and assessment of cross-reactivity risk. *Pediatr Allergy Immunol.* 24:270–275.
12. Bansal, A.S., Sanghvi, M.M., Bansal, R.A., & Hayman, G.R. 2014. Variably severe systemic allergic reactions after consuming foods with unlabeled lupin flour: A case series. *J Med Rep.* 8:55.
13. Barouki, R., Gluckman, P.D., Grandjean, P., Hanson, M., & Heindel, J.J. 2012. Developmental origins of non-communicable disease: Implications for research and public health. *Environm Health.* 11:42.
14. Baughan, S.J. 2002. What's under the coat of section 175.300? http://www.khlaw.com/showpublication.aspx?Show=2293.
15. Bellinger, D.C. 2011. A strategy for comparing the contributions of environmental chemicals and other risk factors to neurodevelopment of children. *Environmen Health Perspect.* 120:501–507.
16. Caldwell, K.L., Pan, Y., Mortensen, M.E., et al. 2013. Iodine status in pregnant women in the United States: National Children's Study and National Health and Nutrition Examination Survey. *Thyroid.* 23:927–937.
17. *Report to the U.S. Consumer Product Safety Commission by the Chronic Hazard Advisory Panel on Phthalates and Phthalate Alternatives.* 2014. Bethesda, MD: U.S. Consumer Product Safety Commission.
18. Consumer Product Safety Improvement Act of 2008. Public Law 110–314, 122 Stat. 3016. 15 USC 2051. 2008.
19. *Federal Register*, Vol. 81, No. 1. January 4, 2016, page 5.
20. Flavor and Extract Manufacturers Association. FEMA Flavor Ingredient Library FAQ. http://www.femaflavor.org/sites/default/files/linked_files/Library_FAQ_0.pdf.
21. Flavor and Extract Manufacturers Association. FEMA Flavor Ingredient Library. http://www.femaflavor.org/flavor.
22. Food Additive Amendment of 1958. July 28, 1958. Mr. Williams, from the Committee on Interstate and Foreign Commerce. 85th Congress, House of Representatives, Report No. 2284.

23. Hall, R.L., & Merwin, E.J. 1981. The role of flavors in food processing. *Food Technol.* 35:46.

24. Hallagan, J.B., & Hall, R.F. 2009. Under the conditions of intended use: New developments in the FEMA GRAS program and the safety assessment of flavor ingredients. *Food Chem Toxicol.* 47:267–278.

25. Investigation of the Use of Chemicals in Foods and Cosmetics. June 30, 1952. Mr. Delaney, from the Select Committee to Investigate the Use of Chemicals in Food and Cosmetics. 82d Congress, House of Representatives, Report No. 2356.

26. Kim, E. 2013, September 1. Processed food: A 2-million-year history. *Scientific American.*

27. Maffini, M.V., & Neltner, T.G. 2015. Brain drain: The cost of neglected responsibilities in evaluating cumulative effects of environmental chemicals. *J Epidemiol Commun Health.* 69:496–499.

28. Maffini, M.V., Alger, H.M., Bongard, E.D., & Neltner, T.G. 2011. Enhancing FDA's evaluation of science to ensure chemicals added to human food are safe: Workshop proceedings. *Compr Rev Food Sci Food Saf.* 10:321–341.

29. Maffini, M.V., Alger, H.M., Olson, E.D., & Neltner, T.G. 2013. Looking back to look forward: A review of FDA's food additives safety assessment and recommendations for modernizing its program. *Compr Rev Food Sci Food Saf.* 12:439–453.

30. Maffini, M.V., Trasande, L., & Neltner, T.G. 2016. Perchlorate and diet: Human exposures, risks, and mitigation strategies. *Curr Environ Health Rep.* 3:107–117.

31. Martinez Steele, E., Galastri Baraldi, L., da Costa Louzada, M.L., Moubarac, J.C., Mozaffarian, D., & Monteiro, C.A. 2016. Ultra-processed foods and added sugars in the US diet: Evidence from a nationally representative cross-sectional study. BMJ Open 6:e009892.

32. Matthews, J. 2011. *2011 Food and Health Survey: Consumer Attitudes Toward Food Safety, Nutrition and Health.* Washington, DC: International Food Information Council Foundation.

33. Miodovnik, A., Eduwards, A., Bellinger, D.C., & Hauser, R. 2014. Developmental neurotoxicity of ortho-phthalate diesters: Review of human and experimental evidence. *Neurotoxicology.* 41:112–122.

34. Moubarac, J.C., Parra, D.C., Cannon, G., & Monteiro, C.A. 2014. Food classification systems based on food processing: Significance and implications for policies and actions. A systematic literature review and assessment. *Curr Obes Rep.* 3:256–272.

35. National Academy of Sciences, National Research Council Committee on the Health Risks of Phthalates. 2008. *Phthalates and cumulative risk assessment: The tasks ahead.* Washington DC: The National Academies Press.

36. Natural Resources Defense Council et al. Filing of Food Additive Petition. Docket ID: FDA-2015-F-0714. https://www.regulations.gov/#!searchResults;rpp=25;po=0;s=FDA-2015-F-0714;fp=true;ns=true.

37. U.S. Food and Drug Administration. 2014. FDA Response to Natural Resources Defense Council's October, 2013, Freedom of Information Request No. 2013-8042: GRN-257, p. 206, www.nrdc.org/food/files/chemicals-in-food-FoIA-Main.pdf.

38. Neltner, T.G., Alger, H.M., Leonard, J.E., & Maffini, M.V. 2013. Data gaps in toxicity testing of chemicals allowed in food in the United States. *Reprod Toxicol.* 42:85–94.

39. Neltner, T.G., Alger, H.M., O'Reilly, J.D., Krimsky, S., Bero, L.A., & Maffini, M,V. 2013. Conflicts of interest in approvals of additives to food determined to be generally recognized as safe: Out of balance. *JAMA Intern Med.* 173:2032–2036.

40. Neltner, T.G., Kulkarni, N.R., Alger, H.M., et al. 2011. Navigating the US food additive regulatory program. *Compr Rev Food Sci Food Saf.* 10:342–368.

41. Neltner, T.G., Maffini, M.V. 2014. *Generally Recognized as Secret: Chemicals Added to Food in the United States.* Natural Resources Defense Council report. https://www.nrdc.org/sites/default/files/safety-loophole-for-chemicals-in-food-report.pdf.

42. Nixon, R.M. 1969, October 30. Special Message to the Congress on Consumer Protection. http://www.presidency.ucsb.edu/ws/index.php?pid=2299.

43. Public Law 85–929, 72 Stat. 1784, 21 USC §348. 1958.

44. Rose, S.R., & Brown, R.S. 2006. Update of newborn screening and therapy for congenital hypothyroidism. *Pediatrics.* 117:2290–2303.

45. Rubin, B.S., Lenkowski, J.R., Schaeberle, C.M., Vandenberg, L.N., Ronsheim, P.M., & Soto, A.M. 2006. Evidence of altered brain sexual differentiation in mice exposed perinatally to low, environmentally relevant levels of bisphenol A. *Endocrinology.* 147:3681–3691.

46. Select Committee on GRAS Substances (SCOGS). 1982. *Insights on Food Safety Evaluation.* Appendix, p 50. Springfield, VA: National Technical Information Service, U.S. Department of Commerce.

47. Shibko, S.I., & Blumenthal. H. 1973. Toxicology of phthalic acid esters used in food-packaging material. *Environ Health Perspect.* 3:131–137.

48. Swan, S.H., Liu, F., Hines, M., et al. 2010. Prenatal phthalate exposure and reduced masculine play in boys. *Int J Androl.* 33:259–269.

49. Swan, S.H. 2008. Environmental phthalates exposure in relation to reproductive outcomes and other health endpoints in humans. *Environ Res.* 108:177–184.

50. Trasande, L., Zoeller, R.T., Hass, U., et al. 2016. *Andrology.* 4:565–572.

51. U.S. Food and Drug Administration. GRAS Substances (SCOGS) database. http://www.fda.gov/food/ingredientspackaginglabeling/gras/scogs.

52. U.S. Food and Drug Administration. 2014. FDA Response to Natural Resources Defense Council's October, 2013, Freedom of Information Request No. 2013-8042: GRN-262, -263, -264, p. 218. www.nrdc.org/food/files/chemicals-in-food-FoIA-Main.pdf.

53. U.S. Food and Drug Administration. 2002. *Guidance for Industry: Preparation of Food Contact Notifications for Food Contact Substances—Toxicology Recommendations.* Silver Spring, MD: U.S. FDA.

54. U.S. Food and Drug Administration. 2005. Threshold of Regulation (TOR) Exemptions. TOR No. 2005-006: Sodium perchlorate monohydrate. http://www.accessdata.fda.gov/scripts/fdcc/?set=TOR&id=2005-006.

55. U.S. Food and Drug Administration. 2015, June 16. News release: The FDA takes steps to remove artificial *trans* fats in processed foods. http://www.fda.gov/NewsEvents/Newsroom/PressAnnouncements/ucm451237.htm.

56. U.S. Food and Drug Administration. 2016. Reference 4 Memorandum from P. Rice to P. Honigfort, July 27, 2015 re Indirect Food Additives: Paper and Paper Board Components. Docket FDA-2015-F-0714. https://www.regulations.gov/#!documentDetail;D=FDA-2015-F-0714-0016.

57. U.S. Food and Drug Administration. 2016. Final rule. Indirect Food Additives: Paper and Paperboard Components. Docket FDA-2015-F-0714. https://www.regulations.gov/#!documentDetail;D=FDA-2015-F-0714-0010.

58. U.S. Food and Drug Administration. 2013. *Food Labeling Guide.* http://www.fda.gov/Food/GuidanceRegulation/GuidanceDocumentsRegulatoryInformation/LabelingNutrition/ucm2006828.htm#background.

59. U.S. Food and Drug Administration. 2014. FDA Response to Natural Resources Defense Council's October, 2013, Freedom of Information Request No. 2013-8042: GRN-225, p. 197. www.nrdc.org/food/files/chemicals-in-food-FoIA-Main.pdf.

60. U.S. Food and Drug Administration. 2008. *GRAS Notices: GRN-257,* gamma-*Amino butyric acid.* Silver Spring, MD: U.S. FDA.

61. U.S. Food and Drug Administration. History of the GRAS List and SCOGS Review.http://www.fda.gov/Food/IngredientsPackagingLabeling/GRAS/SCOGS/ucm084142.htm.

62. Vogel, S. 2012. *Is it Safe?: BPA and the Struggle to Define the Safety of Chemicals.* Oakland, CA: University of California Press.

63. Watson, E. 2013. Researcher files lawsuit vs FDA after it ignored his petition calling for ban on artificial *trans* fats. *Food Navigator.*

64. World Health Organization. 2008. Assessment of Iodine Deficiency Disorders and Monitoring Their Elimination: A Guide for Programme Managers. 3rd ed. Geneva, Switzerland: WHO.

65. World Health Organization. 2014. *Global Status Report on Noncommunicable Diseases.* Geneva, Switzerland: WHO.

12

Classic Toxicology vs. New Science: Unique Issues of Endocrine-Disrupting Chemicals

LAURA N. VANDENBERG

Key Concepts

- Endocrine-disrupting chemicals (EDCs) interfere with one or more actions of hormones (e.g., binding, synthesis, secretion, transport, metabolism). Most EDCs identified to date are agonists or antagonists of estrogen, androgen, or thyroid hormone receptors.
- A large body of literature shows associations between EDC exposures and human diseases, and animal laboratory studies have shown that low doses of EDCs can disrupt developmental end points, reproduction, and metabolism.
- The methods that have traditionally been used to determine whether an environmental chemical is toxic have failed in the evaluation of EDCs because traditional screening programs are too insensitive and rely on assumptions that do not hold true for this class of compounds.
- Important issues have been raised about the evaluation of EDCs, including what makes a study good for safety assessment, the effects of EDCs at low doses, determination of chemical potency, nonmonotonic dose responses, and the level of evidence needed to determine whether harm has occurred.
- Improvements are needed, including better evaluations of EDC safety, changes in risk assessment that account for nonlinear dose responses, and inclusion of public health costs in cost-benefit analyses.

Introduction

Numerous scientific reports have concluded that many endocrine-related diseases and disorders are increasing in prevalence.[8] These conditions include infertility (i.e., male, female, and idiopathic); birth defects involving the male genital tract; neurobehavioral disorders, including attention deficit hyperactivity disorder and autism; asthma and autoimmune disorders; endocrine-related cancers of the breast, ovary, prostate, testes, and uterus; early puberty in females; aspects of metabolic syndrome, including obesity and type 2 diabetes; preterm birth and low birth weight; and gestational diabetes. Improved detection and changes in diagnostic criteria may account for some of these increases.

Because genetic changes are not sufficient to explain the increases in disease incidence observed over 3 to 4 decades, other environmental factors have been proposed to have etiologic roles. Changes in diet and exercise patterns are likely to be involved in some of these diseases, but these behavioral changes are not sufficient to account for the increases in disease incidences that have been observed in developed and developing nations.[45] For this reason, exposures to environmental chemicals have been investigated in controlled laboratory studies and in human populations. Environmental compounds, particularly chemicals that can mimic or disrupt the actions of hormones, can induce many of these conditions in laboratory animals. Epidemiologic studies also suggest associations between chemical exposures and disease outcomes.

This chapter describes the class of compounds called *endocrine-disrupting chemicals* (EDCs) and reviews how they are identified and why current methods of evaluation have failed to protect human and wildlife populations from harm. Suggestions are given for better risk assessment of chemicals to reduce disease burden through improved regulatory decision making. With better chemical safety assessments, many diseases of concern can be prevented.

The Early History of Endocrine-Disrupting Chemicals

In the 1960s, with the publication of Rachel Carson's book *Silent Spring*, the public became aware that exposures to chemicals in the environment could affect the health of wild animals with devastating effects. Carson used animal examples to illustrate the possibility that the widespread use of these compounds could also cause harm to human health. Carson pointed out that many chemicals used as pesticides altered metabolism and function of the nervous systems of exposed animals.

Perhaps one of the greatest causes for concern raised in *Silent Spring* was the ability of these compounds to bioaccumulate in the tissues of exposed creatures, which also contributed to compounding of the chemicals in the food chain. Pesticides that were applied to pests at the bottom of the food chain were detected in and affecting the health of creatures at the top of the food chain. Carson's work highlighted the problem in birds of prey, which were never the target of the applied pesticides but were drastically affected. Adverse effects included egg shell thinning (which contributed to decreased fecundity), neuromuscular diseases, wasting, and death. Carson documented that the chemical effects were most profound on developing creatures (e.g., embryos, hatchlings) rather than their parents.

After the publication of *Silent Spring*, environmental health scientists and wildlife biologists continued to describe the effects of environmental compounds on wildlife. One researcher, Theo Colborn, documented the effects of several chemicals on the health of wildlife in the Great Lakes area. Working with the World Wildlife Fund, Colborn wrote about the connections between environmental chemicals and disruptions of the endocrine system. Taking a broad approach, Colborn concluded that animals were affected by even low-level exposures to environmental chemicals in a variety of ways, including thyroid problems, diminished reproduction, altered neurobehaviors, and metabolic changes such as wasting. She pointed out that each of these factors is controlled by the endocrine system.

In 1991, Colborn summoned a group of 21 scientists with varied training and a diversity of backgrounds, including cancer biology, medicine, ecology, endocrinology, law, reproductive physiology, toxicology, wildlife conservation, and management, to the Wingspread Conference Center in Racine, Wisconsin. Each of the invited participants was asked to discuss his or her findings on the effects of environmental chemicals on a range of end points in cultured cells, laboratory animals, or human patients. The Wingspread meeting participants discussed the effects of environmental chemicals on sexual differentiation, reproductive function, neurobehavioral development, and autoimmune diseases. They drew parallels between the effects observed in wildlife and the health outcomes induced by developmental exposures to synthetic hormones, including diethylstilbestrol, a potent pharmaceutical estrogen.

By the end of the meeting, the scientists had agreed to write a consensus statement summarizing the state of the science on environmental chemicals. They wrote, "We are certain of the following: A large number of man-made chemicals that have been released into the environment, as well as a few natural ones, have the potential to disrupt the endocrine system of animals, including humans."[21] This was the first time that the term *endocrine disruptor* was used, and Colborn and other Wingspread participants became the leaders in their study, continuing to use approaches from a range of scientific fields.

Defining Endocrine Disruptors

Since the term *endocrine disruptor* was first used, many definitions have been proposed by various groups and agencies. One of the first definitions, used by EPA scientists beginning in 1996, categorized an endocrine disruptor as "an exogenous agent that interferes with the synthesis, secretion, transport, binding, action, or elimination of natural hormones in the body, which are responsible for the maintenance of homeostasis, reproduction, development, and/or behavior."[39] Other groups subsequently defined endocrine disruptors using different language, including the World Health Organization (WHO) and International Programme on Chemical Safety (IPCS): "An exogenous substance or mixture that alters function(s) of the endocrine system and consequently causes adverse effects in an intact organism, its progeny, or subpopulations. A potential endocrine disruptor is an exogenous substance or mixture that possesses properties that might be expected to lead to endocrine disruption in an intact organism, its progeny, or (sub)populations."[22] In 2012, scientists associated with The Endocrine Society simplified these definitions, writing that EDCs were "compounds or mixtures of compounds that interfere in some way with hormone action."[80]

Not only are different definitions used by different regulatory agencies in different jurisdictions, the definitions have different requirements for determining whether a chemical should be considered an EDC.[79] For example, the WHO/IPCS definition of an EDC involves a three-step process: a compound must induce an adverse effect, it must have a demonstrated endocrine mechanism of action, and there must be a plausible link between the adverse effect that is observed and the endocrine mechanism of action. Contrasted with the U.S. EPA's definition, which requires only that a compound be demonstrated to disrupt one or more actions of natural hormones in the body, the WHO/IPCS definition has very different data and evidence requirements for drawing conclusions about the endocrine-disrupting potential of an emerging compound.[10] There has been significant controversy about the use of these definitions because use of one can lead to the characterization of a compound as an EDC, but use of a different definition can prevent its identification as an EDC.

There is also significant debate about the definition and use of the term *adverse.*[6,68] For example, the U.S. EPA defines an *adverse effect* as "any effect resulting in anatomical, functional, or psychological impairment that may affect the performance of the whole organism." Groups have found that the term typically relates to overt signs of toxicity (e.g., significant loss of body weight, altered organ weight) that are separated from signs of disease. Some effects of chemicals that the general public would describe as adverse (e.g., migraine headaches, obesity, gastrointestinal distress) have been dismissed as nonadverse by regulatory agencies such as the U.S. Food and Drug Administration (FDA).[46]

Environmental health scientists, experts from The Endocrine Society, and other biomedical professionals have pushed for the FDA and other regulatory agencies to accept 21st century science. Many of these groups have argued that the FDA must acknowledge that a narrow view, focused solely on overt signs of toxicity (e.g., death, severe loss of body weight, palpable tumors), is not sufficient to evaluate chemical safety.[23,27,28,59,75,80]

State of the Science for Endocrine-Disrupting Chemicals

With more than 80,000 chemicals in commerce, tests to determine which compounds should be classified as EDCs have been limited by financial and logistical constraints. Despite restrictions to comprehensive testing, the FDA identified more than 1000 chemicals as actual or putative EDCs based on their ability to bind to three hormone receptors: estrogen, androgen, and thyroid hormone.[64] This has also proved to be a limitation because many hormone and receptor components of the endocrine system have not been evaluated.

It is anticipated that the chemicals found in the FDA's Endocrine Disruptor Knowledge Base are only a fraction of the total number of compounds with endocrine-disrupting properties. For example, chemicals that bind to the peroxisome proliferator–activated receptor-γ (PPARγ) alter differentiation of mesenchymal stem cells, biasing them toward the adipocyte lineage, increasing adiposity, and inducing obesity.[30,34,35] Some chemicals can interfere with glucocorticoid and mineralocorticoid receptors. EDCs that act through mechanisms other than receptor binding (e.g., interfering with hormone synthesis or plasma transport) are also not represented in the FDA's Endocrine Disruptor Knowledge Base and are unlikely to be identified by the screening assays currently in use by regulatory agencies around the world.

EDCs, including compounds identified by the FDA, EPA, and other agencies, are used in a range of industry and consumer products, including insecticides, herbicides, plasticizers, industrial chemicals, detergents, preservatives, personal care products, flame retardants, and resins. Human exposures to many of these compounds have been documented in biomonitoring studies. Exposures to other compounds are anticipated based on their use (e.g., foods, personal care products, and pesticides used in and around homes).

Numerous reports have summarized the state of the science concerning EDCs. A report published in February 2013 by the United Nations Environment Programme (UNEP) and WHO, entitled "State of the Science of Endocrine-Disrupting Chemicals–2012,"[77] was an update of the IPCS/WHO 2002 report, "Global Assessment of the State of-the-Science of Endocrine Disruptors." Using the available evidence, the 2013 UNEP/WHO report drew several key conclusions:

- Based on data generated in controlled laboratory studies, chemicals can contribute to endocrine disorders. Many of these diseases have been observed in humans and wildlife.
- Wildlife populations have been affected by EDC exposures, with negative effects on growth and reproduction.
- The methods that are widely used and accepted for identifying EDCs examine only limited end points and capture only a small fraction of the known spectrum of endocrine-disrupting effects. The evaluative methods are likely to be underestimating the harmful effects of EDCs.
- The increased risk of diseases due to EDC exposures may be significantly underestimated by regulatory agencies around the world.

Controversy Generated by Manufactured Doubt

After publication of the 2013 UNEP/WHO report[77] and other large-scale reviews of the EDC literature,[23,43,67,80] criticisms were raised about the way in which conclusions were drawn. Critics of these reports condemned the use of narrative reviews rather than a systematic approach employing prespecified criteria for the selection of studies to be included. They suggested that the science was not conclusive, accused the UNEP/WHO authors of ignoring studies that did not support their conclusions, and implied that the authors did not have the expertise to evaluate the literature.[4,24,44]

The strong critiques of state-of-science documents have come from individuals with ties to industries and with financial stakes in preventing action against EDCs.[29] For example, an investigative reporter found that undisclosed conflicts of interest were identified for almost all authors of a criticism of the UNEP/WHO report. These conflicts included accepting large sums of money to consult for the pesticide industry, chemical manufacturers, and others.[31,32]

The concept of manufactured doubt has its roots in the actions taken by the tobacco industry. Long after their own scientists and physicians knew about the links between tobacco use and serious diseases, including lung cancer, numerous tobacco companies colluded to cast doubt on studies conducted by academics or scientists affiliated with government agencies. They produced conflicting studies and manipulated data to compete with widespread scientific and medical consensus. It has been suggested that the chemical industry is co-opting many of the same techniques to prevent action against EDCs.[7,52] Many of the attacks on state-of-science documents and other influential scientific pieces can be described as carefully crafted examples of manufactured doubt, designed to prevent regulatory action and protect consumer products and company profits.

Challenges to Identifying Endocrine-Disrupting Chemicals

To determine whether chemicals have endocrine-disrupting activity, the EPA developed the Endocrine Disruptor Screening Program (EDSP) based on the Food Quality Protection Act (FQPA) passed by Congress in 1996. The EDSP includes assays that are split into two tiers. Tier 1 includes in vitro and in vivo assays that allow identification of chemicals that have the potential to interact with estrogen, androgen, and thyroid systems. Other aspects of the endocrine system are not evaluated in the EDSP assays, and it has been argued that evaluations of thyroid hormone end points are very limited.[78,80] The end points evaluated in tier 1 are not necessarily considered *adverse* according to the EPA's definition, but chemicals that are identified as *positive* in tier 1 assays are further evaluated using the assays in tier 2. Tier 2 involves more complex tools to evaluate whether chemicals induce adverse effects, as defined by the EPA.

In tier 1, the 11 assays employed can ascertain whether chemicals interfere with estrogen, androgen, or thyroid hormone signaling. There are three cell-fraction in vitro assays: the estrogen receptor binding assay, the androgen receptor binding assay, and the aromatase assay (i.e., aromatase converts androgens to estrogens). There are two whole-cell in vitro assays: the estrogen receptor transcriptional assay and the steroidogenesis assay, which evaluates a compound's ability to induce the production of estradiol or testosterone, or both. There are six whole-animal in vivo tests: the uterotrophic assay, which evaluates the ability of compounds to act as estrogens; the Hershberger assay, which evaluates the ability of compounds to act as androgens or anti-androgens; the pubertal female assay, which evaluates interactions between chemicals and thyroid and estrogen signaling pathways; the pubertal male assay, which evaluates effects of chemicals on thyroid and androgen pathways; the fish short-term reproduction assay, which focuses on the hypothalamic-pituitary-gonadal axis; and the amphibian metamorphosis assay, which evaluates thyroid hormone disruption. The mixture of in vitro and in vivo assays is meant to provide evaluative tools to determine whether the metabolites of chemicals have endocrine-disrupting properties in addition to the test compound itself.

Tier 2 assays are more complex and use formalized test guidelines that are internationally recognized and validated by groups including the EPA and the Organisation for Economic Co-operation and Development (OECD). Test guidelines use internationally approved methods to examine end points that are widely acknowledged to represent toxicologically relevant (adverse) effects. For example, in a standard one-generation assay, adult male and female rodents are exposed to a test compound for 2 weeks before mating. Exposures continue through mating, pregnancy, and lactation; after weaning, the offspring continue to be exposed through puberty and adulthood.

Traditional measures of toxicity are assessed in the parental generation, including body weight, weights of organs, measures of clinical chemistry (e.g., serum cholesterol, measures of oxidative stress), and reproductive measures (e.g., time to pregnancy, length of pregnancy, number of live pups, sex of offspring). Other developmental measures are evaluated in the offspring, including the incidence and type of birth defects and overt signs of neurotoxicity (e.g., seizures, abnormal posture), body weights, organ weights, and measures of clinical chemistry. Gross morphology of organs is evaluated at the time of euthanasia, and some minor histopathologic evaluations are conducted. In a standard two-generation assay, exposures continue as the F1-generation offspring are mated, and the F2-generation offspring (i.e., grandchildren) are also evaluated.

By definition, the end points included in guideline assays have been replicated in laboratories around the world.[62] Their highly reproducible nature is their major advantage, but there are many concerns about guideline assays, including those that have been included in the EDSP (i.e., tier 1 and tier 2).[48,49,80] For example, in contrast to the assumption that these assays are highly reproducible, there was significant variability in the responses observed in participating contract laboratories when the uterotrophic assay (i.e., EDSP tier 1 assay widely used to assess estrogenic activity) was validated.[37] During validation, 10 laboratories tested nonylphenol on the immature rat and used subcutaneous dosing.[37] One laboratory identified the lowest observed effective concentration (LOEC) as 35 mg/kg/day, five as 80 mg/kg/day, and one as 100 mg/kg/day. Three other laboratories were unable to identify a LOEC; one failed to include the highest dose, another did not conduct the study appropriately (i.e., forgot to weigh the animals), and the third found no effect at any of the five doses administered (up to 100 mg/kg/day).

Other issues with variations in EDSP tier 1 assays suggest other problems. For example, the shape of the dose-response curve can differ significantly between replicates produced by the same laboratory for guideline studies such as the steroidogenesis assay.[66] Several end points were rejected from inclusion in guideline assays (i.e., tools to evaluate serum hormone concentrations) because contract laboratories reported unacceptably high levels of interassay variability.[13] This issue is highly concerning in the context of clinical assays that are used to measure blood hormone levels. They have been used since the 1960s and are conducted worldwide with strict performance standards in clinical laboratories. However, researchers in contract laboratories continue to argue that these assays are too complicated and there are too many reproducibility issues to include hormone assays in guideline study protocols.[13] This provides important insight into the skill level in commercial toxicology laboratories.

Although the end points examined in tier 2 guideline studies are typically taken as reasonably adequate indictors of toxicity,[63] they have proved to be poor predictors of endocrine-disrupting properties and endocrine diseases.[80] There are also concerns that these kinds of end points do not adequately map to relevant human diseases. For example, there is no end point regularly included in a tier 2 test guideline that evaluates reproductive senescence, asthma, autism, or endometriosis. There are also concerns that tier 2 evaluations do not examine whether chemical exposures sensitize animals to subsequent environmental challenges, even though it is widely accepted that an increased responsiveness to secondary stressors would be considered adverse. Tier 2 assays also do not appropriately evaluate whether EDCs contribute to cancers, metabolic diseases, or other conditions that have raised concern about the safety of EDCs in human populations.[48,49,70,73] Guideline studies typically examine a limited number of very high doses based on the maximum tolerated dose that causes adverse effects but does not result in death, making it difficult to determine the true nature of a dose-response curve.

The EDSP tier 1 and tier 2 assays cannot be considered state-of-the-art science. Some assays, such as the rodent uterotrophic assay, were developed more than 80 years ago.[16,26] There have been strong calls for the development and use of evaluative tools that rely on modern scientific knowledge from the fields of endocrinology and toxicology. For example, a series of high-throughput methods were developed for the U.S. National Toxicology Program and the EPA's screening programs, called Tox21 and ToxCast, respectively.[3,11,15,25,38,41] These approaches use a large number of assays, typically requiring cell fractions or whole cells, although some involve whole organisms (e.g., zebrafish embryos).

The assays developed are designed to measure the ability of test compounds to act as nuclear hormone receptor agonists or antagonists. A small number of assays also evaluate steroidogenesis end points. Although some of the assays appear to improve on the EDSP tier 1 assays (i.e., those that evaluate estrogen and androgen receptors[56,57]), other assays that evaluate additional nuclear receptors (i.e., 9-*cis* retinoic acid receptor and the peroxisome proliferator–activated receptor[36]) have significant flaws that must be addressed before these high-throughput methods are used to screen thousands of compounds. Although the EPA has proposed a series of ToxCast assays to replace the estrogenic assays in the EDSP tier 1,[14] additional improvements are needed before these assays can be relied on for detecting EDCs and making regulatory decisions.[36]

Validated screening methods are available only for a very limited number of endocrine end points. Databases compiled by the FDA estimate that at least 1000 chemicals may have endocrine-disrupting properties, but these are limited to compounds that act as agonists and antagonists of the estrogen, androgen, and thyroid hormone receptors. Most EDCs that have been identified are hormone receptor agonists or antagonists, but the classification of compounds as endocrine disruptors must also include compounds that act by altering hormone production, release, transport, metabolism, or elimination,[39] and additional tools must be developed to probe each of these hormone actions.

Studying Endocrine-Disrupting Chemicals: Operating at the Interface of Scientific Fields

Continued interest in EDCs is driven by hundreds of striking epidemiologic studies showing associations between EDC exposures and adverse outcomes in human populations. Many of these associations have been followed by laboratory animal studies. It is widely acknowledged that the study of EDCs, like the study of many other environmental factors, operates at the intersection of observational studies (i.e., epidemiologic and wildlife) and experimental studies, which typically use cultured cells and laboratory animals, although intervention studies from human and wildlife populations are occasionally available.

Less acknowledged is the importance of different scientific disciplines and approaches in experimental laboratory studies. Although endocrinologists seem to be the likely participants in scientific debate and discussion about EDCs, they are often excluded from the regulatory decision-making process.[28,68] The underlying scientific principles understood by toxicologists and endocrinologists are quite different and can be at odds with each other. Understanding these driving forces is essential to identify common ground between the disciplines and allow progress to be made on chemical regulations for which there is not common ground.

PRINCIPLES OF TOXICOLOGY

The field of toxicology was developed for determining the hazards associated with chemical exposures. Several principles guide the study of chemical exposures.

Relationship Between Dose and Effect. The observed toxicologic response is expected to be positively associated with the amount of exposure, with a monotonic (and oftentimes linear) relationship observed between the two factors. This relationship is sometimes referred to as "the dose makes the poison" meaning that higher exposures are expected to be associated with worse health outcomes. The effect that is examined can be quantal (e.g., life or death, tumor or no tumor) or continuous (e.g., organ weight, measures of fecundity). Effects can be characterized as acute (i.e., rapidly developing), subacute (i.e., less severe than acute), or chronic (i.e., progressing at a slow and varying rate). Because a monotonic relationship is assumed across the entire dose range, the ability to use linear extrapolation from very high to very low doses is a core assumption.[67]

Characterization of Exposures. Exposures can be separated in toxicologic experiments based on duration (i.e., acute, subacute, subchronic, and chronic). They also can be differentiated based on the route of exposure (i.e., oral, intravenous, intramuscular, dermal, inhalation, or subcutaneous). In the evaluation of chemicals for the purposes of regulatory toxicology, the default exposure route for all chemicals is by (oral) intragastric gavage, regardless of whether the chemical is used as a food additive or an additive in cosmetics.[71] Calculations of human exposures are typically based on models, not data, because there are few chemicals for which all routes of exposure are documented.[70] This occurs because confidentiality laws protect corporations from having to provide this information for most chemicals.

Absorption, Distribution, Metabolism, and Excretion. Compounds are studied and understood based on their absorption, distribution in the body, metabolism, and excretion from the body (ADME). ADME can be influenced by the physiologic state of the individual (e.g., a young person with diminished metabolic capacities) and the physiochemical properties of the compound (e.g., lipophilic versus hydrophilic substances). Traditionally, toxicologic studies have not focused on sensitive periods in development and have focused on relatively short-term exposures to assess health hazards in early adulthood.

Tissue-Specific Sensitivities. Although some toxicants induce general toxic effects, many induce effects that are tissue or organ specific. Some specificity is based on the route of exposure (e.g., lungs as the entry point for exposures to aerosols), the chemical's accumulation in a specific tissue, enzymes in specific organs that metabolize a compound to a more active form, specific receptors in a tissue or organ, and other factors, including physiologic sensitivities (e.g., changes in the production of metabolizing enzymes during pregnancy).

KEY ENDOCRINE PRINCIPLES

EDCs can be studied and understood using the toxicologic principles described here, and they can be examined considering the principles of endocrinology.[5,28,49,68,80] Five major principles dictate the study of hormones:

1. **Hormones coordinate the tissues of the body.** Although the endocrine system is often thought of as a mediator of homeostasis, it is more accurate to consider the changing role of hormones in the coordination of body tissues from conception until death. Hormones are responsible for proper functioning of virtually all organs of the body, and they are essential for reproduction, embryonic and fetal development, and puberty. Hormonal changes also play a role in aging.
2. **Receptor binding is required for hormone signaling.** Hormones act by highly specific interactions with receptors. Hormones have high affinity for their own receptors, allowing cells that express these receptors to be responsive to the hormone, whereas cells that do not express the receptor are unaffected. However, as the concentration of a hormone increases, it can bind to other receptors, which would not normally occur within the physiologic range of the hormone. This receptor cross-talk is expected when very high doses of hormones, hormonally active drugs, or hormonally active EDCs are administered.
3. **Hormones are potent signaling molecules**. Hormones act at exceptionally low doses, typically in part-per-billion or part-per-trillion

concentrations. There is a nonlinear relationship between the hormone concentration and the percentage of receptors that are occupied, and there is a nonlinear relationship between the number of receptors that are occupied and the biologic effect. Modulation of the biologic response to a hormone is influenced by three factors: concentration of the hormones in blood or target tissues, number of receptors, and expression of unique co-regulatory proteins that have a significant impact on potency.

4. **Hormones can permanently alter organisms if exposures occur during critical periods of development**. It has been known for many decades that the effects of hormones are life stage dependent. One hormone can have different effects on adults than on developing embryos, fetuses, or neonates, even if the level of exposure is the same. The effects of hormones on adults are called *activational* because the individual responds only during the period of exposure. The effects of hormones during development are called *organizational* because they can permanently alter the identity and function of cells, tissues, and organs.

5. **Nonlinear and nonmonotonic dose responses are common**. Hormones rarely exhibit linear relationships between dose and effect if a sufficient range of doses is evaluated. Instead, nonlinear and nonmonotonic dose responses are common. Several mechanisms are responsible for nonlinear responses, including receptor downregulation, receptor desensitization, activation of endocrine negative feedback loops, and competition between overlapping biologic responses that are each monotonic. For EDCs, nonmonotonic dose-response relationships should be expected and not considered as exceptions.

COMPETING APPROACHES OF ENDOCRINOLOGY AND TOXICOLOGY

Although the principles of toxicology and endocrinology can be relevant to the study and hazard assessments of EDCs, some of the principles from the two fields are in conflict with each other. For this reason, risk assessments that only consider the perspectives from one scientific field are likely to be at odds with evaluations that consider the alternative field. In this section, we discuss the issues that are disputed between the fields of toxicology and endocrinology. The issues are important to the evaluation of chemical safety, particularly EDC safety.

Issue 1: What are the Necessary Components of a Good Study? Regulatory toxicology has relied on a method developed by industry scientists to determine whether a study is deemed of high enough quality to be included in a risk assessment evaluation. This method, called the Klimisch score, evaluates studies based on their adherence to good laboratory practices (GLP).[40] GLP involves are record-keeping methods that were developed in response to widespread fraud in contract and industry toxicology laboratories. It is a resource-intensive means of ensuring that fraud has not occurred, but it does not ensure that studies are well designed or conducted.[48] Because academic laboratories are rarely equipped or provided the funding to conduct studies according to GLPs, the Klimisch method typically awards the highest quality scores to industry-funded studies. When risk assessments identify a single key study on which to base their evaluations, this often means that a GLP-compliant, industry-funded study is considered the best for making regulatory decisions.[10]

Endocrinologists and environmental health scientists reject the Klimisch score,[10,48,79] instead raising a number of study design issues that should be considered when assessing the quality of experimental EDC studies. First, to ensure that the experimental system was capable of responding to hormones, there must be a positive (significant) effect of the test chemical or a known positive control. Second, studies should include a positive control that shows significant effects at low doses. If no effects are observed in the low-dose range for the positive control, it suggests that the experimental system (or animal species or animal strain) is not appropriate for the assessment of hormones or EDCs. Third, negative controls, which are treated the same way as the test group (with the exception of the compound administered), are required and should be run concurrently with the test chemical. Negative control groups should account for all other variations in the experiment, including housing conditions, feed, water, environmental stresses, and handling. In a controlled laboratory experiment, the negative control should remain truly unexposed to the compound of interest. This can be challenging for many EDCs, which can be found in environmental media, feed, and water. However, if no effects of the test compound are observed and the negative control group is contaminated (even with low levels of the compound), the result could confound data analysis, and the study must be considered to have failed.[33]

Issue 2: Can We Prioritize EDCs by Levels of Exposure? Biomonitoring studies have revealed blood, urine, and tissue concentrations of EDCs typically in the part-per-trillion and part-per-billion range, although some values are as high as parts per million.[17–19,76] Although these studies indicate that exposures are occurring, it has been argued that exposures are so low that they are inconsequential. Although it can be argued that the presence of a chemical is not sufficient evidence that harm will occur from exposures, it similarly cannot be concluded that exposures are too low to cause concern. This is especially true for compounds that interact with the endocrine system; because hormones are active at very low concentrations, compounds that similarly interact with the endocrine system (e.g., EDCs) are also expected to act at low doses. Large amounts of data support this presumption.[65] In endocrine studies, the parts-per-million (i.e., 1 μg/mL) serum concentration range of a chemical is seen for hormones such as estradiol, which is a million times higher than the bioactive concentration in women. However, this very low concentration is typically considered safe for estrogenic EDCs even though they are bioactive in the parts-per-trillion range.[69]

Issue 3: Can We Prioritize EDCs by Their Relative Potency or Ignore Certain EDCs Because of Weak Properties? EDCs that mimic endogenous hormones are often described by comparing their binding affinity with the binding affinity of the natural hormone (e.g., chemical X is a weak estrogen compared to 17β-estradiol, the endogenous ligand). *Binding affinity* describes the concentration of the ligand that is required to occupy 50% of the receptors. *Potency* describes the concentration of a compound that is required to produce a biologic effect at a given intensity. The affinity of a hormone or an EDC for the receptor is a constant, whereas the potency of a hormone depends on the end point being examined. This means that descriptors of the potency of an EDC based on one assay (e.g., compound Y is a weak estrogen in the uterotrophic assay) cannot predict its potency in another assay (e.g., compound Y is a potent estrogen in a fetal tissue during organogenesis).

Potency can be used to prioritize compounds for regulatory action, as has been proposed by some toxicologists,[4] but to do so, endocrinologists argue that the most sensitive end points should be used for prioritization. For example, the EDC bisphenol A (BPA) has been described as very weak compared with 17β-estradiol. It has a binding affinity for the estrogen receptor that is approximately 1/10,000th that of the endogenous estrogen. In the uterotrophic assay, BPA must be administered at doses 10,000 to 50,000 times higher than that of 17β-estradiol to induce the same effect. For other end points, BPA appears to have equipotency to 17β-estradiol. Endocrinologists argue that if these more sensitive end points were used, BPA would not be classified as a weak estrogen.[69,80] Unfortunately, the most sensitive end points are not included in GLP guideline-compliant studies funded by industry and accepted by regulatory agencies such as the FDA.

Issue 4: Can We Predict Safe Doses by Studying Only Very High Doses? The toxicologic dogma that the dose makes the poison does not hold true for many vitamins, essential nutrients, pharmaceuticals, or hormones. Nonmonotonic dose responses are defined by a dose-response curve in which the slope of the line changes sign (i.e., positive to negative or vice versa) along the range of tested doses[42] (Fig. 12.1). These dose-response shapes are common for hormones and EDCs.[67] The mechanisms responsible for these curves have been described by endocrinologists. Many of the same end points shown to produce nonmonotonic responses after endogenous hormone treatments also display nonmonotonic dose responses after EDC exposures.

Nonmonotonic dose responses challenge the traditional methods of regulatory toxicology and risk assessment. In experiments conducted as part of a typical chemical risk assessment, three high doses usually are administered to animals. The lower end of these limited number of doses (typically in the 1 mg/kg body weight range) produce few or no overt signs of toxicity and are used as points of departure from which safe doses are calculated. For example, a guideline study might find no effects of a chemical at dose X on body weight, organ weight, or the incidence of gross malformations. A risk

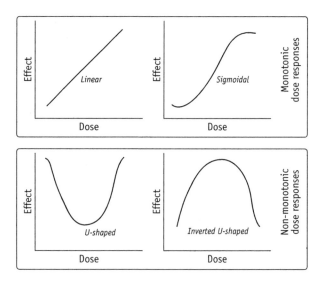

FIGURE 12.1. Examples of monotonic and nonmonotonic dose-response curve shapes. Linear and sigmoidal curves are classified as monotonic dose responses because the sign of the slope does not change (i.e., the direction of change does not reverse). Both of the two monotonic curves shown here have a positive slope. Nonmonotonic curves are often described as biphasic, U-shaped, or inverted U-shaped, although they also can have more complicated shapes.

assessor then takes dose X and divides it by a set of uncertainty factors (using the assumption that linear extrapolation is valid) to account for a number of uncontrolled variables (e.g., genetic diversity within the population, concerns for vulnerable populations such as children, extrapolations from animals to humans). The final calculated dose, called the *reference dose* in the United States or the *tolerable daily intake dose* in the European Union (EU) and elsewhere, is anticipated to be safe for humans, although it is never directly tested.

When nonmonotonic dose responses are seen, the doses that are anticipated to be safe can instead induce harm.[67] A striking example of this is the estrogenic drug tamoxifen. At high doses, tamoxifen inhibits proliferation of breast cancer cells, but there is a large body of literature on tamoxifen flare, which shows that low doses of this drug stimulate proliferation of the same cells.[2,53] If tamoxifen were treated like an environmental chemical, using the traditional toxicologic approach would place the calculated safe dose directly in the middle of the flare reaction (i.e., stimulation of metastatic cancer cells).[55,67] Similar examples of non-monotonicity have been observed for other EDCs.

Issue 5: When Must Effects Manifest to be Considered Evidence of Harm? The fields of toxicology and endocrinology acknowledge that there are vulnerable periods of development, during which animals are more sensitive to chemicals with specific characteristics. For example, the effects of teratogens are severe and profound when exposures occur during embryonic or fetal development, but they can have much less severe effects when exposures occur during adulthood. A classic example, thalidomide, highlights this age-specific effect.[47,72] The effects of teratogen exposures are apparent and visible at birth, often manifesting as severe birth defects. However, thalidomide, an angiogenesis inhibitor and antineoplastic agent, is used safely to treat erythema nodosum leprosum, multiple myeloma, and other diseases in adults.

EDCs are not teratogens; individuals exposed to EDCs during development can have a normal appearance at birth, with adverse effects manifesting only at puberty or in adulthood. The developmental origins of health and disease (DOHaD) theory proposes that many diseases that typically develop in adulthood (e.g. cancer, metabolic syndrome) originate much earlier in life.

One of the earliest examples of DOHaD was observed in women who were prescribed diethylstilbestrol (DES) during pregnancy. This potent synthetic estrogen was mistakenly thought to prevent spontaneous abortion. Although the mothers were relatively unharmed by exposures (there is some evidence that they had a moderately increased risk of breast cancer), the DES daughters exposed in utero had much more severe health outcomes, including increased incidence of rare vaginal cancers, malformations of the female reproductive tract, infertility, altered timing of menopause, and more than 40 years after exposure as a fetus, increased risk of breast cancer.[60] These outcomes were not apparent until the exposed daughters reached puberty, attempted to become pregnant, or reached the age at which menopause occurs. Physicians delivering these babies did not notice any abnormality on gross external examination, which is the only outcome used in standard toxicologic testing for risk assessments.

The tragic history of DES and emerging examples of nonpharmaceutical EDCs indicate that the harm from exposures can often take months to manifest in exposed laboratory animals and decades to manifest in exposed humans.[20,51] For example, pregnant mice exposed to very low doses of BPA during pregnancy exhibited diabetes 4 months postpartum.[1] Diseases with a long latency should not be dismissed, even when the temporal relationship to EDC exposures can require extensive efforts to establish.

A Proposed Path Forward

EDCs challenge many of the classic approaches in toxicology, including the expectation of a linear dose-response curve, the belief in using linear extrapolation to calculate a threshold safe dose that is never tested for safety, and the end points used to evaluate harm. Many groups are dedicated to improving how EDCs are evaluated, with the ultimate goal of improving the health of the public by the reduction of EDC exposures. One such effort aims to improve premarket testing of compounds using more appropriate evaluative tools, such as moving beyond guideline end points to include sensitive, state-of-the-art assays.

A group of environmental health scientists and green chemists developed the tiered protocol for endocrine disruption (TiPED), a series of assays to evaluate endocrine-disrupting properties. The TiPED approach can be used to assess the safety of chemicals before their use or to evaluate compounds that are already on the market.[58] Using TiPED, chemicals are evaluated with in silico assays (e.g., quantitative structure-activity relationships), followed by in vitro screening methods, followed by medium-throughput in vivo evaluations (e.g., fish assays), and then in vivo assays that incorporate guideline and nonguideline end points. What distinguishes TiPED from other evaluative approaches (e.g., EDSP tier 1 and tier 2 assays) is that the assays are ordered from least complex or expensive to most complex or expensive. Chemists are encouraged to redesign their chemical as soon as it receives a positive response in any assay. If the positive response is obtained in an early assay (including in silico assays), the chemist saves time and money by not continuing to test the compound (hoping for a better response) but rather focusing on the compounds with few or no hazards identified.

The TiPED approach also addresses the need to identify and use the most appropriate, disease-oriented, predictive, sensitive end points. Efforts to improve guideline assays have been undertaken in collaborations across government agencies and academic laboratories in the United States[12] Although some of these efforts have been hampered by technical and experimental constraints (e.g., contamination of negative control animals[33]), the ultimate goal is to determine whether end points that have previously revealed effects of low doses of EDCs can be added to traditional guideline studies. It does appear that this can be done, although it would be best to involve government agencies (e.g., the U.S. National Toxicology Program) without a particular stake in the study's outcomes (i.e., agencies that are not responsible for the regulation of the chemical being studied) instead of the EPA or FDA. These agencies have assured the American public that chemicals that have never been tested for health effects are safe.[50] Regulatory agencies are likely concerned that acknowledging that an unknown number of chemicals (and EDCs in particular) are not safe at the exposures predicted from traditional toxicologic testing would lead to widespread distrust of any future risk assessments that they conducted.

Other simple steps can be taken to improve how risk assessments are conducted. One is to increase the use of systematic review criteria, including transparent and disclosed methods for data selection and analysis.[74] Risk evaluations should no longer be made based on one key study, but rather they should incorporate all available data.[9] It is common for risk assessments to use unpublished (and unavailable to the public) industry studies in chemical risk assessments, but this practice should not be allowed because there is no method for independent analysis of the quality of the data.

When cost-benefit analyses are conducted for EDCs and other environmental hazards, the cost of inaction should be evaluated. Current analyses of the costs of regulating chemicals evaluate only the costs to industry, calculating the economic consequences of removing a chemical from the market, and these estimates by industry have been shown to be grossly inflated (see Pope and Dockery's estimates related to the costs of regulating air pollutants[54]). The cost to public health and the environment of keeping the chemical on the market and the savings in health care costs that could be realized by eliminating exposures to the chemical are ignored. An analysis of the annual costs of EDCs on health outcomes in the EU was estimated as €157 billion,[61] making the cost of inaction very high. The public is generally unaware that cost-benefit analysis limited only to costs for a few corporations, not public health costs, is a determining factor in whether chemicals are or are not regulated.

Conclusions

Hundreds of environmental epidemiologic studies have suggested associations between EDC exposures and disease outcomes in human populations. Although individual studies may have limitations, as a body of literature, they cannot be dismissed or ignored. They highlight that the traditional approaches that have been used to prioritize chemicals for regulation and the methods used to calculate safe levels of exposure are flawed.

Issues discussed in this chapter underscore how traditional means of risk assessment and regulation have failed to protect the public from EDCs. They include conflation of the potency of hormone-mimicking chemicals with binding affinity, an inability to detect and acknowledge nonmonotonic dose responses, failure to identify sensitive disease-oriented end points, flaws in guideline studies, ignorance of low-dose effects, heavy reliance on GLPs, and the failure to use systematic review criteria.

Although not systematically investigated, chemicals that are not EDCs may also be affected by these flaws. EDCs provide a compelling case for why change is needed in current regulatory practices. A greater awareness of the limitations of current chemical risk assessment approaches and the need for vigilance with regard to exposure to endocrine-disrupting chemicals is critical for maintaining a healthy population.

REFERENCES

1. Alonso-Magdalena, P., Vieira, E., Soriano, S., et al. 2010. Bisphenol A exposure during pregnancy disrupts glucose homeostasis in mothers and adult male offspring. *Environ Health Perspect.* 118:1243–1250.
2. Arnold, D.J., Markham, M.J., & Hacker, S. 1979. Tamoxifen flare. *JAMA.* 241:2506.
3. Attene-Ramos, M.S., Miller, N., Huang, R., et al. 2013. The Tox21 robotic platform for the assessment of environmental chemicals: From vision to reality. *Drug Discov Today.* 18:716–723.
4. Autrup, H., Barile, F.A., Blaauboer, B.J., et al. 2015. Principles of pharmacology and toxicology also govern effects of chemicals on the endocrine system. *Toxicol Sci.* 146:11–15.
5. Beausoleil, C., Ormsby, J.N., Gies, A., et al. 2013. Low dose effects and non-monotonic dose responses for endocrine active chemicals: Science to practice workshop. Workshop summary. *Chemosphere.* 93:847–856.

6. Bergman, A., Andersson, A.M., Becher, G., et al. 2013. Science and policy on endocrine disrupters must not be mixed: A reply to a "common sense" intervention by toxicology journal editors. *Environ Health*. 12:69.

7. Bergman, A., Becher, G., Blumberg, B., et al. 2015. Manufacturing doubt about endocrine disrupter science: A rebuttal of industry-sponsored critical comments on the UNEP/WHO report "State of the Science of Endocrine Disrupting Chemicals 2012." *Regul Toxicol Pharmacol*. 73:1007–1017.

8. Bergman, Å., Heindel, J., Jobling, S., Kidd, K., & Zoeller, R. (eds.). 2013. *The State-of-the-Science of Endocrine Disrupting Chemicals—2012*. World Health Organization and United Nations Environment Programme. http://www.who.int/iris/bitstream/10665/78101/1/9789241505031_eng.pdf.

9. Beronius, A., Hanberg, A., Zilliacus, J., & Ruden, C. 2014. Bridging the gap between academic research and regulatory health risk assessment of endocrine disrupting chemicals. *Curr Opin Pharmacol*. 19:99–104.

10. Beronius, A., & Vandenberg, L.N. 2016. Using systematic reviews for hazard and risk assessment of endocrine disrupting chemicals. *Rev Endocr Metab Disord*. 16:273–287.

11. Betts, K.S. 2013. Tox21 to date: Steps toward modernizing human hazard characterization. *Environ Health Perspect*. 121:A228.

12. Birnbaum, L.S., Bucher, J.R., Collman, G.W., et al. 2012. Consortium-based science: The NIEHS's multipronged, collaborative approach to assessing the health effects of Bisphenol A. *Environ Health Perspect*. 120:1640–1644.

13. Borrell, B. 2010. Toxicology: The big test for bisphenol A. *Nature*. 464:1122–1124.

14. Browne, P., Judson, R.S., Casey, W.M., Kleinstreuer, N.C., & Thomas, R.S. 2015. Screening chemicals for estrogen receptor bioactivity using a computational model. *Environ Sci Technol*. 49:8804–8814.

15. Bucher, J.R. 2013. Regulatory forum opinion piece: Tox21 and toxicologic pathology. *Toxicol Pathol*. 41:125–127.

16. Bulbring, E., & Burn, J.H. 1935. The estimation of oestrin and of male hormone in oily solution. *J Physiol*. 85:320–333.

17. Calafat, A.M., Kuklenyik, Z., Reidy, J.A., Caudill, S.P., Tully, J.S., & Needham, L.L. 2007. Serum concentrations of 11 polyfluoroalkyl compounds in the U.S. population: Data from the National Health and Nutrition Examination Survey (NHANES). *Environ Sci Technol*. 41:2237–2242.

18. Calafat, A.M., Ye, X., Wong, L.Y., Bishop, A.M., & Needham, L.L. 2010. Urinary concentrations of four parabens in the U.S. population: NHANES 2005–2006. *Environ Health Perspect*. 118:679–685.

19. Calafat, A.M., Ye, X., Wong, L.Y., Reidy, J.A., & Needham, L.L. 2008. Urinary concentrations of triclosan in the U.S. population: 2003–2004. *Environ Health Perspect*. 116:303–307.

20. Cohn, B.A., La Merrill, M., Krigbaum, N.Y., et al. 2015. DDT exposure in utero and breast cancer. *J Clin Endocrinol Metab*. 100:2865–2872.

21. Colborn, T., vom Saal, F.S., & Soto, A.M. 1993. Developmental effects of endocrine-disrupting chemicals in wildlife and humans. *Environ Health Perspect*. 101:378–384.

22. Damstra, T., Barlow, S., Bergman, A., Kavlock, R.J., & Van der Kraak, G. (eds.). 2002. Global assessment of the state-of-the-science of endocrine disruptors. Geneva, Switzerland: International Programme on Chemical Safety.

23. Diamanti-Kandarakis, E., Bourguignon, J.P., Guidice, L.C., et al. 2009. Endocrine-disrupting chemical: An Endocrine Society scientific statement. *Endocr Rev.* 30:293–342.

24. Dietrich, D., von Aulock, S., Marquardt, H.W., et al. 2013. Open letter to the European Commission: Scientifically unfounded precaution drives European Commission's recommendations on EDC regulation, while defying common sense, well-established science, and risk assessment principles. *Arch Toxicol.* 87:1739–1741.

25. Dix, D.J., Houck, K.A., Martin, M.T., Richard, A.M., Setzer, R.W., & Kavlock, R.J. 2007. The ToxCast program for prioritizing toxicity testing of environmental chemicals. *Toxicol Sci.* 95:5–12.

26. Dorfman, R.I., Gallagher, T.F., & Koch, F.C. 1936. The nature of the estrogenic substance in human male urine and bull testis. *Endocrinology.* 19:33–41.

27. Gore, A.C., Chappell, V.A., Fenton, S.E., et al. 2015. EDC-2: The Endocrine Society's Second Scientific Statement on Endocrine-Disrupting Chemicals. *Endocr Rev.* 36:E1–E150.

28. Gore, A.C., Heindel, J.J., & Zoeller, R.T. 2006. Endocrine disruption for endocrinologists (and others). *Endocrinology.* 147:S1–S3.

29. Grandjean, P., & Ozonoff, D. 2013. Transparency and translation of science in a modern world. *Environ Health.* 12:70.

30. Heindel, J.J., vom Saal, F.S., Blumberg, B., et al. 2015. Parma consensus statement on metabolic disruptors. *Environ Health.* 14:54.

31. Horel, S. 2016, June 8. Endocrine disruptors: Brussels' industry-linked scientists sow doubt. *Environ Health News.* http://www.environmentalhealthnews.org/ehs/news/2016/june/endocrine-disrupters-final-maneuvers-by-brussels2019-industry-linked-scientific-community.

32. Horel, S., & Bienkowski, B. 2013, September 23. Special report: Scientists critical of EU chemical policy have industry ties. *Environ Health News.* http://www.environmentalhealthnews.org/ehs/news/2013/eu-conflict.

33. Hunt, P.A., Vandevoort, C.A., Woodruff, T., & Gerona, R. 2014. Invalid controls undermine conclusions of FDA studies. *Toxicol Sci.* 141:1–2.

34. Janesick, A., & Blumberg, B. 2011. Endocrine disrupting chemicals and the developmental programming of adipogenesis and obesity. *Birth Defects Res C.* 93:34–50.

35. Janesick, A., & Blumberg, B. 2012. Obesogens, stem cells and the developmental programming of obesity. *Int J Androl.* 35:437–448.

36. Janesick, A.S., Dimastrogiovanni, G., Vanek, L., et al. 2016. On the utility of ToxCast and ToxPi for identifying new obesogens. *Environ Health Perspect.* 1224:1214–1226.

37. Kanno, J., Onyon, L., Peddada, S., Ashby, J., Jacob, E., & Owens, W. 2003. The OECD program to validate the rat uterotrophic bioassay. Phase 2: Dose-response studies. *Environ Health Perspect.* 111:1530–1549.

38. Kavlock, R., Chandler, K., Houck, K., et al. 2012. Update on EPA's ToxCast program: Providing high throughput decision support tools for chemical risk management. *Chem Res Toxicol.* 25:1287–1302.

39. Kavlock, R.J., Daston, G.P., DeRosa, C., et al. 1996. Research needs for the risk assessment of health and environmental effects of endocrine disruptors: A report of the U.S. EPA-sponsored workshop. *Environ Health Perspect.* 104:715–740.

40. Klimisch, H.J., Andreae, M., & Tillmann, U. 1997. A systematic approach for evaluating the quality of experimental toxicological and ecotoxicological data. *Regul Toxicol Pharmacol.* 25:1–5.

41. Knudsen, T.B., Houck, K.A., Sipes, N.S., et al. 2011. Activity profiles of 309 ToxCast chemicals evaluated across 292 biochemical targets. *Toxicology.* 282:1–15.

42. Kohn, M.C., & Melnick, R.L. 2002. Biochemical origins of the non-monotonic receptor-mediated dose-response. *J Mol Endocrinol.* 29:113–123.

43. Kortenkamp, A., Martin, O., Faust, M., et al. 2011. *State of the Art Assessment of Endocrine Disruptors: Final Report.* Brussels, Belgium: The European Commission. http://ec.europa.eu/environment/chemicals/endocrine/pdf/sota_edc_final_report.pdf.

44. Lamb, J.C., Boffetta, P., Foster, W.G., et al. 2014. Critical Comments on the WHO-UNEP State of the Science of Endocrine Disrupting Chemicals—2012. *Regul Toxicol Pharmacol.* 69:22–40.

45. Lind, L., Lind, P.M., Lejonklou, M.H., et al. 2016. Uppsala Consensus Statement on Environmental Contaminants and the Global Obesity Epidemic. *Environ Health Perspect.* 124:A81–A83.

46. Maffini, M.V., Alger, H.M., Bongard, E.D., & Neltner, T.G. 2011. Enhancing FDA's evaluation of science to ensure chemicals added to human food are safe: Workshop proceedings. *Comp Rev Food Sci Food Saf.* 10:321–341.

47. Matthews, S.J., & McCoy, C. 2003. Thalidomide: A review of approved and investigational uses. *Clin Ther.* 25:342–395.

48. Myers, J.P., vom Saal, F.S., Akingbemi, B.T., et al. 2009. Why public health agencies cannot depend upon "good laboratory practices" as a criterion for selecting data: The case of bisphenol-A. *Environ Health Perspect.* 117:309–315.

49. Myers, J.P., Zoeller, R.T., & vom Saal, F.S. 2009. A clash of old and new scientific concepts in toxicity, with important implications for public health. *Environ Health Perspect.* 117:1652–1655.

50. Neltner, T.G., Alger, H.M., Leonard, J.E., & Maffini, M.V. 2013. Data gaps in toxicity testing of chemicals allowed in food in the United States. *Reprod Toxicol.* 42:85–94.

51. Newbold, R.R. 2004. Lessons learned from perinatal exposure to diethylstilbestrol. *Toxicol Appl Pharmacol.* 199:142–150.

52. Oreskes, N., Carlat, D., Mann, M.E., Thacker, P.D., & vom Saal, F.S. 2015. Viewpoint: Why disclosure matters. *Environ Sci Technol.* 49:7527–7528.

53. Plotkin, D., Lechner, J.J., Jung, W.E., & Rosen, P.J. 1978. Tamoxifen flare in advanced breast cancer. *JAMA.* 240:2644–2646.

54. Pope, C.A. 3rd, & Dockery, D.W. 2006. Health effects of fine particulate air pollution: Lines that connect. *J Air Waste Manag Assoc.* 56:709–742.

55. Reddel, R.R., & Sutherland, R.L. 1984. Tamoxifen stimulation of human breast cancer cell proliferation in vitro: A possible model for tamoxifen tumour flare. *Eur J Cancer Clin Oncol.* 20:1419–1424.

56. Rotroff, D.M., Dix, D.J., Houck, K.A., et al. 2013. Using in vitro high throughput screening assays to identify potential endocrine-disrupting chemicals. *Environ Health Perspect.* 121:7–14.

57. Rotroff, D.M., Martin, M.T., Dix, D.J., et al. 2014. Predictive endocrine testing in the 21st century using in vitro assays of estrogen receptor signaling responses. *Environ Sci Technol.* 48:8706–8716.

58. Schug, T.T., Abagyan, R., Blumberg, B., et al. 2013. Designing endocrine disruption out of the next generation of chemicals. *Green Chem.* 15:181–198.

59. Schug, T.T., Heindel, J.J., Camacho, L., et al. 2013. A new approach to synergize academic and guideline-compliant research: The CLARITY-BPA research program. *Reprod Toxicol.* 40:35–40.

60. Soto, A.M., Vandenberg, L.N., Maffini, M.V., & Sonnenschein, C. 2008. Does breast cancer start in the womb? *Basic Clin Pharmacol Toxicol.* 102:125–133.

61. Trasande, L., Zoeller, R.T., Hass, U., et al. 2015. Estimating burden and disease costs of exposure to endocrine-disrupting chemicals in the European Union. *J Clin Endocrinol Metab.* 100:1245–1255.

62. Tyl, R.W. 2009. Basic exploratory research versus guideline-compliant studies used for hazard evaluation and risk assessment: Bisphenol A as a case study. *Environ Health Perspect.* 117:1644–1651.

63. Tyl, R.W. 2010. In honor of the Teratology Society's 50th anniversary: The role of Teratology Society members in the development and evolution of in vivo developmental toxicity test guidelines. *Birth Defects Res C.* 90:99–102.

64. U.S. Food and Drug Administration. 2010. Endocrine Disruptor Knowledge Base. http://www.fda.gov/ScienceResearch/BioinformaticsTools/EndocrineDisruptor. Knowledgebase/ucm135074.htm.

65. Vandenberg, L.N. 2014. Low-dose effects of hormones and endocrine disruptors. *Vitam Horm.* 94:129–165.

66. Vandenberg, L.N., & Bowler, A.G. 2014. Non-monotonic dose responses in EDSP tier 1 guideline assays. *Endocr Disrupt.* 2:e964530.

67. Vandenberg, L.N., Colborn, T., Hayes, T.B., et al. 2012. Hormones and endocrine-disrupting chemicals: Low-dose effects and nonmonotonic dose responses. *Endocr Rev.* 33:378–455.

68. Vandenberg, L.N., Colborn, T., Hayes, T.B., et al. 2013. Regulatory decisions on endocrine disrupting chemicals should be based on the principles of endocrinology. *Reprod Toxicol.* 38C:1–15.

69. Vandenberg, L.N., Ehrlich, S., Belcher, S.M., et al. 2013. Low dose effects of bisphenol A: An integrated review of in vitro, laboratory animal and epidemiology studies. *Endocr Disrupt.* 1:e25078.

70. Vandenberg, L.N., Hunt, P.A., Myers, J.P., & Vom Saal, F.S. 2013. Human exposures to bisphenol A: Mismatches between data and assumptions. *Rev Environ Health.* 28:37–58.

71. Vandenberg, L.N., Welshons, W.V., vom Saal, F.S., Toutain, P.L., & Myers, J.P. 2014. Should oral gavage be abandoned in toxicity testing of endocrine disruptors? *Environ Health.* 13:46.

72. Vargesson, N. 2009. Thalidomide-induced limb defects: Resolving a 50-year-old puzzle. *Bioessays.* 31:1327–1336.

73. vom Saal, F.S., Nagel, S.C., Timms, B.G., & Welshons, W.V. 2005. Implications for human health of the extensive bisphenol A literature showing adverse effects at low doses: A response to attempts to mislead the public. *Toxicology.* 212:244–252; author reply 253–244.

74. Whaley, P., Halsall, C., Agerstrand, M., et al. 2016. Implementing systematic review techniques in chemical risk assessment: Challenges, opportunities and recommendations. *Environ Int.* 92–93:556–564.

75. Woodruff, T.J., Zeise, L., Axelrad, D.A., et al. 2008. Meeting Report. Moving upstream: Evaluating adverse upstream end points for improved risk assessment and decision-making. *Environ Health Perspect.* 116:1568–1575.

76. Woodruff, T.J., Zota, A.R., & Schwartz, J.M. 2011. Environmental chemicals in pregnant women in the United States: NHANES 2003-2004. *Environ Health Perspect.* 119:878–885.

77. World Health Organization and United Nations Environment Programme. 2012. *State of the Science of Endocrine Disrupting Chemicals—2012.* 229 PP. http://unep.org/pdf/9789241505031_eng.pdf.

78. Zoeller, R.T. 2010. Environmental chemicals targeting thyroid. *Hormones.* 9:28–40.

79. Zoeller, R.T., Bergman, A., Becher, G., et al. 2014. A path forward in the debate over health impacts of endocrine disrupting chemicals. *Environ Health.* 13:118.

80. Zoeller, R.T., Brown, T.R., Doan, L.L., et al. 2012. Endocrine-disrupting chemicals and public health protection: A statement of principles from the Endocrine Society. *Endocrinology.* 153:4097–4110.

13

Sustainable Chemistry: Addressing Low-Dose Adverse Effects Through Contaminant Remediation and Design of Safe Products for Our Future

GENOA R. WARNER AND TERRENCE J. COLLINS

Key Concepts

- Unsustainable chemical products and processes are causing irreversible degradation and putting life at risk.
- Synthetic chemicals that are endocrine disruptors are top-priority health and environmental threats.
- Green science, sustainable chemistry, and integrative environmental medicine are sibling fields involved in solving chemical sustainability problems.
- Sustainable chemistry embraces design, stewardship, and regulatory approaches.
- Health and environmental performances must become equivalent to the technical and cost performances in the value propositions of commercial chemicals.
- The framework for strategic sustainable development should be considered for organizing collaborations addressing chemical sustainability problems.

Introduction

In 1991, the U.S. Environmental Protection Agency (EPA) gave birth to a new field with a call for proposals aimed at promoting design for the environment in chemistry. The Agency later named the field *green chemistry* and defined it as "the design of chemical products and processes that reduce or eliminate the use or generation of hazardous substances."[71] Although the term *hazardous substance* is broader, most chemical hazards result from toxicity, and toxic substances are the focus of this chapter.

The EPA emphasizes that "green chemistry applies across the life cycle of a chemical product, including its design, manufacture, use, and ultimate disposal. Green chemistry is also known as sustainable chemistry."[71] The Organisation for Economic Co-operation and Development (OECD) has also drafted definitions of sustainable chemistry.[53] A 2001 essay in *Science* provided insight into what sustainable chemistry had to become.[17] We consider sustainable chemistry to be broader than what green chemistry has become today. Carnegie Mellon University has housed the first Institute for Green Science for many years. We apply the following definition: Green science engages multidisciplinary, transsectorial, and cross-cultural collaborations to prioritize the future good through the design, stewardship, and regulation of products and processes to protect life and to build the technologic dimension of a sustainable civilization. Sustainable chemistry, which aims to produce chemical products and processes with high technical, cost, health, and environmental performances, is a vital component of green science.

It is particularly appropriate that a U.S. agency gave birth to the field of green chemistry. Solving sustainability challenges through green science and sustainable chemistry has much to do with helping to "form a more perfect Union, establish Justice, insure domestic Tranquility, provide for the common defense, promote the general Welfare, and secure the Blessings of Liberty to ourselves and our Posterity."[20] Society and the technologic world are very different today from the time of the founders of the United States. The stage of justice has expanded from the qualities of the interactions of men and women to include the interactions of society and technologies with the environment and with all living things,[35] and this especially includes chemical technologies.

We can be grateful for the innumerable benefits of chemical products and processes that have improved our lives, but negative effects are almost always discerned long after the initial commercialization when the producing industries and society have become accustomed to the technical and economic benefits. The resulting dependencies are often enormous and hard to escape, even when it is essential to do so for establishing forms of justice necessary for a good future. Some of the negative health and environmental effects are so serious that they have moved transgenerational justice to the center of the ethical stage of civilization. The quality of future life depends vitally on adapting development to account for scientific understanding of the detrimental effects of incumbent technologies. Green science is needed to build and foster appropriate metrics for sustainable chemical products and processes.

Developed deliberately, with appropriate scientific skepticism and the future good as the lodestar, green science and sustainable chemistry can produce concrete examples of transgenerational justice as powerful guides for developing a sustainable world. Green science, sustainable chemistry, and integrative environmental medicine are closely related fields, and close collaborations can do much to advance the pursuit of sustainability. In this chapter, we refer to this collective set as *sibling sustainability fields.*

In 1987, the Brundtland Commission defined sustainable development as "development that meets the needs of the present without compromising the ability of future generations to meet their own needs."[83] In its famous report, "Our Common Future," this opening definition was followed immediately with two qualifications: "It contains within it two key concepts: The concept of 'needs,' in particular the essential needs of the world's poor, to which over-riding priority should be given; and the idea of limitations imposed by the state of technology and social organization on the environment's ability to meet present and future needs."

Insight into the Brundtland Commission's definition and qualifica-tions offers powerful guidance for the builders of the sibling sustainability fields. First, the duality in the definition should be considered. It is innate to human nature to take care of the needs of the present. It is not innate to take care of the needs of the future, largely because humanity has never had a pressing need to prioritize the future welfare beyond the intergen-erational obligations of the living. The temporal and spatial reach of human powers has had relatively little impact on the ecosphere until recently. As Hans Jonas eloquently taught us, responsibility is a correlate of power.[35] The novelty, impacts, and spatial and temporal reach of science and technology have outpaced our competence to ascertain and correct for the downsides. With many chemical technologies, near-term benefits often paralyze actions that are inspired by the long-term view or camouflage the longer-term and often irreversible damage to the ecosphere. Acquiring competence for guid-ing science and technology so that the present is built "without compromis-ing the ability of future generations to meet their own needs" has taken on epic ethical and practical significance.

Second, in addressing "the essential needs of the world's poor," it is impor-tant for practitioners not to forget that the sibling sustainability fields are elite enterprises. For example, scientific elites preside over the collection and analysis of data on sustainability and are more aware than any other group of what is at stake. It is much easier for rich elites than for most people to minimize the impacts on their families of the endocrine disruptors (EDs) extensively discussed in earlier chapters. Rich elites can buy more expensive, pesticide-free, or minimally contaminated foods and acquire the knowledge and practices for avoiding toxic chemicals in their daily lives. For the urban poor in particular, these possibilities usually are out of reach.[26] In their work to reduce and eliminate EDs, the elites involved should lift the burdens off everyone's shoulders while answering the most important question mankind has ever faced: Is a large, technologically powerful human population sustainable on the earth?[16,19]

Third, in addressing the state of technology, it is undeniable that some commercial chemicals are EDs, which by the agency of low-dose toxicity[76] are imposing heavy limitations on the environment's ability to meet present and future needs.

We must also consider the world's energy needs. In its addiction to fossil carbon and nuclear technologies, the energy sector continues to hinder sustainability. The global society is continuing to expand fossil sources while much safer renewable alternatives are in hand.[13] Inadequate energy policies in many jurisdictions are driving a steady and deadly erosion of the future good. Many American power brokers celebrate the diligence of the United States in doing so, as can be seen in the current political attitude that expanding fossil fuel drilling is good for the United States. People gripped in this short-term pattern of unsustainable energy thinking and action seem unable to grasp the dangers of their advocacy and actions, which extend all the way to extinction.

In addressing "the state of ... social organization," forcing lethal technologies on the world by elites who make fortunes in the process is indicative of the most fundamental flaw undermining sustainability.[19] For as long as misdirected elite power controls the world, it seems that change agents will be up against virtually omnipotent people who are incapable of caring about the future good. Correcting this problem is the biggest ethical and political challenge required for sustainability.[19]

The chemical enterprise has sometimes imposed heavy limitations on the present and future good by the way its leaders have acted in dealing with discoveries of toxicity in their products.[31,45,68] Responsibility is a correlate of power and entails for the powerful in chemistry an obligation to prioritize transgenerational justice whenever the realization strikes that valuable chemical products once considered to be benign are clearly harmful. Key roles for green science and sustainable chemistry entail making this obligation less threatening and more easily operational.

Qualities of the Sibling Sustainability Fields

Because the pedagogic content of integrative environmental medicine, green science, and sustainable chemistry is being produced in real time, it is appropriate to consider a list of skills and habits that can best equip young scientists for success in the pursuit of sustainability.

1. The generality implicit in the definition of green chemistry and explicit in the definition of green science gives sustainability chemists and green scientists carte blanche to follow the mission in any way that imagination may suggest and technical virtuosity may enable. There is sometimes a mistaken impression that green chemistry involves chemical synthesis—what goes into, goes on in, and comes out of reaction vessels—to the exclusion of other areas. The term *sustainable chemistry* is gaining popularity in part to escape this inadequacy of green chemistry.[19,53]

2. Wherever possible, green scientists and especially chemists need to understand the mechanism of the toxicity they are designing against because this knowledge can be mapped most effectively onto the structures of chemicals to deliver the deepest form of design insight. Research partnerships between scientists in the appropriate toxicity areas are vital.[78,81]

3. The importance of any project in green science can be measured by the seriousness of the toxicity problem that is being designed against. It is critical to prioritize work on the higher shelves of the Chemistry and Sustainability (C&S) bookcase.

4. The challenges for achieving sustainable development in the chemical sector are both technical and cultural. The cultural challenges are the more difficult ones. The history of the chemical industry is replete with products for which toxicity problems that were not obvious at the commercial launching have manifested later. Toxicity has often surfaced deep into the merchandizing lives of very valuable products. The academic identification of toxic substances in commerce as the focus of green alternative design projects naturally promotes a parallel case for removing the product from the marketplace and for avoiding regrettable substitutions of equally toxic, less-studied alternatives.[52,78,84] This can create tension that scales with the gravity of the toxicity issue and the value of the product in the marketplace. For a sustainable civilization, the chemical industry must figure out how to effectively steward or eliminate by design the adverse health and environmental impacts of its products and processes. The sibling sustainability fields are creatively embracing this tension, and possibilities abound for win-win-win advances for industry-society-environment as illustrated in later discussions of the Tiered Protocol for Endocrine Disruption (TiPED).[60] Turning a blind eye toward costly

toxicity challenges to avoid this stress can only doom green science and sustainable chemistry to irrelevancy.

5. Green stewardship is vital. Many toxic chemicals bring such high value to people that society will perhaps never wish to abandon them. Often, as in the case of drugs, bioactivity is the principal component of the technical performance that then manifests as low-dose adverse effects when the used product is released into the environment. An example is the synthetic estrogen in birth control pills.[47] In these cases, the development of green stewardship technologies can provide solutions by preventing a toxic chemical from being released into the environment after the benefit of its use has been accomplished.

6. Chemists cannot go it alone in developing effective sustainable chemistry. Design against toxicity is by definition a communal endeavor involving experts from multiple branches of science. Sustainable chemistry must become the broadest multidisciplinary collaborative space in all of chemistry, with deep collaborations across the sibling sustainability fields.

7. In communicating with the world, it is important for green scientists to emphasize and remain true to the highest-order goal of their mission, which is to use their personal powers and skills to protect life from chemical toxicity. Such a demanding goal, when authentically articulated and pursued, has the gravity to inspire young people and hold together loyal multidisciplinary partnerships needed as foundations for pursuing the mission effectively.

Performances

In the economic world, a value proposition is a business or marketing statement that a company uses to summarize why a consumer should buy a product or service or an investor invest in its economic potential. It aims to persuade potential customers and investors that a product or service can add value or solve a problem effectively and better than the competition. When considering the intellectual framework of how to address toxicity in commercial chemicals, the place to begin is recognition of the importance of value propositions and acknowledgment that traditional value propositions that emphasize technical and cost performances are inadequate for any sector deploying chemicals in products and processes.

When sustainability is considered, four performance parameters should be recognized as embedded in the real value propositions of all chemical products and processes. They are the technical performance, the economic performance, the health performance, and the environmental performance.[19] In the sustainability domain, both present and future goods must be considered, not just the former as has been the tradition.

Chemical products and processes have brought immense benefits to mankind according to the traditional definition of a value proposition. Throughout the 19th and 20th centuries, the technical and economic performances were the principal components of chemical product value propositions. In 1856, William Henry Perkin invented the first commercial synthetic dye, which he called *mauveine*. In doing so, he effectively launched the corporate chemical enterprise as we know it today. Mauveine, also known as aniline purple, is made from coal tar. It entered commerce in 1857 accompanied by rapidly growing profits up and down the supply, demand, and use chains of the highly desirable materials it enabled. Mauveine's value was quickly reminted in companion dyes, producing a growing color palate. In the second part of the 19th century, colored clothing became less and less emblematic of wealth as the general population gained access to cheaper synthetically dyed clothing.

There can be little doubt that the commercial dye industry contributed significantly to the self-confidence and joie de vivre of ordinary people. Later, it was found that some of the dyes in the mauveine line (i.e., azo dyes) were carcinogens, and ongoing use has been restricted.[3] Today, more than 10,000 dyestuffs exist.

Since Perkin, the chemical enterprise has been driven by the dynamic that chemicals delivering desirable properties at low cost are the functional equivalents of goldmines for advancing economic development and prosperity. Moreover, the development and prosperity have allowed chemists and industrialists to enjoy a profound and appropriate sense of accomplishment in contributing to the general welfare.

High-value chemicals tend to be emphasized much more than low-value chemicals in chemical education, and modern chemistry textbooks tend to be founded on the pure and applied science of products and processes with high economic and technical performances. However, life is based on chemicals and chemical processes, and any chemical released to the environment can perturb the chemistry of life. Every commercial chemical has health and environmental performances. They may be very good or very bad. Some of the most valuable commercial chemicals have been discovered to possess large negative health and environmental performances, but this information rarely turns up in chemistry textbooks.

How can health and environmental performances be better incorporated into the value propositions of commercial chemicals and into the basic knowledge and motivations of chemists? It is easy to characterize the performance balance needed to move toward sustainability. In thinking about the current average weighting of the four performances embedded in the net value propositions of chemicals in commerce, we have settled on the guestimate shown in Figure 13.1A. Embedded technical and cost performances dominate value propositions about equally. Health performance is given short shrift (except for pharmaceuticals and pesticides). Environmental performance barely features. We emphasize that this apportioning is a qualitative and not a quantitative estimate; there is a big spread in the values for different technologies. We advance these average guestimates as a starting point for thinking about balancing all four performances in creating sustainable chemical products and processes. The process of building a sustainable chemical enterprise involves moving from the performance balance of Figure 13.1A to that of Figure 13.1B.

The fact that health and environmental performances are not securely embedded across the value propositions of most products and processes has cast shadows over the remarkable contributions of the chemical enterprise in building the global civilization. There are three approaches by which society can overcome this performance imbalance. First, through green design,

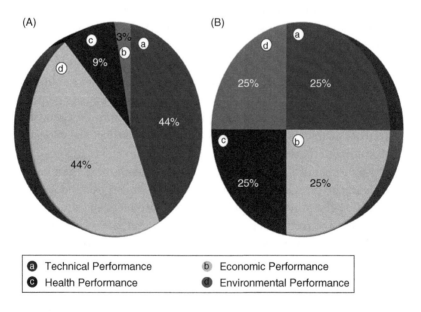

FIGURE 13.1. The four performance parameters of chemical technologies. (A) Investigator's estimates of the relative performance priorities in the value propositions of nonpharmaceutical chemical products in commerce. (B) The reasonable distribution of the relative performance priorities in the value proposition of sustainable chemical products in commerce.

sustainability oriented chemists in partnership with scientists from the sibling sustainability fields can build high health and environmental performances into new chemical products. Second, advanced stewardship tools that are designed to be inherently safe can be developed and commercialized for mitigating low health and environmental performance chemicals that society continues to need (e.g., drugs); development must also be an undertaking of siblings to be successful. The work in our Institute for Green Science in oxidation catalysis (discussed later) is an example of both approaches in action. Third, regulatory, communication, and legal tools are essential assets for resisting the continued use of chemicals with low health and environmental performances.

Green scientists may have different points of view about which of the approaches should be prioritized. It has been asserted that "green chemistry does not have a regulatory bone in its body."[32] Although this may be true of the design phase, following in the footsteps of environmental health sciences, all three approaches should be embraced, taught, and advanced in building the sibling sustainability fields. A key goal of academic green science is to educate competent leaders who know how to make transformative progress toward real-world sustainability, and teaching students the different content and powers of all three approaches is a better way to equip them to be leaders than teaching only one approach. This tripartite strategy is entirely facts based and deliberately blind to politics, which leads to more realistic assessments of the problems that are the most pressing and solutions that can most effectively protect the future good, such as green design of replacements, green stewardship of problem chemicals, and regulatory and legal actions to constrain unsustainable products and processes.

Common and ubiquitous chemicals are disrupting the development of living things, and this serious problem requires immediate action. In response, environmental health scientists and green chemists have collaborated to produce a simple, common sense strategy called the *Tiered Protocol for Endocrine Disruption* (TiPED)[60] for building health and environmental performances into the value propositions of new chemicals. Once this strategy is accepted, it will be apparent that it is not as hard to incorporate health and environmental performances into value propositions as many once thought.

Codifying and Prioritizing the Sustainability Challenges of Chemistry

The case for building a more perfect union among the sibling sustainability fields can be highlighted by an examination and prioritization of the chemical problem spaces associated with sustainability. In the 25 years since 1991, the efforts to redirect chemistry to advance sustainability have attracted considerable attention and public interest. There are many active academic research groups, a deepening and authentic engagement of industry, and important work by nonprofit groups that are assessing, reporting on, and educating about toxic products and processes.

In the Institute for Green Science at Carnegie Mellon University, this burgeoning activity is codified using an organizational tool called the *Chemistry and Sustainability (C&S) Bookcase* (Fig. 13.2), so named because of the course in which it was developed.[19]

The C&S Bookcase collects and codifies "books" in green science. Each book defines a chemically related sustainability project, examines the cultural and technical history, explains why research and development are needed for advancing sustainability, and details the progress that has been made in achieving solutions.

The bookcase has six shelves, with each representing an important area of related challenges for green science scholarship and research. The shelves are ordered by integrating (1) the importance to sustainability, (2) the technical and cultural difficulties of conducting research in the area, (3) the challenges for building requisite collaborative programs, and (4) the barriers to progress from the pushback of power that safeguards the economic interests of

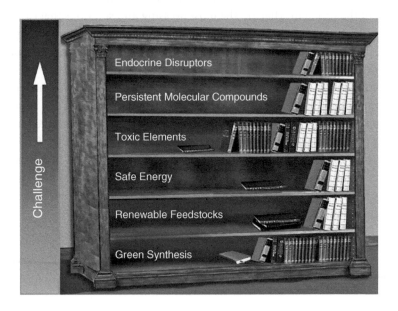

FIGURE 13.2. The chemistry and sustainability bookcase ranks the chemical research problems that are most relevant to sustainability.

existing unsustainable products and processes. According to these criteria, the least challenging set of problems is placed on the first or bottom shelf (not to imply that these are unimportant), progressing to the most challenging set on the sixth or top shelf.

The order of topics has been developed with the idea that it will create a healthy debate about the prioritization and cast light on the diversity of research opportunities that green science presents. The C&S Bookcase is dynamic; shelves can be reordered, extra shelves can be added, and books are updated as new knowledge or changing consensus requires. All shelves are associated with integrative environmental medicine, and include precautionary analysis, laboratory research, and in-field and clinical relevancies, showing that much educational and research ground is shared in common with sustainable chemistry. The book collection is growing as chemists and collaborators expand the literature of problems defined and solutions achieved.

SHELF 1: GREEN SYNTHESIS

Most research in green chemistry is focused on the first shelf in the area of green synthesis. This is the most comfortable space in green science for chemists to focus because the technical skills required are typically those acquired through classical training in chemistry. To give an idea of how chemists think about reducing and eliminating hazards on shelf 1, Anastas and Warner's Principles of Green Chemistry,[4] which encompass and guide this area of research, are presented in Box 13.1.[71]

It is important to conduct research on how to clean up industrial processes or to design safer chemicals. This work can reduce the costs of treating waste. It can help to avoid polluting the land, air, and water. It can reduce occupational exposures and better protect fenceline communities. It can help weakly regulated jurisdictions, where chemical waste is more likely to find its way into a river or landfill than to be treated effectively. However, the broader impact of shelf 1 solutions on global sustainability will likely be less than those on higher shelves, because shelf 1 problems are contained within reaction vessels and are never meant to escape from chemical plants into the open environment. The Presidential Green Chemistry Challenge Awards of the EPA have become markers of progress in green chemistry. Most awards have been given for work on shelves 1 and 2.

The more serious chemical challenges of sustainability are associated with chemicals in products for which the results of commercial activity ensure broad exposures of people and the environment. Because some of these common chemicals are being found to elicit low-dose adverse effects,

Box 13.1 Anastas and Warner's Principles of Green Chemistry

1. **Prevent waste.** Design chemical syntheses to prevent waste. Leave no waste to treat or clean up.
2. **Maximize atom economy.** Design syntheses so that the final product contains the maximum proportion of the starting materials. Waste few or no atoms.
3. **Design less hazardous chemical syntheses.** Design syntheses to use and generate substances with little or no toxicity to humans or the environment.
4. **Design safer chemicals and products.** Design chemical products that are fully effective but have little or no toxicity.
5. **Use safer solvents and reaction conditions.** Avoid using solvents, separation agents, or other auxiliary chemicals. If they must be used, choose safer ones.
6. **Increase energy efficiency.** Run chemical reactions at room temperature and pressure whenever possible.
7. **Use renewable feedstocks.** Use starting materials (i.e., feedstocks) that are renewable rather than depletable. The source of renewable feedstocks is often agricultural products or the wastes of other processes. The source of depletable feedstocks is often fossil fuels (e.g., petroleum, natural gas, coal) or mining operations.
8. **Avoid chemical derivatives.** Avoid using blocking or protecting functional groups or temporary modifications if possible. Chemical derivatives use additional reagents and generate waste.
9. **Use catalysts, not stoichiometric reagents.** Minimize waste by using catalytic reactions. Catalysts are effective in small amounts and can carry out a single reaction many times. They are preferable to stoichiometric reagents, which are used in excess and carry out a reaction only once.
10. **Design chemicals and products to degrade after use.** Design chemical products to break down to innocuous substances after use so that they do not accumulate in the environment.
11. **Analyze in real time to prevent pollution.** Include in-process, real-time monitoring and control during syntheses to minimize or eliminate the formation of byproducts.
12. **Minimize the potential for accidents.** Design chemicals and their physical forms (i.e., solid, liquid, or gas) to minimize the potential for chemical accidents, including explosions, fires, and releases into the environment.

From U.S. Environmental Protection Agency (EPA). 2016. Basics of Green Chemistry. https://www.epa.gov/greenchemistry/basics-green-chemistry.

without ongoing and expanding collaborations among researchers in the sibling sustainability fields, the fate of sustainable chemistry could be to miss the most important sustainability challenges, particularly those on the top three shelves. This would mean that the chemical enterprise never evolves to become adequately sustainable, resulting ultimately in our civilization never becoming sustainable.

SHELF 2: RENEWABLE FEEDSTOCKS

The second shelf entails challenges associated with converting biomass into chemical feedstocks and higher-value products. In this space, chemists and collaborators are working to derive the materials of the everyday economy from recently dead biomass rather than fossilized plant matter such as mined oil, methane, and coal. Shifting from fossil to renewable feedstocks offers the potential for recycling carbon dioxide from the atmosphere instead of adding to it. Renewable chemical processes often are energy intensive. As renewables conquer the energy landscape, the energy density of processes on this and other shelves should become of less concern to sustainability.

Shelf 2 green science is a large and growing area with much promise for sustainability. As an example of the type of advances that have been made, Bristol-Myers Squib (BMS), an American pharmaceutical company headquartered in New York City, received a 2004 Presidential Green Chemistry Challenge Award for developing a sustainable source of the anticancer drug Taxol (Box 13.2). Before this development, Taxol was extracted from the bark of yew trees to treat cancer patients. The BMS approach uses plant cell fermentation to give more cost-effective access to Taxol while protecting yew trees.[73]

SHELF 3: SAFE ENERGY

The third shelf describes the research and development space where chemists work to advance sustainable energy. The term *safe* has been chosen because so much of the energy economy of today is unsafe and even inimical to a sustainable future. This space is so large and important to sustainability but also somewhat separated from the toxicity issues that are the prime concern in this book that we can only qualitatively frame the familiar problems and praise renewable energy trajectories in general.

The conceptual relationship, *risk = hazard × exposure*, has played an important role in guiding green chemistry and green science thinking. The

Box 13.2 Presidential Green Chemistry Challenge: 2004 Green Synthetic Pathways Award

Bristol-Myers Squibb (BMS) received the award for development of a green synthesis for Taxol manufacture using plant cell fermentation and extraction. Paclitaxel, the active ingredient in the anticancer drug Taxol, was first isolated and identified from the bark of the Pacific yew tree, *Taxus brevifolia*, in the late 1960s by Wall and Wani under the auspices of the National Cancer Institute (NCI). The utility of paclitaxel to treat ovarian cancer was demonstrated in clinical trials in the 1980s. The continuity of supply was not guaranteed because yew bark contains only about 0.0004% paclitaxel. Isolating paclitaxel required stripping the bark from the yew trees, killing them in the process. Yews take 200 years to mature and are part of a sensitive ecosystem.

The complexity of the paclitaxel molecule makes commercial production by chemical synthesis from simple compounds impractical. Published syntheses involve about 40 steps, with an overall yield of approximately 2%. In 1991, the NCI signed a collaborative research and development agreement with BMS in which the company agreed to ensure a supply of paclitaxel from yew bark while it developed semisynthesis of paclitaxel from the naturally occurring compound 10-deacetylbaccatin III (10-DAB).

10-DAB contains most of the structural complexity (i.e., eight chiral centers) of the paclitaxel molecule. It occurs in the leaves and twigs of the European yew, *Taxus baccata*, at approximately 0.1% by dry weight and can be isolated without harm to the trees. *T. baccata* is cultivated throughout Europe, providing a renewable supply that does not adversely impact the sensitive ecosystem. The semisynthetic process is complex, however, requiring 11 chemical transformations and 7 isolations. The semisynthetic process also poses environmental concerns, requiring 13 solvents along with 13 organic reagents and other materials.

BMS developed a more sustainable process using the latest plant cell fermentation (PCF) technology. In the cell fermentation stage of the process, calluses of a specific *Taxus* cell line are propagated in a wholly aqueous medium in large fermentation tanks under controlled conditions at ambient temperature and pressure. The feedstock for the cell growth consists of renewable nutrients: sugars, amino acids, vitamins, and trace elements. BMS extracts paclitaxel directly from plant cell cultures, purifies it by chromatography, and isolates it by crystallization. By replacing leaves and twigs with plant cell cultures, BMS improved sustainability of the paclitaxel supply, allowed year-round harvest, and eliminated solid biomass waste.

Compared with semisynthesis from 10-DAB, the PCF process has no chemical transformations, which eliminated six intermediates. During its first 5 years, the PCF process eliminated an estimated 71,000 pounds of hazardous chemicals and other materials. The PCF process eliminates 10 solvents and 6 drying steps, saving a considerable amount of energy. BMS now manufactures paclitaxel using only plant cell cultures.

From U.S. Environmental Protection Agency. 2016. Presidential Green Chemistry Challenge: 2004 Greener Synthetic Pathways Award. https://www.epa.gov/greenchemistry/presidential-green-chemistry-challenge-2004-greener-synthetic-pathways-award.

value of the relationship can be seen from consideration of the shelf 3 challenges. The incumbent giants of fossil and nuclear fuels differ substantially at the molecular and atomic level in how hazard and exposure are apportioned to risk. Each militates against sustainability in a different way. In the carbon energy sector, the hazard function associated with a single carbon dioxide or methane molecule is miniscule; after all, carbon dioxide is the principal waste gas of all aerobic life and methane of anaerobic life. However, because of the immensity of fossil fuel–related releases of carbon dioxide, methane, and other warming gases, the exposure function has become so large as to increase the risk to the point that the chance for a good future for human civilization is rapidly dissipating.[44] In the nuclear sector, the hazard associated with heavy metal radioactive isotopes is so great that releases cannot be tolerated, requiring that exposures be maintained at or close to zero for tens of thousands of years.

Some scholars, including climate scientists, have become so worried about the climate impacts of fossil fuels that they have advocated for a rapid expansion of nuclear energy.[30] The problems with this approach have been explained.[58] As demonstrated by the aftermath of the Fukushima Daiichi disaster, the risks of nuclear power have introduced a whole new challenge space for integrative environmental medicine through radioactive contamination of water and the food chain. It would be much better for the world if these research projects did not need to exist.

If there is a reason for optimism concerning sustainability in the energy sector, it is the expansion that is taking place of safe, cost-effective, and job-rich renewable energy technologies.[13] Renewable technical solutions have advanced so far that the barriers to adoption are more cultural and political than technical. The best strategy for sustainability-concerned scientists, while analyzing and trying to react to the environmental and health assaults of fossil carbon and nuclear energy, is to support the renewables revolution in any way possible.

SHELF 4: TOXIC ELEMENTS

Shelf 4 encompasses elemental pollutants mined and refined from the earth's crust that are persistent and toxic in the ecosphere.[17] They are biologically uncommon elements such as heavy metals, and releases from mining and incorporation into commercial products have caused widespread exposure that has proved disastrous for human and environmental h ealth. On this shelf, the roles for green science and sustainable chemistry are to develop replacement technologies that eliminate toxic elements and to craft stewardship processes that reduce exposures. Integrative environmental medicine has key collaborative roles to play in assessing the safety of the alternative technologies and the ongoing need to clarify exposures and the mechanisms of toxicity.

Extensive evidence exists to prove that industrial leaders have often opted to pursue economic interests at the known expense of human health, leading to widespread cover-ups of massive health damage over many decades. For example, industry, academic, and governmental protectionism of lead in household paint and gasoline resulted in extensive and unnecessary poisoning of workers, consumers, and especially children. U.S. history is replete with propaganda and tactics with which doubt was manufactured and scientists and government officials were recruited to keep lead exposures high for many decades after the dangers were clear.[45] It took very few people to create and perpetuate this massively damaging malfeasance, which serves as a warning that the science of toxic compounds must be treated with absolute integrity as a necessary condition for a sustainable civilization.

Toxic elements such as heavy metals in batteries and electronics are often deliberately used in distributive technologies. The organoarsenic compound roxarsone has been used in chicken feed, which leads to arsenic-contaminated meat and organs.[51] Toxic elements are also dispersed unintentionally in ways that lead to human exposures. One example is the cadmium and arsenic contamination of superphosphate fertilizer, which in combination with glyphosate herbicide, has been associated with fatal kidney disease in farming communities in Sri Lanka and Central America.[5,34] Another is the arsenic contamination of drinking water wells in Bangladesh arising from well-intentioned efforts to help the Bangladeshi people escape microbial-contaminated surface waters.[65]

All fossil carbon industries are major sources of toxic elements. Heavy metals, radioactive elements, and other uncommon elements are often brought to the earth's surface during hydraulic fracturing for natural gas.[66,80] Coal burning releases toxic elements into the atmosphere that partition among the various compartments of the environment.[46] Radioactive elements occasionally escape nuclear power plants to produce extensive contamination.[37] For many reasons, these technologies are all incompatible with a sustainable future. Scientists in the sibling sustainability fields have multiple challenges in recognizing, studying, mitigating, and replacing the toxic technologies.

SHELF 5: PERSISTENT MOLECULAR COMPOUNDS

Shelf 5 includes all persistent organic pollutants (POPs) that are of special concern because of their recalcitrance in the environment.[68] Widespread use of any chemical that nature cannot break down on a reasonable timescale has a high probability of resulting in unexpected toxicity.[17]

The class of POPs includes persistent bioaccumulative toxic compounds (PBTs), which carry known added bioaccumulation and toxicity burdens. There is much collaborative work to be done on this shelf by the sibling sustainability fields. PBTs are among the most serious threats to sustainability from the chemical enterprise. Bioaccumulation is easily approximated using the surrogate of the octanol-water partition coefficient (K_{ow}). Toxicity is much more difficult to evaluate; it usually takes many toxicity assays to begin to understand how particular compounds are toxic. This is especially true for compounds that exhibit low-dose adverse effects,[27,76] and joint efforts in the sibling sustainability fields to avoid toxicity in new products and processes are essential for the future good. Extensive interactions have led to the TiPED assay protocol for dealing with the most challenging toxicants. Currently, there is no adequate measure for persistence, making the development of a persistence parameter a high priority for sustainable chemistry.

On shelf 5, sustainable chemists can try to design nonpersistent substitute compounds that deliver the technical and cost advantages of PBTs and then collaborate with researchers in integrative environmental medicine to subject successful candidates to appropriate toxicity testing. The persistence factor means that legacy pollutants may not go away over prolonged periods. Chemists can work to develop more effective technologies for degrading PBTs in environmental media. This is a major technical mission in the oxidation catalysis program of the Institute for Green Science.[33]

It is worth reflecting on legacy chemicals. The toxicity of PBTs has often manifested years or decades after commercialization began for chemicals such as dioxins, polychlorinated biphenyls (PCBs), organochlorine pesticides including dichlorodiphenyltrichloroethane (DDT), and brominated fire retardants. Many PBTs are organohalogens with high lipophilicity, causing bioaccumulation in fatty tissue and biomagnification up the food chain. PBTs can be transported through air and water, causing contamination far from the sites of initial releases. High levels of PBTs have been found in the bodies of high-trophic-level animals such as polar bears that live in remote locations.[43,50]

Some PBTs, such as brominated fire retardants, are industrial products. Others, such as the highly toxic dioxins, are unintended chemical byproducts.[70] Although regulatory tools effectively terminated the use of DDT and PCBs in the United States more than 40 years ago, dioxins are still produced as side products in industrial reactions, in the burning of organochlorine compounds, and through environmental photochemical reactions.[42] The carcinogenicity and developmental toxicity of dioxins is evident from the effects of the Seveso accident in Italy[68] and the human consequences of the spraying of Agent Orange and other dioxin-tainted agents in the Vietnam War.[55]

In 2001, the international Stockholm Convention on Persistent Organic Pollutants was formalized to restrict the production and use of an initial "dirty dozen" list of POPs, manage hazardous waste, and identify new POPs.[70] Polybrominated diphenyl ethers (PBDEs) are one class of chemicals that has been added to the Stockholm Convention since it took effect in 2004.

SHELF 6: ENDOCRINE DISRUPTORS

The sixth shelf represents the most insidious form of toxicity for anthropogenic chemicals that has been discovered. Certain common chemicals can disrupt the hormonal control of homeostasis and especially of development.[21,27,76] Along with green chemistry, the field of endocrine disruption science emerged in 1991 into the broader scientific consciousness with a workshop held at the Wingspread Conference Center in Racine, Wisconsin, in July of that year. The resulting consensus statement presented the collective wisdom of the attendees, beginning with the assertion that "We are certain of the following: a large number of man-made chemicals that have been released into the environment, as well as a few natural ones, have the potential to disrupt the endocrine system of animals, including humans."[8] The attendees also summarized what they could estimate with confidence, what the models of the day predicted, what the many uncertainties were in their predictions, what their collective judgment was, and what they considered was needed to improve predictive capabilities for EDs. The designating terms *endocrine disruptor* and *endocrine disruption* were introduced in the statement.

Reading the Wingspread statement today leaves us in awe of the far-sighted thinking and multidisciplinary virtuosity of its authors. In its construction and content, the statement serves as a premier example of practical wisdom in which steps are identified for understanding, evaluating, and reacting to the phenomena of endocrine disruption. The statement also serves as a landmark in applied sustainability ethics because it charts a course for the research establishment and the chemical enterprise that is a critical constitutive element of transgenerational justice. In 1996, "Our Stolen Future" was published to set endocrine disruption on course for international recognition as one of the greatest problem areas of green science and sustainable chemistry.

EDs are of particular concern because low-dose adverse effects can occur at environmentally relevant concentrations.[76] This means the famous adage condensed from Paracelsus' writing of "the dose makes the poison" is invalid; effects may be more pronounced or manifest at different end points at lower doses than at the high doses used in traditional toxicology testing. Biological hormones program reproduction and development in animals, and these are crucial processes that EDs jeopardize. Study of the actions of EDs has attracted a vibrant multidisciplinary community drawn from the disciplines of zoology, endocrinology, biology (i.e., developmental, cell, pathologic, integrative, amphibian, regenerative, and evolutionary biology), biochemistry, toxicology (i.e., environmental, ecologic, and molecular), epidemiology, pharmacology, neuroscience, sustainable chemistry, ecologic risk assessment, environmental regulations and policies, and the nonprofit environmental communications and advocacy worlds. Engagement of this remarkable talent pool with chemical design is creating effective guidance for the chemical industry to follow in incorporating health and environmental performances into their products and processes for the benefit of current and future generations.[78]

Unfortunately, the technical versatility of some high-profile EDs magnifies their value to a very special status, leading to incorporation into multiple products and processes. These chemicals create their own economies, in which new products and processes founded on high multifunctional technical and cost performances are limited only by the collective research ingenuity of the producers.

Bisphenol A (BPA) is among the most widely incorporated chemicals in a diversity of products and processes, including many that contribute to food and medical devices.[77] In the paradigm controlled by technical and cost performances, BPA is archetypical of a chemical that keeps on giving, a goldmine in which new and apparently inexhaustible veins have been discovered and mined with high frequency over many decades. People engaged in the chemical economy of BPA likely cannot imagine life without it. They look to a future in which the product space and production volume will continue to evolve and increase.

In 2016, there is something entirely questionable about this 19th and 20th century dynamic because BPA is an ED.[79] Manufacturers of products containing BPA have somewhat yielded to consumer pressure by incorporating alternatives with analogous functions, but many of these structurally similar chemicals have similar endocrine-disrupting properties.[57] The staying power of BPA and its structural analogues in commerce illustrates the deep cultural, political, and technical barriers that shelf 6 encompasses.

Challenges and Solutions

At the core of the burgeoning green science endeavor resides the challenge of optimizing collaborations between the sibling sustainability fields to most effectively promote sustainability. We find several stellar efforts helpful for catalyzing interdisciplinary action and developing pedagogic materials. Substantial multidisciplinary, transsectorial, and cross-cultural activity to build a collaborative space for addressing toxic chemicals, especially EDs, has been underway for more than a decade under the leadership of John Peterson Myers, Founder and Chief Scientist of the nonprofit Environmental Health Sciences and a leader of the exceptional daily newsletter *Environmental Health News* (EHN).[24] The Collaborative of Health and the Environment (CHE) shares with its diverse membership emerging scientific research on various environmental factors that can contribute to disease and disability, fosters interdisciplinary and inclusive collaboration among diverse constituencies interested in those links, and facilitates effective actions to improve health across the life span.[14]

The Endocrine Disruption Exchange (TEDX) focuses specifically on the technical content and collaborative space of protecting health from endocrine disruption.[23] The U.S. National Institute of Environmental Health Sciences (NIEHS) has been leading in supporting scientific studies that have advanced our understanding of endocrine disruption.[61] In a similar vein, much work has been done in Europe to try to come to grips with EDs. Andreas Kortenkamp at Brunel University has led efforts to build effective regulatory policies; he and others are deeply disappointed in the current European Union regulatory approaches.[31,38] The clean-tech website CleanTechnica provides daily clarion calls on development in renewable energy.[13]

Because many forces come into play when valuable products and processes are identified as EDs, dealing with the disputes reasonably, especially at the global level, is challenging. How can all the sustainability-concerned scholars in the world be helped to unite to make the best of their good will, vision, and desire to more effectively confront transgenerational injustice and their multitude of skill sets across diverse fields? How can figuring out what to do about endocrine disruption be guided to achieve effective results in protecting life?

Given their future-distorting powers over life, we think no one should be able to participate in important policy considerations over EDs and other important sustainability matters without first agreeing to abide by a common set of rules and a framework for engagement. The rules and framework should acknowledge the priority of the future good and protect it from being overwhelmed by the needs of the present. The ideas that worked in Sweden and elsewhere to organize the process of tackling sustainability problems may help in providing the rules and a suitable framework.

A Framework for Strategic Sustainable Development

Another important sibling sustainability field encompasses the development of systematic leadership. Leaders in this area, Karl-Henrik Robèrt and Göran Broman at the Blekinge Institute of Technology, have for more than a decade been teaching sustainability based on the framework for strategic sustainable development (FSSD).[56] The FSSD is a comprehensive model for planning in complex systems. It was founded on a set of three material sustainability principles and five social sustainability principles (Box 13.3).[10]

We think the FSSD principles are excellent for guiding the development of sustainable chemistry to protect life. FSSD thinking and language effectively captures the concept that nature has boundaries that society is overstraining with its technologies and activities and prescribes a common-sense framework for approaching and solving the many associated problems. Although progress in the sibling sustainability fields on understanding and reacting to low-dose adverse effects has been inspirational, we think the FSSD, with its emphasis on well-designed operational procedures, communication, and consensus building across disciplines, sectors, and cultures, is worth considering as an organizational framework for collaborative work.

The FSSD can also serve as a methodology for guiding the deliberations of regulatory agencies about sustainability challenges such as endocrine disruption to achieve optimal results. As Broman and Robèrt point out, when people engage with the FSSD, the true character of the challenge and the self-benefit of proactivity become clearer; the sustainable potential of various materials and practices becomes possible to assess; trade-offs can be managed strategically; system boundary setting can be guided by the purpose of reaching sustainability; collaboration across disciplines, departments, organizations, and sectors can be better facilitated; unknown problems can more easily be avoided; selection, development, and combination of other forms of support can be better guided; and education and research for sustainable development can be better organized.[10]

To see what Broman and Robèrt are suggesting, imagine that a diverse set of people from different disciplines, sectors, and cultures gather to discuss how to deal with EDs. If all stakeholders were represented, the diversity of strongly held positions would be considerable. For collaborative research, FSSD approaches can help in easily optimizing the meetings and plans. To meet the full potential of a regulatory FSSD exercise, the responsible agency must insist that the principles and structure be honored in all proceedings. In FSSD exercises, each participant first is required to agree that the Box 13.3

Box 13.3 Framework for Strategic Sustainable Development

The framework for strategic sustainable development (FSSD) is based on several sustainability principles. In a sustainable society, nature is not subject to systematically increasing the following:

1. *Concentrations of substances extracted from the Earth's crust.* This means limited extraction and safeguarding so that concentrations of lithospheric substances (e.g., fossil carbon, metals) do not increase systematically in the atmosphere, the oceans, the soil, or other parts of nature.
2. *Concentrations of substances produced by society.* This means using conscious molecular design, limited production, and safeguarding so that concentrations of societally produced molecules and nuclides (e.g., nitrogen oxides, chlorofluorocarbons) do not increase systematically in the atmosphere, the oceans, the soil, or other parts of nature.
3. *Degradation by physical means.* This means that the area, thickness, and quality of soils; availability of fresh water; biodiversity; and other aspects of biologic productivity and resilience are not systematically deteriorated by mismanagement, displacement, or other forms of physical manipulation (e.g., overharvesting of forests, overfishing).

and people are not subject to structural obstacles to the following:

4. *Health.* This means that people are not exposed to social conditions that systematically undermine the possibilities to avoid injury and illness (e.g., dangerous working conditions).
5. *Influence.* This means that people are not systematically hindered from participating in shaping social systems (e.g., suppression of free speech).
6. *Competence.* This means that people are not systematically hindered from learning and developing competence (e.g., obstacles to education).
7. *Impartiality.* This means that people are not systematically exposed to partial treatment (e.g., discrimination).
8. *Meaning making.* This means that people are not systematically hindered from creating individual or common meaning (e.g. suppression of cultural expression).

Other than these principles, the FSSD is not prescriptive.

Modified from Broman, G.I., & Robèrt, K.H. 2015. A framework for strategic sustainable development. *J Clean Prod.* 2015:1–15.

principles are foundational to sitting at the negotiating table. To participate, each also needs to agree that clashing points of view will be evaluated by scrutinizing their fidelity to the principles. If a participant's argument cannot be substantiated based on the principles, he or she has to stop making it.

The participants then move to agree on definitions and identities in the five stages of the FSSD: the sustainability *system* under consideration, determination of *success* within the system (i.e., critical vision), *strategic guidelines* for approaching this success, needed *actions* following the principled guidelines, and *tools* that enable the actions. This can lead to the discovery of creative guidelines, identification of data gaps, and launching of research to create missing tools. The goals are always to identify what success in the system should look like and to chart a course to ensure that it is reached with appropriate measurement throughout the course.

How can the global community deal with sustainability challenges effectively if everyone goes their own way? How can people work together without fearing they may lose their autonomy? FSSD exercises can help scientists, industrialists, and regulators from multiple jurisdictions to answer these questions. If the value we perceive in the FSSD were to become evident to others upon experimentation, it would assist in building a common approach for analyzing and advancing sustainability challenges across the board and across the globe. Commonly shared expectations and commitments are critical for pursuing sustainability.

Box 13.4 offers a preliminary attempt to organize the developing collaborative space of the sibling sustainability fields around the logic and dynamics of the FSSD. In a meeting of appropriate parties, it would serve as little more than a starting point, but we hope our colleagues will consider the FSSD as a useful organizing edifice for uniting their efforts.

EDUCATION

To guide the design process, sustainable chemists need to know much more about human toxicity and ecotoxicity than chemists usually do. Various educational efforts are underway that highlight endocrine disruption, but much more needs to be done. This area has been recently reviewed.[19]

ASSESSMENT

Assessment tools are critical for differentiating unsustainable from sustainable products and processes. The approaches that are being developed and

Box 13.4 Adaptation of the Framework for Strategic Sustainable Development for Advancing the Interfaces of Integrative Environmental Medicine, Green Science, and Sustainable Chemistry

The following covers all levels of interactions among the sibling sustainability fields:

1. **System.** The system level is the collective of all living things.
2. **Success.** The success level captures the mission to be pursued within the system. Success equates with maintaining the vitality of all life and the ongoing viability of everything required to sustain it.
3. **Strategic guidelines.** This level captures the guidelines used for approaching the principled vision within the system. The sibling sustainability fields seek to understand the adverse effects of chemicals on the system and to act correctively in ways that adhere to the framework for strategic sustainable development (FSSD) principles. Examples of existing guidelines include (1) the Chemistry and Sustainability (C&S) bookcase, which serves as a principled guideline for ranking chemical sustainability challenges according to the seriousness of the hazards and the difficulty of acting to achieve success[19]; (2) the technology sustainability compass, which is a guideline explicitly based on FSSD principles that is used to compare the sustainability character of technologies[19]; (3) the four performances concept, which serves as a strategic guideline for rating actions according to their ability to bring sustainability directed balance to value propositions[19]; and (4) Anastas and Warner's principles of green chemistry, which serve as guidelines for research and development on the green synthesis shelf.[4]
4. **Actions.** The action level includes the concrete actions that have been prioritized by the FSSD after development of group consensus on the strategic plan, using the strategic guidelines and the vision to inspire, inform, and scrutinize the possible actions. We propose the following starting points. Sustainable chemistry covers all commercial chemistry. The actions required vary considerably where there is more commonality of required actions within each shelf of the C&S bookcase than between them. Optimal actions can be discerned by their promise to elevate the health and environmental performances of chemical products and technologies without sacrificing economic and technical performances. These actions, for example, take the form of partnerships developed from the sibling sustainability fields to (1) advance the design of verifiably sustainable products and processes, (2) further the development and deployment of safe stewardship methods that prevent useful but toxic chemicals from being released after use, (3) support regulatory action that reduces or eliminates toxic compounds from commerce, and (4) create joint educational programs that equip people to understand what chemical sustainability requires of them and the different elements of society.
5. **Tools.** The tools level includes methods, tools, and other forms of support that are often required for decision making, monitoring, and disclosures of

the actions to ensure they are chosen in line with the strategic guidelines to arrive step by step at the defined success in the system. This level includes (1) theoretical and experimental toxicity assessment tools that are capable of identifying and monitoring over the full lifetimes the impacts of chemical products and technologies on the system as prescribed by the Tiered Protocol for Endocrine Disruption (TiPED); (2) epidemiologic analyses that associate adverse effects with particular chemicals using biomarkers of cause and effect; (3) sustainable products and technologies that can replace unsustainable incumbents; (4) safe remediation methods for preventing releases of toxic chemicals and purifying ecospheric compartments; (5) online approaches to public education that highlight adverse impacts of chemicals on health and the environment and the development of solutions; and (6) regulations that impel disclosures of the toxicities that lower the health and environmental performances of current and potential commercial chemicals or that restrict the uses of toxic substances.

deployed vary according to the stage in the life cycle of the product. For EDs, the TiPED[60] was developed for use in precommercialization chemical design. The TiPED originated from the efforts of a team of environmental health scientists and green chemists and took shape over 4 years to serve as a tool for detecting low-dose adverse effects of chemicals, especially those associated with the disruption of hormone action.

The TiPED includes five levels of interrogation for a proposed chemical product, from computational analysis based on modeling and structure activity relationships, to in vitro and in vivo screening, to whole-animal assessments. The multifaceted approach examines a wide variety of endocrine pathways and end points to identify endocrine disruption and other potential hazards in chemical products before they are marketed. The in silico and in vitro tiers and zebrafish analyses on tier 4 are affordable and accessible, and many TiPED assays provide feedback to the designer on how a target molecule has failed, guiding further design.

The TiPED is a living protocol. New assays can be incorporated as the state of knowledge on endocrine disruption broadens. Another way to think about the TiPED is that the developers of new chemicals are essentially approaching willing environmental health scientists and asking, "By the end points over which you preside scientifically, what tests does my chemical have to pass to convince you that it is not an ED?" All answers are collected in the TiPED, the use of which is managed by the nonprofit Advancing Green Chemistry[2] to help scientists and industry analyze for low-dose adverse effects typically elicited by EDs.

Chemicals that have already entered the public sphere with entrenched uses and profits are the easiest to study due to the environmental contamination that signaled the presence of low-dose adverse effects. It is much more difficult to remove them from commerce than it is to steer new chemicals that are EDs away from commercial development. The American system of chemical regulation has typically followed the model of produce first, test later, while providing the EPA with extremely limited powers to ban or restrict toxic chemicals from commerce.[74]

The Frank R. Lautenberg Chemical Safety for the 21st Century Act has become law, and changes can be anticipated.[72] An immense body of academic studies on the properties of endocrine-disrupting chemicals exists, but government definitions and screening programs have set unrealistically high burdens of proof to effectively identify and regulate EDs.[1,27,38] To organize scientific studies on the wide variety of end points and effects of EDs on humans, wildlife, and the environment, the field is moving toward development of systematic review processes similar to those used in clinical medicine.[9] Its application in environmental health will help guide risk assessment. A group of leading ED researchers have released a framework for the systematic review and integrated assessment (SYRINA) of EDs. SYRINA provides a uniform method for evaluating evidence and supporting decision making.[75]

Further assessment of chemicals already commercialized is performed by the nonprofit group Clean Production Action. Their GreenScreen for Safer Chemicals method compiles available toxicity data to allow buyers, regulators, and industry to choose among chemicals already in use to find the least harmful alternative for a specific application.[28] For chemicals that are in consumer products, especially personal care products, the nonprofit Environmental Working Group (EWG) has developed licensing criteria based on the collective understanding of unsafe chemicals of key regulatory agencies around the world. Producers who formulate personal care products according to the EWG criteria are able to label their product with the EWG VERIFIED mark.[25]

STEWARDSHIP

Improved environmental management is required to mitigate the effects of EDs and other toxic commercial chemicals. Although we hope for the eventual restriction of some of these chemicals, others such as pharmaceuticals serve vital roles in society. Technologies that deactivate these drugs after they are no longer useful and have been released to water are a key aspect of the stewardship required to build a sustainable society.

At the Institute for Green Science at Carnegie Mellon University, we have designed and developed small-molecule mimics of oxidizing enzymes called TAML activators. The design program was started in 1980 with the long-term goal of enabling cost-effective water disinfection using hydrogen peroxide to replace chlorine to escape carcinogenic chlorinated disinfection byproducts.[15,18,36,59]

Peroxidase enzymes and their cousins (i.e., cytochrome P450 enzymes that make peroxide in situ) are deployed broadly in living things to oxidize organic chemicals for various purposes, including detoxification. TAML activators are designed to function like the active centers of these enzymes, but without the amino acid milieu, making them ≤1% the size of the peroxidase enzymes while being competitively reactive. TAML/peroxide has exceptionally potent disinfection properties. Moreover, TAML processes offer new approaches for removing organic micropollutants such as EDs and other PBTs, which have toxic effects at small concentrations, from water.[6,7,11,12,29,39–41,47–49,63,64,67]

For water treatment applications,[62] TAML and peroxide approaches are strong competitors with ozone and other technologies in technical, cost, and environmental performances. At low parts per billion (ppb), TAML activators catalyze the oxidative destruction of micropollutants in wastewater at environmentally relevant low (parts per billion to parts per trillion) concentrations using hydrogen peroxide or other oxidants at low (parts per million) concentrations.

TAML/peroxide-based water purification was tested by collaborators at Brunel University for remediating London municipal wastewater to produce the following estimate of costs and efficacy by the leading scientist, Professor Rak Kanda (personal communication, 2016): "Compared with ozone plants, TAML plants are estimated to be 3 to 5 times lower in operating costs, significantly lower in capital costs, and 2 to 3 times lower in energy use." Switzerland regulated a reduction of micropollutant concentrations in its municipal effluents. This is being managed over a decade or so by the end-of-pipe addition of ozone or activated carbon plants to about 100 of the country's estimated 700 water treatment plants.[82] Ozone is the cheaper option. It was evaluated by the EU for the same purpose, but it was considered too expensive to adopt.[54] TAML/peroxide is a potential candidate technology to fill this role. TAML approaches are already cheaper than ozone, and recent advances in the technology ensure increased efficiencies and further reduced costs.

In vitro and in vivo TiPED assays have revealed no biologic toxicity of the TAML activators that are candidates for commercialization.[22,69] Extensive studies of the breakdown products of the catalysts (which have limited lifetimes) and target pollutants have been performed to gain added confidence that this technology would not introduce added toxicity if released into the natural environment.[47]

Engagement of the universities is key for expanding green science as a force in the pursuit of sustainability.[19] Effective partnerships between chemists and environmental health scientists have pushed the frontiers of chemical design for the environment in remarkable ways. Immense potential exists for collaborative work to improve our ability to build the chemical dimension of a sustainable civilization.

In field building over the past 15 years, researchers at the Institute for Green Science have experienced the immense privilege of engaging with molecular toxicologists, environmental health scientists, sustainability strategists, public health scientists, and water engineers to advance our shared mission, interest, goals, and accomplishments. The overarching importance of endocrine disruption and low-dose adverse effects on the future of sustainable chemistry, transgenerational justice, and the future good must receive recognition. We look forward to a bright future for collaboration in the sibling sustainability fields of green science, sustainable chemistry, and integrative environmental medicine and to systematic leadership toward sustainability.

REFERENCES

1. Ågerstrand, M., Bero, L., Beronius, A., et al. 2016. Open letter in response to the proposed criteria for identification and regulation of endocrine disrupting chemicals, under the PPP and Biocides Regulations. http://policyfromscience.com/wp-content/uploads/2016/07/Open-Letter-to-Andriukaitis-about-EDC-Criteria.pdf.

2. Advancing Green Chemistry [website]. http://advancinggreenchemistry.org/.

3. Ahlström, L.H., Eskilsson, C.S., & Björklund, E. 2005. Determination of banned azo dyes in consumer goods. *Trends Anal Chem.* 24:49–56.

4. Anastas, P.T., & Warner, J.C. 1998. *Green Chemistry: Theory and Practice.* New York, NY: Oxford University Press.

5. Bandara, J.M., Wijewardena, H.V., Liyanege, J., Upul, M.A., & Bandara, J.M. 2010. Chronic renal failure in Sri Lanka caused by elevated dietary cadmium: Trojan horse of the green revolution. *Toxicol Lett.* 198:33–39.

6. Banerjee, D., Markley, A.L., Yano, T., et al. 2006. "Green" oxidation catalysis for rapid deactivation of bacterial spores. *Angew Chemie Int Ed.* 45:3974–3977.

7. Beach, E.S., Malecky, R.T., Gil, R.R., Horwitz, C.P., &Collins, T.J. 2011. Fe-TAML/hydrogen peroxide degradation of concentrated solutions of the commercial azo dye tartrazine. *Catal Sci Technol.* 1:437–443.

8. Bern, H., Blair, P., Brasseur, S., et al. 1992. Statement from the work session on chemically-induced alterations in sexual development: The wildlife/human

connection. In Colborn, T., & Clement, C. (eds.). *Chemically-Induced Alterations in Sexual and Functional Development: The Wildlife/Human Connection*, pp 1–8. Princeton, NJ: Princeton Scientific.

9. Beronius, A., & Vandenberg, L.N. 2016. Using systematic reviews for hazard and risk assessment of endocrine disrupting chemicals. *Rev Endocr Metab Disord.* 16:273–287.

10. Broman, G.I., & Robèrt, K.H. 2015. A framework for strategic sustainable development. *J Clean Prod.* 2015:1–15.

11. Chahbane, N., Popescu, D.-L., Mitchell, D.A., et al. 2007. FeIII-TAML-catalyzed green oxidative degradation of the azo dye Orange II by H2O2 and organic peroxides: Products, toxicity, kinetics, and mechanisms. *Green Chem.* 9:49–57.

12. Chanda, A., Khetan, S.K., Banerjee, D., Ghosh, A., & Collins, T.J. 2006. Total degradation of fenitrothion and other organophosphorus pesticides by catalytic oxidation employing Fe-TAML peroxide activators. *J Am Chem Soc.* 128:12058–12059.

13. CleanTechnica [website]. http://cleantechnica.com/.

14. The Collaborative on Health and the Environment [website]. http://www.healthandenvironment.org/.

15. Collins, T. 1994. Designing ligands for oxidizing complexes. *Acc Chem Res.* 27:279–285.

16. Collins, T. 1997. Green chemistry. In *Macmillan Encyclopedia of Chemistry*, vol 2, pp 691–697. New York, NY: Simon & Schuster.

17. Collins, T. 2001. Toward sustainable chemistry. *Science.* 291:48–49.

18. Collins, T.J. 2002. TAML oxidant activators: A new approach to the activation of hydrogen peroxide for environmentally significant problems. *Acc Chem Res.* 35:782–790.

19. Collins, T.J. 2015. Review of the twenty-three year evolution of the first university course in green chemistry: Teaching future leaders how to create sustainable societies. *J Clean Prod.* 140(Pt 1):93–110.

20. Constitution of the United States of America. 1789. Preamble.

21. Diamanti-Kandarakis, E., Bourguignon, J.-P., Giudice, L.C., et al. 2009. Endocrine-disrupting chemicals: An Endocrine Society scientific statement. *Endocr Rev.* 30:293–342.

22. Ellis, W.C., Tran, C.T., Roy, R., et al. 2010. Designing green oxidation catalysts for purifying environmental waters. *J Am Chem Soc.* 132:9774–9781.

23. The Endocrine Disruptor Exchange (TEDX) [website]. http://endocrinedisruption.org/.

24. Environmental Health News [website]. http://www.environmentalhealthnews.org/.

25. EWG Verified [website]. http://www.ewg.org/ewgverified/.

26. Gochfeld, M., & Burger, J. 2011. Disproportionate exposures in environmental justice and other populations: The importance of outliers. *Am J Public Health.* 101:S53–S63.

27. Gore, A.C., Chappell, V.A., Fenton, S.E., et al. 2015. Executive summary to EDC-2: The Endocrine Society's second scientific statement on endocrine-disrupting chemicals. *Endocr Rev.* 36:E1–E150.

28. GreenScreen For Safer Chemicals [website]. http://www.greenscreenchemicals. org/.
29. Gupta, S.S., Stadler, M., Noser, C.A., et al. 2002. Rapid total destruction of chlorophenols by activated hydrogen peroxide. *Science* 296:326–328.
30. Hansen, J., Emanuel, K., Caldeira, K., & Wigley, T. 2015, December 3. Nuclear power paves the only viable path forward on climate change. *The Guardian.* https://www.theguardian.com/environment/2015/dec/03/nuclear-power-paves-the-only-viable-path-forward-on-climate-change.
31. Horel, S. 2014, September 25. Endocrination: New film exposing lobby battles on endocrine disrupting chemicals. *YouTube.* https://www.youtube.com/watch?v=plnFVYGTJM8.
32. Horton, B. 1999. Green chemistry puts down roots. *Nature.* 400:797–799.
33. The Institute for Green Science [website]. http://igs.chem.cmu.edu/.
34. Jayasumana, C., Fonseka, S., Fernando, A., et al. 2015. Phosphate fertilizer is a main source of arsenic in areas affected with chronic kidney disease of unknown etiology in Sri Lanka. *SpringerPlus* 4:90.
35. Jonas, H. 1984. *The Imperative of Responsibility: In Search of an Ethics for the Technological Age.* Chicago, IL: University of Chicago Press.
36. Khetan, S.K., & Collins, T.J. 2007. Human pharmaceuticals in the aquatic environment: A challenge to green chemistry. *Chem Rev.* 107:2319–2364.
37. Kinoshita, N., Sueki, K., Sasa, K., et al. 2011. From the cover: Assessment of individual radionuclide distributions from the Fukushima nuclear accident covering central-east Japan. *Proc Natl Acad Sci U S A.* 108:19526–19529.
38. Kortenkamp, A., Bourguignon, J.-P., Slama, R., et al. 2016. EU regulation of endocrine disruptors: A missed opportunity. *Lancet Diab Endocrinol.* 4:649–650.
39. Kundu, S., Chanda, A., Espinosa-Marvan, L., Khetan, S.K., & Collins, T.J. 2012. Facile destruction of formulated chlorpyrifos through green oxidation catalysis. *Catal Sci Technol.* 2:1165–1172.
40. Kundu, S., Chanda, A., Khetan, S.K., Ryabov, A.D., & Collins, T.J. 2013. TAML activator/peroxide-catalyzed facile oxidative degradation of the persistent explosives trinitrotoluene and trinitrobenzene in micellar solutions. *Environ Sci Technol.* 47:5319–5326.
41. Kundu, S., Chanda, A., Thompson, J.V.K., et al. 2014. Rapid degradation of oxidation resistant nitrophenols by TAML activator and H2O2. *Catal Sci Technol.* 5:1775–1782.
42. Latch, D.E., Packer, J.L., Arnold, W.A., & McNeill, K. 2003. Photochemical conversion of triclosan to 2,8-dichlorodibenzo-p-dioxin in aqueous solution. *J Photochem Photobiol A Chem.* 158:63–66.
43. Letcher, R.J., Bustnes, J.O., Dietz, R., et al. 2009. Exposure and effects assessment of persistent organohalogen contaminants in arctic wildlife and fish. *Sci Total Environ.* 408:2995–3043.
44. Mann, M.E. 2014. False hope. *Sci Am.* 310:78–81.

45. Markowitz, G., & Rosner, D. 2002. *Deceit and Denial: The Deadly Politics of Industrial Pollution*. California/Milbank Books on Health and the Public, book 6. Berkley, CA: University of California Press.
46. McConnell, J.R., & Edwards, R. 2008. Coal burning leaves toxic heavy metal legacy in the Arctic. *Proc Natl Acad Sci U S A*. 105:12140–12144.
47. Mills, M.R., Arias-Salazar, K., Baynes, A., et al. 2015. Removal of ecotoxicity of 17α-ethinylestradiol using TAML/peroxide water treatment. *Sci Rep*. 5:10511.
48. Mitchell, D.A., Ryabov, A.D., Kundu, S., Chanda, A., & Collins, T.J. 2010. Oxidation of pinacyanol chloride by H2O2 catalyzed by Fe III complexed to tetraamidomacrocyclic ligand: Unusual kinetics and product identification. *J Coord Chem*. 63:2605–2618.
49. Mondal, S., Hangun-Balkir, Y., Alexandrova, L., et al. 2006. Oxidation of sulfur components in diesel fuel using Fe-TAML catalysts and hydrogen peroxide. *Catal Today* 116:554–561.
50. Muir, D.C., Backus, S., Derocher, A.E., et al. 2006. Brominated flame retardants in polar bears (*Ursus maritimus*) from Alaska, the Canadian Arctic, East Greenland, and Svalbard. *Environ Sci Technol*. 40:449–455.
51. Nachman, K.E., Baron, P.A., Raber, G., Francesconi, K.A., Navas-Acien, A., & Love, D.C. 2013. Roxarsone, inorganic arsenic, and other arsenic species in chicken: A U.S.-based market basket sample. *Environ Health Perspect*. 121:818–824.
52. National Research Council. 2014. *A Framework to Guide Selection of Chemical Alternatives*. Washington, DC: National Academies Press.
53. Organization for Economic Co-operation and Development. 2016. Sustainable chemistry. http://www.oecd.org/chemicalsafety/risk-management/sustainablechemistry.htm.
54. Owen, R., & Jobling, S. 2012. Environmental science: The hidden costs of flexible fertility. *Nature*. 485:441.
55. RetroReport. 2014. *The Dark Shadow of Agent Orange* [video]. The NY Times, U.S. & Politics Channel. http://www.nytimes.com/video/us/100000002872288/agent-orange.html?smid=pl-share.
56. Robert, K.H., Broman, G.I., & Basile, G. 2013. Analyzing the concept of planetary boundaries from a strategic sustainability perspective: How does humanity avoid tipping the planet? *Ecol Soc*. 18:5.
57. Rochester, J.R., & Bolden, A.L. 2015. Bisphenol S and F: A systematic review and comparison of the hormonal activity of bisphenol A substitutes. *Environ Health Perspect*. 123:643–650.
58. Romm, J. 2016, January 7. Why James Hansen Is Wrong About Nuclear Power. http://thinkprogress.org/climate/2016/01/07/3736243/nuclear-power-climate-change/.
59. Ryabov, A., & Collins, T. 2009. Mechanistic considerations on the reactivity of green FeIII-TAML activators of peroxides. *Adv Inorg Chem*. 61:471–521.
60. Schug, T., Abagyan, R., Blumberg, B., et al. 2013. Designing endocrine disruption out of the next generation of chemicals. *Green Chem*. 15:181–198.

61. Schug, T., Johnson, A., Birnbaum, L., et al. 2016. Endocrine disruptors: Past lessons and future directions. *Mol Endocrinol.* 30:833–847.

62. Schwarzenbach, R.P., Escher, B.I., Fenner, K., et al. 2006. The challenge of micropollutants in aquatic systems. *Science.* 313:1072–1077.

63. Shappell, N.W., Vrabel, M.A., Madsen, P.J., et al. 2008. Destruction of estrogens using Fe-TAML/peroxide catalysis. *Environ Sci Technol.* 42:1296–1300.

64. Shen, L.Q., Beach, E.S., Xiang, Y., et al. 2011. Rapid, biomimetic degradation in water of the persistent drug sertraline by TAML catalysts and hydrogen peroxide. *Environ Sci Technol.* 45:7882–7887.

65. Smith, A.H., Lingas, E.O., & Rahman, M. 2000. Contamination of drinking-water by arsenic in Bangladesh: A public health emergency. *Bull WHO.* 78:1093–1103.

66. Soeder, D.J., & Kappel, W.M. 2009. *Water Resources and Natural Gas Production from the Marcellus Shale.* Fact Sheet 2009-3032. U.S. Geological Survey. https://pubs.usgs.gov/fs/2009/3032/pdf/FS2009-3032.pdf.

67. Tang, L.L., DeNardo, M.A., Gayathri, C., Gil, R.R., Kanda, R., & Collins, T.J. 2016. TAML/H2O2 oxidative degradation of metaldehyde: Pursuing better water treatment for the most persistent pollutants. *Environ Sci Technol.* 50:5261–5268.

68. Thornton, J. 2000. *Pandora's Poison.* Cambridge, MA: MIT Press.

69. Truong, L., DeNardo, M.A., Kundu, S., Collins, T.J., & Tanguay, R.L. 2013. Zebrafish assays as developmental toxicity indicators in the green design of TAML oxidation catalysts. *Green Chem.* 15:2339–2343.

70. United Nations Environment Programme. 2001. Stockholm Convention on Persistent Organic Pollutants. http://chm.pops.int/Portals/0/download.aspx?d=UNEP-POPS-COP-CONVTEXT-2009.En.pdf.

71. U.S. Environmental Protection Agency. 2016. Basics of Green Chemistry. https://www.epa.gov/greenchemistry/basics-green-chemistry.

72. U.S. Environmental Protection Agency. 2016. The Frank R. Lautenberg Chemical Safety for the 21st Century Act. https://www.epa.gov/assessing-and-managing-chemicals-under-tsca/frank-r-lautenberg-chemical-safety-21st-century-act.

73. U.S. Environmental Protection Agency. 2016. Presidential Green Chemistry Challenge: 2004 Greener Synthetic Pathways Award. https://www.epa.gov/greenchemistry/presidential-green-chemistry-challenge-2004-greener-synthetic-pathways-award.

74. U.S. Government Accountability Office. 2005. Chemical Regulation: Options Exist to Improve EPA's Ability to Assess Health Risks and Manage Its Chemical Review Program. GAO-05-458. www.gao.gov/cgi-bin/getrpt?GAO-05-458.

75. Vandenberg, L.N., Ågerstrand, M., Beronius, A., et al. 2016. A proposed framework for the systematic review and integrated assessment (SYRINA) of endocrine disrupting chemicals. *Environ Health.* 15:74.

76. Vandenberg, L.N., Colborn, T., Hayes, T.B., et al. 2012. Hormones and endocrine-disrupting chemicals: Low-dose effects and nonmonotonic dose responses. *Endocr Rev.* 33:1–78.

77. Vandenberg, L.N., Hauser, R., Marcus, M., Olea, N., & Welshons, W.V. 2007. Human exposure to bisphenol A (BPA). *Reprod Toxicol.* 24:139–177.

78. Vandenberg, L.N., Luthi, D., & Quinerly, D. *2017.* Plastic bodies in a plastic world: Multi-disciplinary approaches to study endocrine disrupting chemicals. *J Clean Prod. 140*:373–385.

79. Vandenberg, L.N., Maffini, M.V., Sonnenschein, C., Rubin, B.S., & Soto, A.M. 2009. Bisphenol-A and the great divide: A review of controversies in the field of endocrine disruption. *Endocr Rev.* 30:75–95.

80. Veil, J.A., Puder, M.G., Elcock, D., & Redweik R.J. Jr. 2004. A white paper describing produced water from production of crude oil, natural gas, and coal bed methane. AQNL/EA/RP-112631. Argonne National Laboratory, Environmental Science Division. http://www.evs.anl.gov/publications/doc/ProducedWatersWP0401.pdf.

81. Voutchkova-Kostal, A.M., Kostal, J., Connors, K.A., Brooks, B.W., Anastas, P.T., & Zimmerman, J.B. 2012. Towards rational molecular design for reduced chronic aquatic toxicity. *Green Chem.* 14:1001–1008.

82. Wepf, M. 2015. 100 Water Treatment Plants Must Be Upgraded. Eawag: Swiss Federal Institute of Acquatic Science and Technology. https://www.admin.ch/gov/en/start/documentation/media-releases.msg-id-58567.html.

83. World Commission on Environment. 1987. Our Common Future: Report of the World Commission on Environment and Development. http://www.un-documents.net/our-common-future.pdf.

84. Zimmerman, J.B., & Anastas, P.T. 2015. Toward substitution with no regrets. *Science.* 347:1198–1199.

14

Proactive Approaches to Reduce Environmental Exposures: Avoidance, Lifestyle Changes, and Practical Resources

ALY COHEN

Key Concepts

- Increasing numbers of toxic chemicals are found in water sources, food and food packaging, personal care and cleaning products, building materials, and indoor air, and human exposure to electromagnetic radiation has been increasing steadily.
- Weak chemical legislation has given rise to more than 87,000 commercially available chemicals, and very few have been tested for safety before going to market.
- Exposure to harmful chemicals during vulnerable periods in human development poses the greatest risk to health.
- Limited environmental health training has left clinicians ill equipped to handle the overwhelming burden of disease that continues to rise from chemical and radiation exposures.
- Clinicians often focus on treating symptoms of disease, whereas the focus of this chapter is on approaches to prevent disease.
- The human body has evolved excellent innate detoxification mechanisms that can be harnessed, maximized, and supported through dietary changes, improved sleep, exercise, stress reduction, sauna use, and appropriate supplements to help eliminate many harmful chemicals.
- If given the right information and practical tools, both patients and clinicians can make better choices to reduce chemical and radiation exposures, reduce the chemical body burden, and improve health and well-being.

Introduction

Environmental chemicals have far-reaching molecular and physiologic impacts on human health. The shear enormity of toxins that are woven into the fabric of day-to-day human life makes educating patients a daunting task for physicians. Most of the more than 87,000 chemicals commercially available lack third-party safety testing; either testing is currently unavailable or there is unwillingness to finance these important safety studies, particularly for safety in pregnancy and in infants, children, and other vulnerable groups. Indeed, there appears to be no end in sight for industrialization and chemical utilization, and the current revised chemical safety regulations are inadequate in both the United States and the European Union.

Often, medical educators are left to the "precautionary principle" to guide us to common-sense changes to improve health. This principle was delineated in the Wingspread statement: "When an activity raises threats of harm to human health or the environment, precautionary measures should be taken, even if some cause and effect relationships are not fully established scientifically."[36] The key element is the matter of acting in the face of uncertainty, because hazard data are available for only a very small number of chemicals in commerce. As practitioners, we must use the available science and our own medical training to guide patients to mitigate exposure to an array of chemical and radiation risks, through common-sense information and well-vetted available resources. This chapter discusses practical approaches to limiting chemical exposures in the home and workplace and gives guidance to clinicians on how to integrate chemical awareness and educational resources into the daily workflow of patient care. The goal is to prevent disease rather than just treat symptoms.

Diet

Hippocrates stated in 460 BC, "Let food be thy medicine and medicine be thy food." Yet, modern day physicians still struggle to convey to their patients appropriate concepts of nutrition, caloric intake, and food choice. Add to this discussion information on food additives, preservatives, and synthetic packaging that leaches chemicals into food and beverages, and the challenge to educate patients within a 15-minute visit can be quite frustrating.

Processed foods contribute to body burden of chemicals and to the overwhelming burden of chronic illness in the United States. Ingredients such as sodium, high fructose corn syrup, *trans* fats, and synthetic food additives and preservatives have been shown to increase risk for obesity, diabetes, hypertension, stroke, and heart and liver disease (collectively referred to as metabolic syndrome), as well as immune system disease in both adults and children.[14,68,71,85,92,112,117,133,150,151] Other chemicals in food and food packaging can contribute to endocrine disorders, infertility, neural tube defects, reduced anogenital distance in male offspring (a biomarker of reduced fetal masculinization), decreased sperm count and quality, developmental delay and attention deficit hyperactivity disorder (ADHD), as recognized by the World Health Organization, the Endocrine Society, the American Academy of Pediatrics, and the American Academy of Obstetricians and Gynecologists.[5,26,30,37,155]

Prevention of health effects from environmental toxins not only involves avoidance of chemicals in various foods but also requires intake of appropriate nutrients that may counteract the harmful effects of some chemicals. When humans are nutrient sufficient, they are also better equipped to handle toxin exposures. Folic acid, a water-soluble B vitamin also known as folate or vitamin B_9, is commonly found in green leafy vegetables and has been shown to offset the damaging effects of bisphenol A (BPA) in exposed offspring.[38] Omega-3 fatty acids, which are found in fish, eggs, nuts, oils, chia and flax seeds, and leafy greens, have been shown to offset the toxic effects of BPA, lead, mercury, and dioxin in both human and animal studies.[3,95,100,118]

Appropriate iodine supplementation in pregnancy and nursing can offset the effects of various environmental pollutants such as nitrate, thiocyanate, and perchlorate, which can disrupt normal thyroid function and affect fetal brain development and cognition.[121] Quercetin, an antioxidant flavonoid found in apples and onions, has been shown to be protective against polychlorinated biphenyls (PCBs) and methylmercury in animal studies.[11,120] Children with sufficient intake of iron, calcium, and vitamin C absorb less lead,[74,124,139,159] and studies found that children who were iron deficient were more likely to absorb cadmium, which is associated with adverse health effects.[132,140]

CRUCIFEROUS VEGETABLES

One group of vegetables that requires special attention is the mustard or Brassicaceae family, which have strong detoxification properties. Included in this family are cabbage, Brussels sprouts, broccoli, Chinese broccoli, kohlrabi, kale, collards, and cauliflower. Among other nutrients such as vitamin C, phytochemicals, carotenoids, calcium, and fiber, brassica vegetables contain large amounts of sulfur-containing compounds called glucosinolates, which may be responsible for their detoxification properties. Sulphoraphane is a naturally occurring isothiocyanate found in cruciferous vegetables; it is an inducer of phase II antioxidant and detoxification enzymes with anticancer properties.[9] Through the increase in phase II detoxification, xenobiotic metabolism may affect the elimination or neutralization of carcinogenic and mutagenic factors and consequently inhibit DNA methylation and cancer development. Indole-3-carbinol (I3C), a natural anticancer indolecarbinol from cruciferous vegetables, and DIM (diindolylmethane) have been shown to increase the ratio of the more benign form of estrogen (2-hydroxyestrone) to the more pathologic form (16α-hydroxyestrone), reducing the risk of developing hormone responsive cancers, such as breast, prostate, and ovarian cancers.[1,19,75]

DIETARY RECOMMENDATIONS

Basic diet recommendations include eating whole, unprocessed foods; produce in an array of colors (e.g., carrots, beets, green vegetables, yellow squash, blueberries, strawberries); limited sodium, sugar, *trans* fats, and food additives (e.g., artificial coloring, preservatives, flavoring, emulsifiers/ stabilizers); and produce that is organic and/or cleaned to removed pesticide residue.

Additional dietary recommendations include the following.

Steam and broil foods rather than frying or grilling. Heterocyclic aromatic amines (HCAs), which are potent mutagens/carcinogens, are formed during the cooking of meat at high temperature. The levels of HCAs produced in cooked meats vary depending on the cooking method, time of cooking, and type of meat being cooked. The application of oregano oil, rosemary oil, black pepper, and several other spices during processing may reduce the formation of these (HCA) mutagenic compounds.[50,131] In addition, cooking procedures that release or remove fat from red meat can reduce the total concentrations of these contaminants in the cooked meat.[39] With cruciferous vegetables such as broccoli and cauliflower, cooking sous vide (under vacuum) helps retain the most bioactive compounds, compared with steaming and microwaving, although this often comes at the expense of plastic exposure when using a sous vide oven with plastic interior.[40]

Limit intake of canned foods. Diet can be modulated to reduce exposure to food packaging chemicals such as BPA, a high-volume, synthetic compound found in epoxy resins that line the interior of cans and in plastics used in food packaging. Although humans are exposed to BPA through exposure to thermal paper (e.g., currency, receipts), dust, and contaminated air,[67] the assumed primary means of exposure is through ingestion,[90] primarily due to a lack of information regarding the likely common household products that BPA might be used in (see Chapters 1 and 2). In one crossover study, 75 participants were served canned soup for lunch over a 2-week period, with all other dietary routines maintained. Then, the same 75 participants were served fresh, unpackaged soup for lunch over the following 2-week period. Testing showed a 1000% increase in urinary BPA in participants after the canned food period compared with the fresh, unpackaged soup period.[20]

Food storage options of concern include glazed pottery. According to the Centers for Disease Control and Prevention (CDC), food should not be stored in glazed pottery originating from outside the United States due to potential lead contamination.[23] Safer choices for food storage and preparation include glass bakeware and food-grade 18/8 (18% chromium and 8% nickel) stainless steel (stamped on the bottom of container).

Choose fresh, unprocessed, organic foods. Choosing to eat foods that are truly organic provides the advantage of reducing intake of pesticide, fungicide, and herbicide residues. In addition, one meta-analysis found that organic crops, on average, have higher concentrations of antioxidants and lower concentrations of cadmium than nonorganic comparators across regions and production seasons.[10] If choosing nonorganic produce, check the "Dirty Dozen & Clean Fifteen" list from the Environmental Working Group (EWG) (Table 14.1), which is updated yearly. EWG research has found that people who eat five fruits and vegetables a day from the Dirty Dozen™ list, consume an average of 10 pesticides a day. Those who eat from the "Clean Fifteen" (i.e., the 15 least contaminated conventionally grown fruits and vegetables) ingest fewer than 2 pesticides daily.

Food preparation. Although rinsing of produce reduces levels of pesticides, it does not eliminate them entirely. White vinegar can be added to clean warm water, using a ratio of 1 part vinegar to 4 parts water. Soak and mildly agitate produce for 5 minutes, then rinse with clean water. Peeling of produce also can reduce pesticide ingestion, but many of the best nutritional assets of the produce will likely be wasted with this approach. In general, it is best to instruct patients to eat a variety of colorful fruits and vegetables, rinse all produce, and buy organic whenever possible (see Table 14.1).

Table 14.1. 2016 Shopper's Guide to Pesticides in Produce™

Dirty Dozen™ (Highest Pesticide Levels—Buy These Organic)	Clean Fifteen™ (Lowest in Pesticides)
1. Strawberries	1. Avocados
2. Apples	2. Sweet Corn
3. Nectarines	3. Pineapples
4. Peaches	4. Cabbage
5. Celery	5. Sweet Peas (frozen)
6. Grapes	6. Onions
7. Cherries	7. Asparagus
8. Spinach	8. Mangoes
9. Tomatoes	9. Papayas
10. Sweet Bell Peppers	10. Kiwi
11. Cherry Tomatoes	11. Eggplant
12. Cucumbers	12. Honeydew Melon
Dirty Dozen +	13. Grapefruit
	14. Cantaloupe
Hot Peppers	15. Cauliflower
Kale/Collard Greens	

SEAFOOD AND FRESHWATER FISH

Almost all seafood contains pollutants in varying amounts, including PCBs (polychlorinated biphenyls), polychlorinated dibenzo-*p*-dioxins (PCDDs), polychlorinated dibenzofurans (PCDFs), polychlorinated diphenyl ethers (PBDEs), perfluorinated acids, and mercury. Consuming too much seafood can lead to brain and nervous system effects, especially in a growing fetus, because methylmercury seamlessly crosses the human placenta connecting mother and fetus. Other effects from high mercury levels include defects in fine motor coordination, speech, sleep, and gait and neuropathy. PCBs are highly lipophilic and are concentrated in fat. Mercury is concentrated in muscle.

By cutting away fat (primarily in the skin) before cooking fish and by grilling, broiling, or baking fish, as opposed to sautéing or frying, one can reduce exposure to these chemicals. Choosing fish with lower chemical contaminates is another means of lowering exposure. Larger fish bioaccumulate mercury through the ingestion of smaller fish, which are lower on the food chain. Ingestion of large fish such as shark, swordfish, and tuna should be limited. According to research by the U.S. Environmental Protection Agency (EPA) in 2007, canned tuna accounts for 28% of Americans' exposure to mercury. Based on testing in 2014, Consumer Reports currently disputes the recommendations of the U.S. Food and Drug Administration (FDA) and EPA, which call for pregnant women, breast-feeding mothers, and women trying to become pregnant to consume 8 to 12 ounces of fish per week. They contend that because of its popularity and variable content of mercury, canned tuna should not be consumed at all by pregnant women.[27] This is just one example of the dominance of corporate profits (referred to as cost-benefit analysis) over the public health in decision making by regulatory agencies such as the EPA (see Chapter 11).

Many other fish are safer and can be eaten several times per week without increased health risk. Smaller fish from cold water, for instance, tend to have lower amounts of contaminants; these fish include salmon, mackerel, anchovies, sardines, and herring (SMASH). Smaller fish also retain the same health benefits of larger fish in terms of their long-chain omega-3 fatty acids, docosahexaenoic acid (DHA) and eicosapentaenoic acid (EPA), which have been found to reduce inflammation. Sardines may be an exception to this rule, however, given that new research from Europe shows higher levels of contaminants than previously thought. Sardines are often sourced from shallow waters in close proximity to human activity and effluent waters.[17]

Another recommendation is to avoid most farm-raised fish, which are extremely high in PCBs because of the feed used in cultivating them; it is often composed of other contaminated seafoods that are concentrated with PCBs because they are rich in lipids. According to testing by the EWG and other independent groups, farmed salmon contains 5 to 10 times the PCB level of wild salmon.[45] Freshwater fish may contain contaminants from local manufacturing (e.g., perfluorinated chemicals [PFCs], methylmercury), pesticides, fertilizer, human and animal sewage, and other run-off constituents. Although the EWG considers farmed-raised U.S. haddock and freshwater trout to have low levels of mercury, it is best, considering our constantly changing environments, to have patients contact their state Fish, Game, and Wildlife Department for important fishing advisories before consuming freshwater fish.

To reduce exposure to PCBs, trim the fat (skin) from fish before cooking. Also, choose broiling, baking, or grilling over frying; these cooking methods allow the PCB-laden fat to cook off the fish. When possible, choose wild Alaskan salmon instead of farmed, and eat farmed salmon no more than once a month. Check the resources listed for fish sustainability and safety specific to your patient population.

Web Sites and Smart Phone Apps to Help Choose Healthier Foods

Environmental Working Group smartphone apps: Food Scores, Dirty Dozen, Healthy Living

Monterey Bay Aquarium smartphone app: Seafood Watch

SeafoodWatch.org: The Super Green List

EWG's Seafood Calculator: http://www.ewg.org/research/ewg-s-consumer-guide-seafood/seafood-calculator

EWG's Consumer's Guide to Seafood: http://www.ewg.org/research/ewgs-good-seafood-guide/executive-summary

FDA: Fish: What Pregnant Women and Parents Should Know http://www.fda.gov/downloads/Food/FoodborneIllnessContaminants/Metals/UCM400358.pdf

Water

Water is critical for all human biologic processes, but contaminated water can cause a host of health issues and even irreparable damage. The U.S. Safe Drinking Water Act (SDWA) passed in 1976 was intended to ensure safe drinking water for the public. Under the SDWA, the EPA sets standards for drinking water quality in all of the 160,000 public water systems in the United States. The SDWA does not apply to residential wells, nor does it apply to bottled water, which is overseen by the FDA.

Currently, the SDWA mandates the monitoring and regulation of 91 contaminants in public water, including microorganisms, organic and inorganic contaminants, and several radionucleotides.[147] In addition, several disinfectants used to clean ground and surface water for drinking use, as well as their byproducts, are permitted up to standardized levels. Levels designated as "safe" are based on effects in an adult man who drinks 2 L of water daily. Residential well water in the United States requires no water testing for corrosive or toxic chemicals (e.g., lead, mercury, arsenic, other pesticides) until or unless the property is sold, at which time only limited chemical testing is mandated. Many unregulated and regulated chemicals are now being identified in thousands of homes, hospitals, and schools throughout the United States. In 2015, extremely high levels of lead found in the drinking water in Flint, Michigan, sounded the alarm for thousands of municipalities across the country to take a stronger stance on lead identification and remediation. For many, this attention may have come too late. Fetuses, infants, and children are at greatest risk for the irreversible neurologic effects of lead exposure, and contrary to EPA statements, there are no safe levels of lead in the human body.[6,146]

Other harmful chemicals that are now pervasive in municipality water systems, such as PFCs, can be lowered using carbon filtration but are not listed among the 91 chemicals monitored by U.S. law.[13,21,105]

It is therefore advisable to recommend to patients that additional water filtration (i.e., pitcher, sink, or refrigerator filters that must be maintained and replaced regularly) may limit the exposure to many low-level toxic chemicals. Patients with residential well water should undergo water testing at least once per year for carcinogenic ground contaminants such as arsenic and for heavy metals from plumbing contamination (e.g., lead, copper, mercury). Only reverse osmotic and ion exchange filters can remove lead from tap water adequately. Most water pitchers use granular-activated carbon and resins to bond with and trap contaminants. These filters are effective at improving the taste of water, and many will also reduce lead, chlorinated chemicals, and other contaminants, depending on the filter quality.

Additional recommendations include the following:

- Use glass or stainless steel water bottles.
- Avoid commercial sports bottles, even if labeled "BPA-free"; often BPA is replaced by other harmful plasticizers or epoxy resins such as bisphenol S (BPS) and bisphenol F (BPF).
- Do not reuse plastic water bottles to avoid bacterial contamination and increased leaching of chemicals as the bottles age.
- Avoid water from blue carboy water containers often found in office water coolers; they likely contain BPA.
- Bottled water should be used if elevated levels of harmful chemicals are found in drinking water.

Resources

Private well information and management: http://www.epa.gov/privatewells
Environmental Working Group information on filter options: www.EWG.org
EPA Safe Drinking Water Hotline: https://www.epa.gov/ground-water-and-drinking-water/safe-drinking-water-hotline

---

Sleep

ENCOURAGE QUANTITY AND QUALITY OF SLEEP

The elucidation of sleep and its critical role in the maintenance of health has increased dramatically over the past few decades. Decreased quantity and quality of sleep, whether due to sleep disorders or lack of proper sleep patterns, have been linked to cardiovascular disease risk factors such as hypertension, obesity, diabetes, and dyslipidemia.[18,80,97] Research has revealed that sleep plays a vital role in chemical clearance and that the human brain has a system similar to the lymphatic system which helps to clear waste products and toxins from the fluid in and around the brain.[156]

It is therefore wise to promote quality sleep for patients using the following advice:

Create a routine. Encourage patients to maintain a regular sleep-wake schedule, including on weekends, allowing for 7 to 8 hours of time spent in bed for adults, 9 to 10 hours for teens, and at least 10 hours per night for school-aged children (Table 14.2).[4,22,24] Exposure to morning light is important for reduction of sleepiness and improved psychomotor performance.[109]

Limit screen time. Eliminate computer, smartphone, and tablet use 60 minutes before sleep time. Dim your computer light, use a blue light filter (smartphone apps: f.lux, Midnight, Night Screen, Twilight), or use orange-tinted glasses 1 to 2 hours before sleep to reduce brain stimulation that can interfere with sleep initiation.

Create a comfortable sleep environment. Keep the bedroom cool, between 65° and 70°F; block out all light from windows, under doorways, and from digital clocks, or use an eye mask.

Encourage adequate daily exercise. This allows for the body's natural desire for sleep to occur.

Table 14.2. Sleep Recommendations by Age Group

Age	Recommended Amount of Sleep (hours/day)
Newborns	16–18
Preschool-aged children	11–12
School-aged children	At least 10
Teens	9–10
Adults (including the elderly)	7–8

From Centers for Disease Control and Prevention. 2016. How much sleep do I need? National Heart, Lung, and Blood Institute sleep guidelines. http://www.cdc.gov/sleep/about_sleep/how_much_sleep.html.

Limit use of medicinal sleep aids and stimulants. Reduce prescribing of pharmaceutical sleep medications. Limit alcohol intake, particularly after dinner. Encourage patients to reduce caffeine intake and stop caffeine intake at least 8 to 10 hours before sleep time because of its long half-life.[106]

Reduce stress. Use daily relaxation routines, such as 4-7-8 breathing (4-second inhalation through nose, 7-second hold, 8-second exhalation through the mouth), along with guided meditation (e.g., Relax and Rest, Headspace, and Zen smartphone apps) and journaling.

Reduce toxins. Change out bedding made with synthetic materials (e.g., polyester, rayon) for those made with 100% cotton materials; avoid bedding labeled "wrinkle-free" because it is often treated with formaldehyde and other chemicals. Improve bedroom air quality by reducing off-gassing of synthetic furnishings, floors, walls, or carpeting. Add a high-efficiency particulate air (HEPA) filtration system, and encourage the addition of air-purifying houseplants (e.g., spider plants, peace lilies, Areca palm) into the bedroom. Clear all sources of electromagnetic fields (EMF) from the bedroom (e.g., television, stereo, alarm clocks, lamps) because EMF suppresses endogenous melatonin.[87,134]

Supplement use for sleep. Preferably, supplements should be used only on a short-term basis.

Melatonin. A dose of 0.3 to 0.5 mg orally or sublingually at bedtime can be used, especially for patients with associated circadian rhythm disorder or jet lag. A time-release formulation is often most effective because the peak concentration with short-acting formulations occurs after only about 4 hours. A very-low-dose, 0.2 mg TR (time release) melatonin formulation has been approved in Europe for those older than 55 years of age. It is advised to take the TR formulation 2 hours before bedtime.

Valerian. For adults, a 300 to 900-mg standardized extract of 0.08% valerenic acid can be used, or a tea of 2 to 3 g dried root steeped for 10 to 15 minutes can be taken 30 to 120 minutes before bedtime, for 2 to 4 weeks to assess effectiveness.

Hops. Prepare hops in a 5:1 ethanolic extract and take 1 to 2 mL, 30 to 60 minutes before bedtime.

Explore medical conditions and test or treat appropriately. Diagnose chronic pain, alcohol and drug use, obstructive sleep apnea, restless leg syndrome, severe anxiety/depression, post-traumatic stress disorder (PTSD), heavy metal toxicity, head injury, or other conditions as contributors to insomnia and treat appropriately.

Exercise

Exercise serves many important roles in human physiology, including maintenance of muscle strength and tone, bone development, increased serotonin release, and toxin removal through perspiration and mobilization of lipids (and lipophilic toxic chemicals) from fat. Exercise, in the presence of adequate caloric intake and nutritional status, has also been shown to result in liver hypertrophy and induction of detoxification enzyme systems, increased antioxidant enzymes, and increased glutathione in several organs. Sweating (see next section) has been shown to help eliminate chemicals such as BPA, PCBs, PFCs, and heavy metals.[15,41,86,157]

Sauna and Sweating

In addition to the health benefits of sauna therapy through stress reduction, lowered blood pressure, and decreased pain levels, sauna or steam bathing has been shown to be an effective method for driving toxins out of the human body.[57] The traditional sauna creates surrounding air temperature as high as 160° to 200°F (~70°–90°C) with 25% humidity; in comparison, steam rooms are typically heated to 120° to 130°F at 100% humidity. In response to the heat, blood flow is diverted to the skin to cause cooling while also releasing excess sodium, nitrogen, and toxins. Sweating has been shown to be an effective route of elimination for both metallic toxicants such as mercury and organic toxicants such as hexachlorobenzene.[91,129] It has also been shown to augment the liver's detoxification mechanisms. Studies have shown that subjects exposed to PCBs, solvents, methamphetamines, heavy metals, PFCs (used with waterproof and nonstick products), and flame retardants had clinical improvement after sauna therapy.[52,77,81,123,128,130]

Although appropriate use of sauna therapy is safe for most people, caution should be used in people who have unstable cardiovascular conditions such as recent myocardial infarction or stroke, recent surgery, multiple sclerosis, acute lung infections, or pregnancy complications.[29,57] Lower-temperature infrared sauna, which are typically heated to 120°F, can be a good alternative for people who cannot tolerate conventional sauna or steam room therapy and may offer similar health benefits. Improved clinical results have been seen in patients with rheumatoid arthritis, ankylosing spondylitis, and Sjögren's syndrome.[107,142,149]

Personal Care

Reduction of chemical body burden can be done and begins with what we choose to put onto our skin. The results from the 2015 HERMOSA Intervention Study revealed a dramatic reduction in urinary metabolites of specific phthalates, parabens, triclosan, and benzophenone-3 when 100 Latina teens had their personal care products swapped out for safer versions over a 3-day period.[58]

Human skin acts like a sponge and absorbs the chemicals in personal care products in the same way it might absorb common pharmaceutical drugs purposefully designed to enter the body via the dermal route (e.g., Dramamine, nicotine, and lidocaine patches; nitroglycerin and diclofenac ointments). Choosing safer personal care products requires some knowledge as to what ingredients to avoid, and this can be acquired through the use of technology and available phone apps, such as the EWG's Healthy Living smartphone app and the EWG website: www.ewg.org/SkinDeep. These sites offer easy-to-navigate safety ratings for almost 80,000 products, along with available ingredient data and related health risks.

Here are a few basic recommendations:

- Use fewer products overall, especially during pregnancy. Check safety and ingredients in personal care products used, and change out products containing contaminants for safer options.
- Avoid products with antimicrobial ingredients, such as triclosan (e.g., liquid soap, toothpaste), bactroban, microban, and triclocarban (bar soap), which can result in endocrine disruption and antibiotic resistance.
- Avoid products with "parfume" or "fragrance," which may contain 200 or more undisclosed, proprietary chemicals that may pose allergy and cancer risk, but are considered to be trade secrets.
- Avoid retinyl palmitate or retinol in moisturizing and lip products; they increase the risk of skin cancer.
- Avoid shampoo and conditioner with fragrance, polyethylene glycol (PEG) and polyethylene, ceteareth, DMDM hydantoin, and parabens (e.g., propylparaben, isopropylparaben, butylparaben, isobutylparaben), which confer cancer and developmental risks.
- Avoid nail polish containing formaldehyde, formalin, toluene, and dibutyl phthalate (DBP), which pose allergy, developmental, and cancer risks.

- Avoid personal care products that contain dermal penetration enhancers that increase dermal absorption of toxic chemicals. They break down the protective barrier in the epidermis, which is why they are used in drugs designed for transdermal absorption. Among the most commonly used enhancers are isopropyl myristate, propylene glycol, and various alcohols.[76]

Cleaning Products

Most household cleaning products contain ingredients that have not been tested for human safety. As with personal care products, fragrance or parfume may contain a cocktail of harmful chemicals. Active ingredients listed on the label typically are added chemicals that kill bacteria, viruses, or mold (e.g., triclosan, bactroban, triclocarban, microban). Substances that release 1-4 dioxane and formaldehyde are caustic chemicals that may infiltrate households and get reapplied daily to household surfaces. The word "organic" or "natural" applied to a cleaning product has no legal value unless the product carries the U.S. Department of Agriculture (USDA) Organic label. Many cleaners contain respiratory irritants, allergy triggers, chemicals that may cause chemical burns with skin contact, and chemicals that are highly toxic if ingested by infants or toddlers. It is therefore advisable to recommend that patients use safe cleaning products with known ingredients that are safe for skin contact and air quality.

BUY PRODUCTS THAT ARE SAFE FOR HOUSEHOLD CLEANING

Avoid products that contain ammonia, chlorine bleach, or nonchlorine bleach substitutes such as oxygen bleach, which are corrosive and irritating to skin. Use the EWG website to understand labels and choose safe products sold on the market at accessible, big box stores http://www.ewg.org/guides/cleaners.

MAKE YOUR OWN PRODUCTS

Do-It-Yourself Household Cleaning Products

Ingredients For Homemade Cleaners:

- Salt can be used as an abrasive and to clean pots and pans.
- White vinegar takes off soap scum, breaks up grease and mineral deposits, and acts as a deodorizer.

- Baking soda absorbs odor and is a mild abrasive.
- Lemon juice cuts grease and mineral build-up.
- Organic or pure essential oils (e.g., peppermint, lavender) can be used for fragrance.
- Fragrance-free and color-free liquid soap (not antibacterial soap) may be used.
- Washing soda or sodium carbonate cuts grease but may scratch waxed, fiberglass, or aluminum floors or pots.
- Sodium percarbonate (wear gloves to avoid skin irritation) is a bleach alternative that works well to whiten a tub, a sink, or even clothes without bleach.

Warning: Never mix chlorine bleach with vinegar, ammonia cleaners, or other acidic substances because they can release chloramine and chlorine fumes.

Recipe for All-Purpose Spray Cleaner

Empty spray bottle
2 cups of very hot water
1 teaspoon of liquid castile soap (not antibacterial or with added fragrance or parfume)
1/2 teaspoon of washing soda

Combine all ingredients in the bottle and shake to dissolve the washing soda.

Recipe for Dishwashing Soap

Empty bottle or large jar
2 cups of water
2 tablespoons of liquid castile soap (not antibacterial or with added fragrance or parfume)
1 teaspoon vegetable glycerin

Combine the castile soap and water in the empty container. Add the glycerin, stir, and apply to sponge or add to clean sink with warm water.

Sources for More Household Cleaner Recipes:

The Smart Human: http://thesmarthuman.com/educational-resources/
Healthy Child Healthy World: http://www.healthychild.org/easy-steps/green-spring-cleaning-9-diy-recipes-for-natural-cleaners/
Clean Mama's household cleaner recipes (printable PDF): http://www.cleanmama.net/wp-content/uploads/2013/04/cleaningrecipepic2.png

Clean Air

Air, an essential for human life, should be clean and free of contaminants, even if an odor is not apparent.[56] The fastest route of entry into the human bloodstream, aside from venipuncture, is via inhalation. It should be emphasized to patients that as humans who walk freely in and out of structures and open air space, we *do* have control over the quality and safety of the air we breathe, especially in our homes and work environments. Important, practical changes to furnishings, air filtration, cleaning products, and air freshening activities can greatly mitigate risk of asthma exacerbation, allergy symptoms, and chronic long-term exposure.

Clinicians can share the following simple recommendations to improve air quality for adults, children, and the growing fetus:

Smoking. Tobacco smoke contains 300 or more individual chemicals (e.g., benzene, toluene, BPA, lead, mercury) in each cigarette and filter. The term *first-hand smoke* describes inhalation by the person who is smoking; *second-hand smoke* refers to those inhaling smoke from a smoker nearby; and *third-hand smoke* refers to the residual chemicals that land on furnishings and objects in the environment of a smoker. A recent journal article stated that smoking cessation, along with other lifestyle changes (e.g., weight loss, exercise, reduced alcohol consumption), could prevent roughly half of all cancer deaths in the United States.[136] It is therefore advisable to make every effort possible to reduce cigarette smoke and its residue, especially around pregnant women and children. The lifelong health consequences of developmental exposure to chemicals in cigarette smoke include obesity and other metabolic diseases, respiratory diseases, and cancer.[62]

Furnishings. Many furnishings (e.g., drawer fronts, cabinets, shelving), bought whole or assembled, contain wood made with medium-density fiberboard. This fiberboard, also known as pressboard, often contains urea-formaldehyde resins that off-gas into small spaces such as bedrooms and home offices as formaldehyde, which the National Cancer Institute has identified as a known carcinogen. Without appropriate ventilation, indoor air concentrations can reach extremely high levels, resulting in symptoms of headache, nausea, rash, and confusion. Other sources of formaldehyde include permanent-press or dry-cleaned clothing, draperies, wrinkle-free linens, glues and adhesives, and some cleaning and personal care products. Instruct patients to avoid furniture made of pressboard. If formaldehyde-treated furniture is purchased, it should be aired out for several days before use, in a well-ventilated garage or basement. Alternatively, one can use exterior-grade pressed wood products, which contain lower concentrations of phenol-formaldehyde resins. In addition, polyvinyl chloride (PVC) flooring and wall coverings containing phthalates, which act as allergens, are implicated in respiratory symptoms, asthma, and allergies.

Personal care products. Avoid hair-straightening treatments (e.g., Brazilian, keratin) with constituents containing formaldehyde or breakdown products such as quaternium 15, bronopol (or 2-bromo-2-nitropane-1,3-diol) diazolidinyl urea, DMDM hydantoin, imidazoliidinyl urea, and sodium hydroxymethlglycinate. These products are banned in Canada and the European Union.

Cleaning products. Avoid use of carpet powders, cleaning products with bleach or other lung irritants, and products containing fragrance or parfume. Limonene and other citrus fragrances are often added to cleaning products and should be avoided because of their ability to form formaldehyde when interacting with ozone in air.

Candles and air fresheners. Avoid synthetic candles made with substances such as limonene, which is used to make citrus fragrance. When burned, limonene reacts with ozone in household air to create formaldehyde. Recommend that patients avoid or use fewer scented candles and choose organic candles made with 100% beeswax. Soy candles, although better than typical candles made with petroleum and byproducts, may be adulterated with synthetic fragrance and should also be avoided unless more information about their composition is available.

Air pollution. Discuss with patients and children about increased air pollution exposure from automobile exhaust, and brainstorm ways to limit exposure to idling buses and cars, especially before and after school is in session. Check daily air quality websites and apps to safely manage time spent outdoors.

Resources

EPA website: https://airnow.gov/ allows you to check air quality index forecast and alerts by zip code
EPA smartphone app: Air Now
American Lung Association smartphone app: State of Air

Stress

Although many clinicians might not consider stress to be an environmental "toxin," it plays a major role in the normal functioning of human cellular processes, hormonal feedback, and mechanisms of detoxification.[127] Chronic stress releases cortisol and has been shown to kill memory cells in the hippocampus, reduce immune system function, and even contribute to the development of dementia.[138] Crowe and colleagues showed that greater reactivity to stress predicted a higher risk of dementia in individuals who reported a high incidence of work-related stress, primarily based on how the individual reacted to that stress, not on the work-related stress itself.[8,31] Increased stress can often interfere with food choice and quantity, energy levels, sleep patterns, and social interaction. There is also extensive evidence that stress during pregnancy can have life-long consequences for disease in offspring.[44,59]

Many modalities exist to help to alleviate stress and should be discussed with patients. These include

- Breathing exercises
- Yoga, Tai Chi, and Reiki
- Mindfulness meditation
- Physical activity and exercise
- Expressive activities such as dance, arts and crafts
- Journaling
- Connecting with friends, community and spiritual support
- Connecting with nature and pets/animals
- Seeking guidance through cognitive therapy
- Acupuncture, energy medicine
- Reduction in technology use, noise reduction
- Aromatherapy

Dietary Supplements

Human health and well-being depend on a diet that not only excludes foods and additives that are generally harmful to human health, but includes foods that are nutrient dense and nourishing for effective biologic activities. Besides adequate amounts of protein, complex carbohydrates, and healthy fats, many vitamins and minerals are integral to human health for genomic maintenance and stability. Niacin, folate, magnesium, vitamin B_{12}, and vitamin B_6 are all necessary for effective DNA repair. Niacin is necessary to maintain telomere length; zinc, copper, and manganese for superoxide dismutase maintenance; zinc for proper function of the protective TP53, important for cell cycle regulation; and calcium for regulation of chromosome segregation during mitosis. Methionine metabolism requires selenium, and deficiency can lead to telomere shortening. Antioxidants such as vitamin C and vitamin E prevent DNA damage and lipid peroxidation.[48]

Can too much of a good thing be bad for you? Yes, in fact this is true in the case of many vitamins, minerals, other dietary supplements and hormones. Examples include adverse effects associated with both hypervitaminosis A and hypovitaminosis A, as well as hyperthyroidism and hypothyroidism. Many micronutrients demonstrate U-shaped toxicity curves, meaning that either very low or very high levels can cause harmful health effects. Copper and iron, for instance, have to be maintained at appropriate levels; excess concentrations, beyond the capacity of available protein binding sites, can result in hydroxyl radical generation that may damage lipid membranes and DNA. Glutamine, an amino acid often used to promote a "healthy gut," has been found to cause several health issues when taken chronically.[65] Surveys indicate that about 20% of Americans use at least one herbal supplement, and at least 25% of herbal supplement users take one or more prescription drugs, raising the potential for herb-drug interactions.[12,43] Patients with chronic illnesses use more medications and herbal supplements than the general population, further increasing the risk for interactions.[98,153] A number of herbal preparations from the Indian subcontinent and China have been found to be adulterated or contaminated with molds, fungi, insects, pesticides, and heavy metals, often due to poor sourcing and manufacturing. This dangerous possibility should be discussed with patients and their parents.[113]

It is prudent to be well informed about all substances patients are consuming in order to manage their health. Many herbal and nutritional supplements have been found to bind and/or increase elimination of various toxic substances from the human body. The following sections discuss a few of the supplements that are widely used for this purpose.

Resources

To learn more about herb-drug interactions:

Herb, Nutrient, and Drug Interactions: Clinical Implications and Therapeutic Strategies, by Mitchell Bebel Stargrove, Jonathan Treasure, and Dwight L. McKee (Mosby, 2007)

Memorial Sloan Kettering Cancer Center: About Herbs, Botanicals & Other Products https://www.mskcc.org/cancer-care/treatments/symptom-management/integrative-medicine/herbs

Mayo Clinic: Drugs and Supplements http://www.mayoclinic.org/drugs-supplements

National Institutes of Health, National Center for Complementary and Integrative Health: Herbs at a Glance https://nccih.nih.gov/health/herbsataglance.htm

Cleveland Clinic: Herbal Supplements: Helpful or Harmful http://my.clevelandclinic.
    org/services/heart/prevention/emotional-health/holistic-therapies/
    herbal-supplements
Natural Medicines Comprehensive Database: http://naturaldatabase.therapeuti-
    cresearch.com/home.aspx?cs=&s=ND

MILK THISTLE

Milk thistle (*Silybum marinum*) is an herb that has historically been used to treat liver and biliary disorders. It was famously found to counteract the poisonous effects of amatoxin from the Amanita mushroom, which is found in many parts of the world.[152] Silymarin, a compound in milk thistle, is a flavonoid. Like several other flavonoids (e.g., quercetin, genistein, green tea polyphenols[137]), it works by modulating the cytochrome P450 (CYP450) system in the liver via phase II detoxifying enzyme activation; an increase in these enzymes (e.g., such as UDP-glucuronyl transferase, glutathione-S-transferase, quinone reductase) results in detoxification of many xenobiotics and carcinogens.

Studies have shown positive effects of milk thistle on acute poisonings including organic solvents[141], chronic hepatitis B and C infection, and alcoholic liver disease.[116] An increasing number of clinical trials and animal studies show application in oncology, not only in reducing the long-term hepatic and cardiovascular effects of cancer treatment but also as a chemopreventive agent and possibly for direct cancer treatment.[54] Although flavonoids have been recognized to exert antibacterial, antiviral, anti-inflammatory, antiangiogenic, analgesic, anti-allergic, hepatoprotective, estrogenic, and anti-estrogenic properties, not all flavonoids and their actions are beneficial. The German Commission E currently recommends the use of milk thistle for dyspeptic complaints, toxin-induced liver damage, and hepatic cirrhosis and as a supportive therapy for chronic inflammatory liver conditions.[79]

Although it is generally well tolerated, with rare reports of a mild laxative effect, additional clinical research is needed before its daily use can be recommended in primary prevention of environmental chemical exposures.[64] Safe dosing for daily liver function health is 250 mg once or twice daily (of an extract standardized to provide 80% silymarin).

GLUTATHIONE AND *N*-ACETYL-CYSTEINE

Glutathione (GSH) is a ubiquitous intracellular thiol present in all human tissues. Besides maintaining cellular integrity, GSH has multiple functions including detoxification of xenobiotics and synthesis of proteins, nucleic acids, and leukotrienes. GSH is also involved in regulating the expression of proto-oncogenes and apoptosis, and it is thought that the development of diseases such as cancer and human immune deficiency may be affected by varying levels of cellular GSH. Its depletion in the lung has been associated with the increased risk of lung damage and disease.

Researchers have looked at the therapeutic effects of *N*-acetyl-cysteine (NAC) on the lung damage in smokers and in mice models of acute liver injury from acetaminophen.[33,99] Exogenous delivery of GSH or its intracellular precursor NAC may have benefit as a chemotherapeutic approach.[115] In addition to stimulating glutathione synthesis, NAC enhances glutathione-*S*-transferase activity and promotes liver detoxification by inhibiting xenobiotic biotransformation.[73]

Use of NAC varies based on indication. Safe, daily use of NAC in healthy individuals for routine chemical exposure ranges from 100 to 400 mg. Food sources of cysteine include whey protein, as long as the product is not hydrolyzed or blended, which can denature its structure.

PREBIOTICS AND PROBIOTICS

Humans have been living symbiotically with bacteria for millennia. Human intestines harbor the largest collection of microbes, consisting of between 10 trillion and 100 trillion organisms. Until recently, medicine has largely ignored this intricate microscopic world, which is an integral part of our genetic landscape and of our genetic evolution.

New research has shown the value of probiotic supplementation for reversal and prevention of a whole host of human illnesses, including type 1 diabetes, ADHD, *Clostridium difficile* infection, and obesity. During antibiotic therapy, probiotic use, together with the addition of prebiotic and probiotic foods (Table 14.3), may counterbalance the indiscriminate depletion of various beneficial bacteria, which can take up to a year to repopulate.

Probiotics have been studied as potential detoxification tools for many substances, including heavy metals, BPA, and PCBs.[70] The most commonly

Table 14.3. Prebiotic and Probiotic Foods

Prebiotic Foods	Probiotic Foods
Onions	Sauerkraut
Jerusalem artichokes	Yogurt
Garlic	Kimchi
Leeks	Kombucha tea
Bananas	Kefir
Jicama	Soft cheese
Chicory root	Pickles
Burdock root	Microalgae
Asparagus	Poi
Dandelion greens	Miso soup
Peas	Tempeh
Eggplant	Natto
Chinese chives	Breast milk
Soybeans	
Sugar maple	
Yogurt, cottage cheese, kefir	
Green tea	
Garlic	
Breast milk	

studied probiotics include *Lactobacillus rhamnosus* GG, *Lactobacillus reuteri*, *Saccharomyces boulardii*, and various strains of *Bifidobacterium*; they are commonly used for generalized bowel health and for treatment of irritable bowel syndrome and diarrhea, and are readily available in most pharmacies.

Children and Chemicals

Infants and children spend time at home, in school and daycare centers, in cars and school buses, as well as in recreational and occupational environments (e.g., synthetic turf, swimming pools). Given their vulnerable periods of growth and development, practitioners should advise parents to avoid exposure of their children to chemicals when at all possible. Playing in and around grass and farmland sprayed with pesticides and herbicides should be avoided; if dermal exposure occurs, immediate removal with soap and water should be undertaken.[119] This also applies to the use of pesticides and other toxic chemicals on carpets and elsewhere in the house. Encourage parents to explore the cleaning products used in their children's daycare centers, air quality and air freshener use in school buildings, and pesticide use in playground areas and schoolyards.

Patient Information for Choosing Safer Products

Environmental Working Group website: www.EWG.org
Smartphone apps: Healthy Living, Think Dirty, GoodGuide

Fertility and Pregnancy

Fertility is multifaceted, but environmental chemical exposures should be explored if one experiences the inability to become pregnant despite frequent, carefully timed, unprotected sex for 1 year. Both men and women should be counseled on avoiding chemical exposures before trying to become pregnant. Sperm and eggs take months to develop and their quality and quantity may be affected by various chemicals, medications, and radiation effects, such as those from cell phone use.[2,34,53,88,114,158,160] Chemical exposure of the growing fetus during pregnancy is of particular concern because of the vulnerability of the fetus and the bioavailability of many toxins, which can affect both short- and long-term health outcomes.[28,30,35,63] Cord blood and epidemiologic studies have shown that children are routinely exposed to chemicals via vertical transmission, making it prudent to share with patients not only risks but healthful, preventive measures to reduce xenobiotic exposures.[21,46,51,125,154] Pregnant mothers with specific occupational exposures (e.g., solvents, ethers, cleaning products, radiation) should be counseled appropriately.[82] The following sections describe some specific recommendations.

PERSONAL CARE PRODUCTS

Coach patients on reducing their use of personal care products such as makeup, antiperspirants, creams, lotions, hair dyes, and nail treatments. Help them choose better products using the Healthy Living smartphone app from EWG.

CLEAN FOOD AND WATER

Ask patients about their water source (e.g., tap water, well water, bottled water) and discuss water filtration options or send them to the EWG's water filter guide (see earlier "Water" section). Encourage pregnant patients to eat clean, unprocessed foods; to eat organic produce and dairy products whenever possible; and to wash nonorganic produce well with safe cleaners and/or vinegar.

SEAFOOD CONSUMPTION

In 2014, the FDA and EPA recommended that pregnant and breast-feeding women and women trying to become pregnant should consume between 8 and 12 ounces of fish per week. However, based on intensive testing, *Consumer Reports* disputed this recommendation and does not recommend consumption of any fish by pregnant women, particularly canned or fresh tuna. It seems prudent to discuss fish consumption with all pregnant patients and those trying to become pregnant and to share important resources for healthier fish options.

Resources

Monterey Bay Aquarium: Seafood Watch smartphone app and website www.MontereyBayAquarium.org/search?term=seafood+watch
EWG's Consumer Guide to Seafood and Calculator www.EWG.org/seafood
Consumer Reports: Choose the Right Fish to Lower Mercury Risk Exposure (August, 2014)
FDA: Fish: What Pregnant Women and Parents Should Know http://www.fda.gov/downloads/Food/FoodborneIllnessContaminants/Metals/UCM400358.pdf

CLEAN AIR

Encourage patients to stop smoking and to avoid second- and third-hand smoke (see earlier section "Clean Air"). Encourage pregnant patients to remove synthetic air fresheners, candles, cleaning products, carpet sprays and powders, fresh dry cleaning, and other sources of airborne chemicals from their home and workplace. Look up cleaning products and make better product choices using EWG's Guide to Healthy Cleaning (EWG.org/guides/cleaners).

TOYS

Avoid imported toys, costume jewelry, and toys found in discount stores because they are subject to fewer regulations and less oversight for heavy metals such as lead, plasticizers (e.g., phthalates, BPA), and other harmful chemicals. Avoid older, hand-me-down toys manufactured before regulations were instituted for several phthalates (2008)[144] and for lead content in toys (1978).[145]

MOBILE PHONES AND TABLETS

Unfortunately, safety standards for mobile phone use have not been updated in over 19 years, since they were first designed. Tablet testing, used to create standards, was based on use by a 220-pound man sitting 8 inches from the device. Therefore, it makes reasonable sense to tell pregnant women, as well as both men and women looking to conceive, to keep mobile phones a safe distance from the fetus and to avoid carrying cell phones in bras and in pants pockets (see the later section on "Radiofrequency Radiation").

Tools for the Clinician

It is generally believed that the role of the physician is to guide patients toward health and well-being. Limited training on environmental health topics is one reason why many physicians do not share this information with patients; lack of time is another, as physician-patient contact has dramatically decreased over the past several decades. A follow-up visit with a physician today may likely consist of questions on chronic disease management, a brief physical examination, and discussion of pharmaceutical management and safety, all in 15 minutes of allotted time. Topics on prevention, dietary intervention, exercise, environmental health, and other recommendations compete for mention during this short window of time. Now more than ever, physician understanding and willingness to convey to patients the crucial associations between chemicals and disease is of paramount importance.

Humans spend varying amounts time in a plethora of environments that may pose health risks. We spend on average 12 hours per day in our homes and hundreds of hours of our lifetime in automobiles. Children spend more than half of their lives in school and recreational environments, and they may engage in sports, crafting, and other hobbies. The most efficient way to help patients make changes to mitigate exposures is to first obtain a strong environmental history (i.e., home, work, school, hobby, and recreational exposures).[25,96,103,104,122] It is especially important to ask parents of small children about occupational exposures to harmful chemicals; often these chemicals can be brought into the home via shoes and clothing. Removing contaminated clothing and shoes outside the home and washing work clothing separately can dramatically reduce cross-contamination.

Resources for Taking an Environmental History:

National Environmental Education Foundation: www.neefusa.org/resource/pediatric-environmental-history

Centers for Disease Control and Prevention: www.cdc.gov/workplacehealthpromotion/

Clinicians can also check environmental factors and sources of pollution that effect their patients by zip code using a tool set up by the EPA: EnviroMapper for Envirofacts http://www.epa.gov/emefdata/em4ef.home

Or check local air quality conditions by state or zip code: http://www.airnow.gov

Asthma home environment assessment checklist (English and Spanish): NEEF Asthma Environmental History Form http://www.neefusa.org/resource/asthma-environmental-history-form

---

Hazardous Chemicals in Healthcare Settings

Healthcare settings are a major source of chemical exposure for both healthcare workers and the patients whom they serve. Use of plastics in medical equipment has revolutionized lifesaving procedures, in large part because of the transparency, flexibility, and versatility of expandable plastic materials. However, along with these benefits comes the added chemical exposure from untested plastic ingredients and those already known to be unsafe. According to the FDA, medical devices that may contain BPA and diethylhexyl phthalate (DEHP)-plasticized PVC include intravenous bags and tubing, catheters, enteral nutrition bags, and respiratory, bypass, and dialysis equipment. For example, blood bags can consist of 70% DEHP. BPA and DEHP readily leach into blood, air, and other fluids with which they are in contact.

Healthcare workers are exposed to harmful chemicals daily, including mercury via blood pressure gauges, thermometers, thermostats, fluorescent lights, and dental amalgams; BPA and phthalates via intravenous bags and tubing, esophageal bougies, Foley catheters, and respiratory tubing; BPA in dental sealants, dental composites, and thermal paper; flame retardant chemicals in hospital and office furniture, bedding, and electronics; PFCs in stain-resistant carpeting and furniture; vinyl in examination gloves; and triclosan and other antimicrobials in hand and equipment sterilizers.

Exposure to chemicals in healthcare settings may be disproportionate. Nurses are at increased risk for chemical and pharmaceutical exposures.[110] For the littlest patients, the neonatal intensive care unit (NICU) is among the most plastic laden of all medical environments. Being in a NICU results in dramatically elevated urine levels of various plasticizers including DEHP and BPA in neonates.[16,49,108,126]

In premature infants, the body burden of plastic chemicals increases exponentially with every needed medical procedure. Underdeveloped organs and reduced phase II glucuronidation pathways greatly limit their detoxification capabilities and increase circulating exposure to plasticizers and other plastic components. In one study, urinary BPA concentrations were highly correlated with DEHP concentrations, suggesting that PVC medical equipment was a significant source of exposure for these two endocrine disrupting plasticizers. Infants with high-intensity exposure to DEHP-containing medical products had an almost nine-fold increased body burden compared to those with low-intensity exposure.[16] In another study, a nursing research team at Simmons College in Boston studied 55 infants, most born prematurely, who spent at least 3 days in a NICU. The urine of newborns who had received treatment with four or more NICU devices contained 36.6 ng/L of BPA on average, a level that was almost three-fold higher than that of the babies treated with three or fewer devices. Roughly one fifth of the babies had been treated with at least four medical devices, but respiratory devices, not intravenous tubing, proved to have the strongest link with elevated BPA levels.[42]

There is something that practitioners can do to mitigate human exposure to dangerous plastic materials in medical devices: change them out for devices containing safer materials that currently exist.[60,61] In 2003, Glanzing Clinic in Vienna, Austria, became the first PVC-free pediatric unit worldwide, and since that time, many European NICUs have followed. In 2013, France passed laws banning the use of tubes containing di-(2-ethylhexyl) phthalate (i.e., DEHP) in pediatric, neonatology, and maternity wards in all of their hospitals. Other phthalates considered for removal included dibutyl phthalate (DBP) and butyl benzyl phthalate (BBP). Unfortunately, another phthalate, diisononyl (DINP), which shows evidence of similar toxicity to DEHP, is beginning to replace DEHP in many PVC products; the cycle of replacing one bad chemical with another bad chemical has a long history in the United States and elsewhere.

Some large and small hospital systems in the United States have successfully reduced their use of DEHP-plasticized medical equipment, including Kaiser Permanente in California and Hawaii, Miller Children's Hospital in California, Lucille Packard NICU in California, Evergreen Hospital NICU in Washington State, and John Muir Medical Center in California.

Hospitals can also limit exposure of harmful chemicals for employees and staff by making simple changes. Hand sanitizers, for instance, often contain the antibacterial, endocrine-disrupting chemical triclosan, and can easily be switched out for safer products containing ethanol and ethyl alcohol. Hand sanitizers contain dermal penetration-enhancing chemicals and touching thermal paper after use of a hand sanitizer will result in very high absorption of BPA from the paper.[67] Vinyl (PVC) examination gloves can be exchanged for unpowdered, nitrile gloves.

For ways in which you can facilitate change in your hospital or healthcare center, contact Health Care Without Harm (https://noharm-uscanada.org/issues/us-canada/alternatives-pvc-and-dehp).

Testing for Toxins

The desire to connect symptoms to a causative agent can be very appealing for both clinicians and patients. However, special care must be taken when testing for toxins because of the vast array of environmental agents with varying physiologic effects, testing expense, variable quality of tests, questionable validity, and unknown clinical significance that may create more questions than answers. Humans can be exposed to dozens, if not hundreds, of industrial chemicals every day, making the timing of testing an additional confounder depending on the persistence of the parent compound or known metabolites. Experimental testing for toxins remains largely unfunded with few exceptions. Only a few hundred chemicals have been tested by the CDC as part of the ongoing National Health and Nutrition Examination Survey (NHANES), at considerable expense; laboratories with this expertise are not available to clinicians or the general public.

Given that screening for chemicals is costly and not routinely available, it is advisable for clinicians to obtain a full environmental health history to ascertain the potential for specific environmental chemicals (e.g., heavy metals, solvents, plasticizers) as a cause for patient's symptoms. Choosing laboratory tests for patients in a thoughtful, methodical manner will better direct resources toward the most appropriate medical recommendations and management.

Detox Protocols

There is a growing body of evidence that reducing exposure and actively eliminating various chemicals from the body can reduce clinical symptoms of disease. Detoxification programs range from juicing, cleanses, and fasts to binding protocols such as chelation therapy, activated charcoal, and bentonite clay ingestion. Given their variable protocols, often unsupervised use, and relative risks, clinicians should discuss these modalities in detail with their patients who employ them.

CLEANSES AND FASTING

Weight loss and even intermittent fasting has many benefits for overall health and longevity. One mechanism that is promoted by intermittent energetic challenges is improved cellular bioenergetics, repair or removal of molecules damaged by oxidative stress, and reduced inflammation.[89,93,94,148] However, because adipose tissue provides storage of toxic lipophilic chemicals, weight loss is associated with increased serum levels as these chemicals are released. In one study, researchers measured levels of chlorinated pesticides in adults undergoing either a calorie-restricted diet or stomach-stapling surgery; they found that the greater the weight loss, the greater the increase in serum pesticide levels.[69] Numerous studies have documented an obesity paradox in which the overweight and obese elderly have a better prognosis than those with ideal body weight. Good prognosis among these elderly persons may reflect the relative safety of storing the harmful lipophilic chemicals, known as persistent organic pollutants (POPs), in adipose tissue rather than in other critical organs. Weight loss in obese elderly patients with higher serum concentrations of POPs may carry some risk.[66] CYP450 enzymes are reliant on adequate precursors as substrate for phase 2 liver detoxification.[55] Complete fasting, juice fasts, and marginally nutrient fasting regimens may result in reduced precursors, leading to highly toxic bioactive intermediates and free radicals, with resulting decrease in phase 2 detoxification activity. Therefore, it is not recommended that patients, particularly those who are chronically ill, follow these types of detoxification methods, especially for prolonged periods.[111]

CHELATION THERAPY

In chelation therapy, a chelator such as ethylenediaminetetraacetic acid (EDTA) or dimercaptosuccinic acid (DMSA) is used to bind with a metal (e.g., mercury, lead, iron) and eliminate it from the body. Heavy metals, similar to many lipophilic environmental chemicals, reside in fat tissue but can be released with rapid weight loss or with chelation therapy. Use of this therapy by medical practitioners for patients with acute, high-dose metal poisoning has proved invaluable, but for the treatment of chronic health disorders (e.g., complications from atherosclerosis), its use has been controversial.

Lead, arsenic, mercury, and cadmium rank among the top 10 substances on the Agency for Toxic Substances and Disease Registry (ATSDR) Priority List of Hazardous Substances.[143] Exposure to metals comes from many sources. Lead is found in residential paint (before 1978), adulterated herbal medicines, gasoline (before the mid-1980s), outdated plumbing, and cigarette smoke; arsenic is found in well water, rice (both organic and conventional), and apple juice; mercury is found in many fish; and cadmium can be found in toys, jewelry, and products from overseas, as well as rechargeable batteries.

Given the pervasiveness of metals in our environment and the known relationships between heavy metal exposure and hypertension, dyslipidemia, atherosclerosis, cardiovascular disease, and kidney disease, interest in chelation therapy has gained traction. Results from the large, double-blinded, placebo-controlled Trial to Assess Chelation Therapy (TACT) study showed that patients who were stable after myocardial infarction (MI) and were taking established evidence-based medical therapy (i.e., statins and aspirin) had a statistically significant reduction in cardiovascular events when treated with a combination of high-dose vitamins and chelation therapy.[84] Even more striking was the finding that post-MI diabetic patients age 50 years or older demonstrated a marked reduction in cardiovascular events with EDTA chelation. There was a 41% reduction in clinical events, including a 43% reduction in deaths over 5 years. The researchers stated that further studies are still needed before routine use of chelation therapy is initiated for all post-MI diabetic patients.[47] Newer studies using TACT data have argued that xenobiotic metal contamination is a modifiable risk factor for atherosclerotic disease and that "prudent public health measures should be taken to fully assess, then minimize the public's exposure to xenobiotic metals."[135] According to some cardiologists, post-MI diabetic patients seeking chelation therapy should not be discouraged from doing so, and high-risk patients in hospitals that offer chelation as a therapeutic choice can be encouraged to undergo therapy.[83] The National Center for Complementary and Integrative Health (NCCIH), run by the NIH, suggests that patients choose an appropriate practitioner if they decide to partake in chelation therapy.[102]

Chelation therapy is not a benign process, however. Side effects include dehydration, hypocalcemia, kidney damage, elevated transaminases, allergic reactions, lowered levels of dietary elements, and even death.[7] Chelation has been studied in small pilot trials for cancer treatment, but no definitive or suggestive data are yet available that would form the basis of treatment for cancer. Chelation therapy has been used to treat autism and behavioral disorders with limited results. As of 2008, 7% of children with autism had undergone chelation therapy[32]; however, a 2015 review and a determination by the NCCIH both concluded that, given its health risks, cost, and lack of clinical evidence for effectiveness, the use of chelation as a treatment for autism spectrum disorders is not supported.[72,78,101]

At this time, evidence does not support the widespread use of chelation therapy for prevention of chronic health diseases or treatment of developmental disorders such as autism spectrum disorder. Certain populations, such as post-MI diabetics, may gain benefit from chelation therapy, but more research is needed before this becomes the standard of care. In cases of acute or chronic poisoning, such as those seen with widespread drinking water contamination, chelation therapy determination and management should be performed under the guidance of a trained medical toxicologist or environmental health physician.

Radiofrequency Radiation

For more information on the health effects of radio frequency radiation, see Chapter 10. Following are some safe cell phone use recommendations.

- Keep devices away from the body, particularly the head, reproductive organs, heart, and pregnant abdomen; choose either wired phone lines, wireless headphones, or speaker phones whenever possible, and keep calls short.
- Do not attach a cell phone to your belt, put it in a pocket, or carry it in your bra. The amount of radiation absorbed by the body decreases dramatically even with a small distance of separation.
- Keep cell phones at least 8 inches from a cardiac pacemaker.
- Turn the device onto airplane mode or turn it off when carrying it next to the body and at night while sleeping.
- Text rather than talk; phones emit less radiation when sending texts than during phone communications, and texting keeps radiation away from the head area.
- Call only when the signal is strong (i.e., more signal bars on screen); fewer signal bars means that the phone must try harder to broadcast its signal to the tower, raising radiation levels.

- Limit children's cell phone use whenever possible. Turn devices to airplane mode when children play with games already downloaded to the phone or tablet.
- Avoid so-called radiation shields such as antenna caps and keyboard covers; they reduce the connection quality and force the phone to transmit greater energy, generating more radiation.
- If looking at computer screens for extended periods, use orange-tinted glasses ("blue-blockers") to protect the retina and reduce blue light exposure and symptoms of extended screen time.
- Adjust phone and computer screen using a blue light filter down-loadable smartphone app (e.g. f.lux, Midnight, Night Screen, Twilight). These programs adjust blue spectrum light emitted from digital devices which can effect circadian rythms and the sleep/wake cycle.
- Clinicians should screen patients for device use and degree of exposure to radiofrequency radiation (RFR); in schools, in the workplace and in homes, given the wide use of WiFi and the addition of smart meters to monitor water and electricity usage.

Resources

BabySafe Project: a group of more than 150 physicians and experts advising practical means to protect pregnancy www.babysafeproject.org
Environmental Health Trust: www.ehtrust.org/resources-to-share/printable-resources/

Summary

As the number of potentially toxic chemicals and radiation sources in the environment continues to increase and government oversight remains limited, patients and clinicians need access to information that could help limit adverse effects from exposures. This chapter offers some best practices and resources for limiting such exposures based on the latest research and use of the precautionary principle. Empowered clinicians are in the best position to guide patients with environmental medicine information, which can greatly impact their health, as well as the health of their children and future generations.

Online Resources

Environmental Working Group www.ewg.org
EWG's Skin Deep Database www.ewg.org/skindeep
The Smart Human http://thesmarthuman.com/
The Endocrine Disruption Exchange www.endocrinedisruption.com
Green Science Policy Institute http://greensciencepolicy.org/
Environmental Defence http://environmentaldefence.ca/
Natural Resources Defense Council www.nrdc.org
U.S. Environmental Protection Agency www.epa.gov
Centers for Disease Control and Prevention www.cdc.gov
Consumer Reports Greener Choices www.greenerchoices.org
U.S. EPA Air Quality: www.AirNow.gov
Association of Occupational and Environmental Clinics (AOEC), Pediatric Environmental Health Specialty Units (PEHSU): http://www.pehsu.net/.
Health Care Without Harm: https://noharm-uscanada.org
American College of Medical Toxicology: www.acmt.net

REFERENCES

1. Acharya, A., Das, I., Singh, S., & Saha, T. 2010. Chemopreventive properties of indole-3-carbinol, diindolylmethane and other constituents of cardamom against carcinogenesis. *Recent Pat Food Nutr Agric.* 2:166–177.
2. Adams, J.A., Galloway, T.S., Mondal, D., Esteves, S.C., & Mathews, F. 2014. Effect of mobile telephones on sperm quality: A systematic review and meta-analysis. *Environ Int.* 70:106–112.
3. Ahmed, H.I., EzzEldin, E., Ahmed, A.A., & Ali, A.A. 2013. The possible protective effects of some antioxidants against growth retardation and malformations induced by bisphenyl-A in rats. *Life Sci J.* 10:1575–1586.
4. Allen, S.L., Howlett, M.D., Coulombe, J.A., & Corkum, P.V. 2015. ABCs of sleeping: A review of the evidence behind pediatric sleep practice recommendations. *Sleep Med Rev.* 29:1–14.
5. American Academy of Obstetricians and Gynecologists. 2013; reaffirmed 2016. Committee Opinion No. 575: Exposure to Toxic Environmental Agents. http://www.acog.org/Resources-And-Publications/Committee-Opinions/Committee-on-Health-Care-for-Underserved-Women/Exposure-to-Toxic-Environmental-Agents.

6. American Academy of Pediatrics Committee on Environmental Health. 2005. Lead exposure in children: Prevention, detection, and management. *Pediatrics.* 116:1036–1046.

7. American College of Medical Toxicology and Agency for Toxic Substances and Disease Registry. 2012. Use and Misuse of Metal Chelation Therapy [conference]. Atlanta, GA, February 29, 2012. http://www.acmt.net/Chelation_Course.html.

8. Andel, R., Crowe, M., Hahn, E.A., et al. 2012. Work-related stress may increase the risk of vascular dementia. *J Am Geriatr Soc.* 60:60–67.

9. Atwell, L.L., Beaver, L.M., Shannon, J., Williams, D.E., Dashwood, R.H., & Ho, E. 2015. Epigenetic regulation by sulforaphane: Opportunities for breast and prostate cancer chemoprevention. *Curr Pharm Rep.* 1:102–111.

10. Baranski, M., Srednicka-Tober, D., Volakakis, N., et al. 2014. Higher antioxidant and lower cadmium concentrations and lower incidence of pesticide residues in organically grown crops: A systematic literature review and meta-analyses. *Br J Nutr.* 112:794–811.

11. Barcelos, G.R., Grotto, D., Serpeloni, J.M., et al. 2011. Protective properties of quercetin against DNA damage and oxidative stress induced by methylmercury in rats. *Arch Toxicol.* 85:1151–1157.

12. Bardia, A., Nisly, N.L., Zimmerman, M.B., Gryzlak, B.M., & Wallace, R.B. 2007. Use of herbs among adults based on evidence-based indications: Findings from the National Health Interview Survey. *Mayo Clin Proc.* 82:561–566.

13. Bartell, S.M., Calafat, A.M., Lyu, C., Kato, K., Ryan, P.B., & Steenland, K. 2010. Rate of decline in serum PFOA concentrations after granular activated carbon filtration at two public water systems in Ohio and West Virginia. *Environ Health Perspect.* 118:222–228.

14. Bullo, M., Casas-Agustench, P., Amigo-Correig, P., Aranceta, J., & Salas-Salvado, J. 2007. Inflammation, obesity and comorbidities: The role of diet. *Public Health Nutr.* 10:1164–1172.

15. Bulow, J. 1983. Adipose tissue blood flow during exercise. *Danish Med Bull.* 30:85–100.

16. Calafat, A.M., Weuve, J., Ye, X., et al. 2009. Exposure to bisphenol A and other phenols in neonatal intensive care unit premature infants. *Environ Health Perspect.* 117:639–644.

17. Cano-Sancho, G., Sioen, I., Vandermeersch, G., et al. 2015. Integrated risk index for seafood contaminants (IRISC): Pilot study in five European countries. *Environ Res.* 143:109–115.

18. Cappuccio, F.P., Taggart, F.M., Kandala, N.B., et al. 2008. Meta-analysis of short sleep duration and obesity in children and adults. *Sleep.* 31:619–626.

19. Caruso, J.A., Campana, R., Wei, C., et al. 2014. Indole-3-carbinol and its *N*-alkoxy derivatives preferentially target ERalpha-positive breast cancer cells. *Cell Cycle.* 13:2587–2599.

20. Carwile, J.L., Ye, X., Zhou, X., Calafat, A.M., & Michels, K.B. 2011. Canned soup consumption and urinary bisphenol A: A randomized crossover trial. JAMA. 306:2218–2220.

21. Centers for Disease Control and Prevention. 2015. Fourth National Report on Human Exposure to Environmental Chemicals. http://www.cdc.gov/biomonitoring/pdf/FourthReport_UpdatedTables_Feb2015.pdf.

22. Centers for Disease Control and Prevention. 2016. How much sleep do I need? National Heart, Lung, and Blood Institute sleep guidelines. http://www.cdc.gov/sleep/about_sleep/how_much_sleep.html.

23. 2016. Environmental Protection Agency 2016. Lead and a Healthy Diet: What You Can Do to Protect Your Child. https://www.epa.gov/sites/production/files/documents/nutrition.pdf

24. Centers for Disease Control and Prevention. 2016. Teen Sleep Habits: What Should You Do? https://www.cdc.gov/media/subtopic/matte/pdf/2011/teen_sleep.pdf.

25. Centers for Disease Control and Prevention. 2016. Workplace Health Promotion: Environmental Assessment. http://www.cdc.gov/workplacehealthpromotion/model/assessment/environmental.html.

26. Collaborative on Health and the Environment. 2011. Toxicant and Disease Database. http://www.healthandenvironment.org/tddb.

27. Consumer Reports. 2014, August. Choose the Right Fish To Lower Mercury Risk Exposure. http://www.consumerreports.org/cro/magazine/2014/10/can-eating-the-wrong-fish-put-you-at-higher-risk-for-mercury-exposure/index.htm.

28. Cordier, S., Bergeret, A., Goujard, J., et al. 1997. Congenital malformation and maternal occupational exposure to glycol ethers. Occupational Exposure and Congenital Malformations Working Group. *Epidemiology.* 8:355–363.

29. Crinnion, W. 2007. Components of practical clinical detox programs: Sauna as a therapeutic tool. *Altern Ther Health Med.* 13:S154–S156.

30. Crinnion, W.J. 2010. Toxic effects of the easily avoidable phthalates and parabens. *Altern Med Rev.* 15:190–196.

31. Crowe, M., Andel, R., Pedersen, N.L., & Gatz, M. 2007. Do work-related stress and reactivity to stress predict dementia more than 30 years later? *Alzheimer Dis Assoc Disord.* 21:205–209.

32. Davis, T.N., O'Reilly, M., Kang, S., et al. 2013. Chelation treatment for autism spectrum disorders: A systematic review. *Res Autism Spect Disord.* 7:49–55.

33. De Flora, S., Izzotti, A., D'Agostini, F., & Balansky, R.M. 2001. Mechanisms of N-acetylcysteine in the prevention of DNA damage and cancer, with special reference to smoking-related end-points. *Carcinogenesis.* 22:999–1013.

34. De Iuliis, G.N., Newey, R.J., King, B.V., & Aitken, R.J. 2009. Mobile phone radiation induces reactive oxygen species production and DNA damage in human spermatozoa in vitro. *PLoS One.* 4:e6446.

35. DeFranco, E., Moravec, W., Xu, F., et al. 2016. Exposure to airborne particulate matter during pregnancy is associated with preterm birth: A population-based cohort study. *Environ Health.* 15:6.

36. deFur, P.L., & Kaszuba, M. 2002. Implementing the precautionary principle. *Sci Total Environ.* 288:155–165.

37. Diamanti-Kandarakis, E., Bourguignon, J.P., Giudice, L.C., et al. 2009. Endocrine-disrupting chemicals: An Endocrine Society scientific statement. *Endocr Rev.* 30:293–342.
38. Dolinoy, D.C., Huang, D., & Jirtle, R.L. 2007. Maternal nutrient supplementation counteracts bisphenol A-induced DNA hypomethylation in early development. *Proc Nat Acad Sci U S A.* 104:13056–13061.
39. Domingo, J.L., & Nadal, M. 2015. Carcinogenicity of consumption of red and processed meat: What about environmental contaminants? *Environ Res.* 145:109–115.
40. Dos Reis, L.C., de Oliveira, V.R., Hagen, M.E., Jablonski, A., Flores, S.H., & de Oliveira Rios, A. 2015. Effect of cooking on the concentration of bioactive compounds in broccoli (*Brassica oleracea* var. Avenger) and cauliflower (*Brassica oleracea* var. Alphina F1) grown in an organic system. *Food Chem.* 172:770–777.
41. Duncan, K., Harris, S., & Ardies, C.M. 1997. Running exercise may reduce risk for lung and liver cancer by inducing activity of antioxidant and phase II enzymes. *Cancer Lett.* 116:151–158.
42. Duty, S.M., Mendonca, K., Hauser, R., et al. 2013. Potential sources of bisphenol A in the neonatal intensive care unit. *Pediatrics.* 131:483–489.
43. Eisenberg, D.M., Davis, R.B., Ettner, S.L., et al. 1998. Trends in alternative medicine use in the United States, 1990–1997: Results of a follow-up national survey. *JAMA.* 280:1569–1575.
44. Entringer, S., Buss, C., & Wadhwa, P.D. 2015. Prenatal stress, development, health and disease risk: A psychobiological perspective. 2015 Curt Richter Award Paper. *Psychoneuroendocrinology.* 62:366–375.
45. Environmental Working Group. 2003. PCBs in Farmed Salmon: Wild Versus Farmed. http://www.ewg.org/research/pcbs-farmed-salmon/wild-versus-farmed.
46. Environmental Working Group. 2005. Body Burden: The Pollution in Newborns. A Benchmark Investigation of Industrial Chemicals, Pollutants and Pesticides in Umbilical Cord Blood. http://www.ewg.org/research/body-burden-pollution-newborns.
47. Escolar, E., Lamas, G.A., Mark, D.B., et al. 2014. The effect of an EDTA-based chelation regimen on patients with diabetes mellitus and prior myocardial infarction in the Trial to Assess Chelation Therapy (TACT). *Circ Cardiovasc Qual Outcomes.* 7:15–24.
48. Fenech, M.F. 2010. Dietary reference values of individual micronutrients and nutriomes for genome damage prevention: current status and a road map to the future. *Am J Clin Nutr.* 91:1438s–1454s.
49. Fischer, C.J., Bickle Graz, M., Muehlethaler, V., Palmero, D., & Tolsa, J.F. 2013. Phthalates in the NICU: Is it safe? *J Paediatr Child Health.* 49:E413–E419.
50. Friedman, M., Zhu, L., Feinstein, Y., & Ravishankar, S. 2009. Carvacrol facilitates heat-induced inactivation of *Escherichia coli* O157:H7 and inhibits formation of heterocyclic amines in grilled ground beef patties. *J Agric Food Chem.* 57:1848–1853.
51. Genuis, S.J. 2009. Nowhere to hide: Chemical toxicants and the unborn child. *Reprod Toxicol.* 28:115–116.

52. Genuis, S.J., Birkholz, D., Ralitsch, M., & Thibault, N. 2010. Human detoxification of perfluorinated compounds. *Public Health.* 124:367–375.

53. Gorpinchenko, I., Nikitin, O., Banyra, O., & Shulyak, A. 2014. The influence of direct mobile phone radiation on sperm quality. *Cent Eur J Urol.* 67:65–71.

54. Greenlee, H., Abascal, K., Yarnell, E., & Ladas, E. 2007. Clinical applications of *Silybum marianum* in oncology. *Integr Cancer Ther.* 6:158–165.

55. Guengerich, F.P. 1995. Influence of nutrients and other dietary materials on cytochrome P-450 enzymes. *Am J Clin Nutr.* 61:651s–658s.

56. Guxens, M., Aguilera, I., Ballester, F., 2012. Prenatal exposure to residential air pollution and infant mental development: Modulation by antioxidants and detoxification factors. *Environ Health Perspect.* 120:144–149.

57. Hannuksela, M.L., & Ellahham, S. 2001. Benefits and risks of sauna bathing. *Am J Med.* 110:118–126.

58. Harley, K.G., Kogut, K., Madrigal, D.S., et al. 2016. Reducing phthalate, paraben, and phenol exposure from personal care products in adolescent girls: Findings from the HERMOSA Intervention Study. *Environ Health Perspect.* 124:1600–1607.

59. Harris, A. & Seckl, J. 2011. Glucocorticoids, prenatal stress and the programming of disease. *Horm Behav.* 59:279–289.

60. Health Care Without Harm. 2008. Alternatives to Polyvinyl Chloride (PVC) and Di(2-Ethylhexyl) Phthalate (DEHP) Medical Devices. https://noharm.org/sites/default/files/lib/downloads/pvc/Alternatives_to_PVC_DEHP.pdf.

61. Health Care Without Harm. 2008. Alternatives to Polyvinyl Chloride (PVC) Medical Devices for the Neonatal Intensive Care Unit (NICU). https://noharm.org/sites/default/files/lib/downloads/pvc/Alternatives_to_PVC_in_NICU.pdf.

62. Heindel, J.J., Blumberg B., Cave M., et al. 2016, October 16. Metabolism disrupting chemicals and metabolic disorders. *Reprod Toxicol.* Epub ahead of print. doi: 10.1016/j.reprotox.2016.10.001

63. Herdt-Losavio, M.L., Lin, S., Chapman, B.R., et al. 2010. Maternal occupation and the risk of birth defects: An overview from the National Birth Defects Prevention Study. *Occup Environ Med.* 67:58–66.

64. Hodek, P., Trefil, P., & Stiborova, M. 2002. Flavonoids: Potent and versatile biologically active compounds interacting with cytochromes P450. *Chem Biol Interact.* 139:1–21.

65. Holecek, M. 2013. Side effects of long-term glutamine supplementation. *JPEN J Parenter Enteral Nutr.* 37:607–616.

66. Hong, N.S., Kim, K.S., Lee, I.K., et al. 2012. The association between obesity and mortality in the elderly differs by serum concentrations of persistent organic pollutants: A possible explanation for the obesity paradox. *Int J Obes.(Lond)* 36:1170–1175.

67. Hormann, A.M., Vom Saal, F.S., Nagel, S.C., et al. 2014. Holding thermal receipt paper and eating food after using hand sanitizer results in high serum bioactive and urine total levels of bisphenol A (BPA). *PLoS One.* 9:e110509.

68. Hu, P., Chen, X., Whitener, R.J., et al. 2013. Effects of parabens on adipocyte differentiation. *Toxicol Sci.* 131:56–70.

69. Hue, O., Marcotte, J., Berrigan, F., et al. 2006. Increased plasma levels of toxic pollutants accompanying weight loss induced by hypocaloric diet or by bariatric surgery. *Obes Surg.* 16:1145–1154.

70. Ibrahim, F., Halttunen, T., Tahvonen, R., & Salminen, S. 2006. Probiotic bacteria as potential detoxification tools: Assessing their heavy metal binding isotherms. *Can J Microbiol.* 52:877–885.

71. Jackson, S.L., King, S.M., Zhao, L., & Cogswell, M.E. 2016. Prevalence of excess sodium intake in the United States—NHANES, 2009-2012. *MMWR Morb MortalWkly Rep.* 64:1393–1397.

72. James, S., Stevenson, S.W., Silove, N., & Williams, K. 2015. Chelation for autism spectrum disorder (ASD). *Cochrane Database Syst Rev.* (5):CD010766.

73. Jan, A.T., Azam, M., Siddiqui, K., Ali, A., Choi, I., & Haq, Q.M. 2015. Heavy metals and human health: Mechanistic insight into toxicity and counter defense system of antioxidants. *Int J Mol Sci.* 16:29592–29630.

74. Jiao, J., Lu, G., Liu, X., Zhu, H., & Zhang, Y. 2011. Reduction of blood lead levels in lead-exposed mice by dietary supplements and natural antioxidants. *J Sci Food Agric.* 91:485–491.

75. Kapusta-Duch, J., Kopec, A., Piatkowska, E., Borczak, B., & Leszczynska, T. 2012. The beneficial effects of Brassica vegetables on human health. *Rocz Panstw Zakl Hig.* 63:389–395.

76. Karande, P., & Mitragotri, S. 2009. Enhancement of transdermal drug delivery via synergistic action of chemicals. *Biochim Biophys Acta.* 1788:2362–2373.

77. Kilburn, K.H., Warsaw, R.H., & Shields, M.G. 1989. Neurobehavioral dysfunction in firemen exposed to polycholorinated biphenyls (PCBs): Possible improvement after detoxification. *Arch Environ Health.* 44:345–350.

78. Klein, N., & Kemper, K.J. 2016. Integrative approaches to caring for children with autism. *Curr Prob Pediatr Adolesc Health Care.* 46:195–201.

79. Klein, S., Rister, R. 1998. *The Complete German Commisssion E Monographs: Therapeutic Guide to Herbal Medicines*, Baltimore, MD: Lippincott Williams & Wilkins.

80. Kohansieh, M., & Makaryus, A.N. 2015. Sleep deficiency and deprivation leading to cardiovascular disease. *Int L Hypertens.* 2015:615681.

81. Krop, J. 1998. Chemical sensitivity after intoxication at work with solvents: Response to sauna therapy. *J Altern Complement Med.* 4:77–86.

82. Kwapniewski, R., Kozaczka, S., Hauser, R., Silva, M.J., Calafat, A.M., & Duty, S.M. 2008. Occupational exposure to dibutyl phthalate among manicurists. *J Occup Environ Med.* 50:705–711.

83. Lamas, G.A. 2015. Cardiology Patient Page. Chelation therapy: A new look at an old treatment for heart disease, particularly in diabetics. *Circulation.* 131:e505–e506.

84. Lamas, G.A., Boineau, R., Goertz, C., et al. 2014. EDTA chelation therapy alone and in combination with oral high-dose multivitamins and minerals for coronary disease: The factorial group results of the Trial to Assess Chelation Therapy. *Am Heart J.* 168:37–44.e35.

85. Lee, W.W. 2007. An overview of pediatric obesity. *Pediatr diab.* 8(Suppl 9):76–87.

86. Leeuwenburgh, C., Hollander, J., Leichtweis, S., Griffiths, M., Gore, M., & Ji, L.L. 1997. Adaptations of glutathione antioxidant system to endurance training are tissue and muscle fiber specific. *Am J Physiol.* 272:R363–R369.

87. Lewczuk, B., Redlarski, G., Zak, A., Ziolkowska, N., Przybylska-Gornowicz, B., & Krawczuk, M. 2014. Influence of electric, magnetic, and electromagnetic fields on the circadian system: Current stage of knowledge. *BioMed Res Int.* 2014:169459.

88. Liu, K., Li, Y., Zhang, G., et al. 2014. Association between mobile phone use and semen quality: A systemic review and meta-analysis. *Andrology.* 2:491–501.

89. Longo, V.D., & Mattson, M.P. 2014. Fasting: Molecular mechanisms and clinical applications. *Cell Metab.* 19:181–192.

90. Lorber, M., Schecter, A., Paepke, O., Shropshire, W., Christensen, K., & Birnbaum, L. 2015. Exposure assessment of adult intake of bisphenol A (BPA) with emphasis on canned food dietary exposures. *Environ Int.* 77:55–62.

91. Lovejoy, H.B., Bell, Z.G. Jr., & Vizena, T.R. 1973. Mercury exposure evaluations and their correlation with urine mercury excretions: 4. Elimination of mercury by sweating. *J Occup Med.* 15:590–591.

92. Manzel, A., Muller, D.N., Hafler, D.A., Erdman, S.E., Linker, R.A., & Kleinewietfeld, M. 2014. Role of "Western diet" in inflammatory autoimmune diseases. *Curr Allergy Asthma Rep.* 14:404.

93. Mattson, M.P. 2014. Challenging oneself intermittently to improve health. *Dose-Response.* 12:600–618.

94. Mattson, M.P. 2015. Lifelong brain health is a lifelong challenge: From evolutionary principles to empirical evidence. *Ageing Res Rev.* 20:37–45.

95. McConaha, M.E., Ding, T., Lucas, J.A., Arosh, J.A., Osteen, K.G., & Bruner-Tran, K.L. 2011. Preconception omega-3 fatty acid supplementation of adult male mice with a history of developmental 2,3,7,8-tetrachlorodibenzo-*p*-dioxin exposure prevents preterm birth in unexposed female partners. *Reproduction.* 142:235–241.

96. McCurdy, L.E., Roberts, J., Rogers, B., et al. 2004. Incorporating environmental health into pediatric medical and nursing education. *Environ Health Perspect.* 112:1755–1760.

97. McEwen, B.S., & Karatsoreos, I.N. 2015. Sleep deprivation and circadian disruption: Stress, allostasis, and allostatic load. *Sleep Med Clin.* 10:1–10.

98. Miller, M.F., Bellizzi, K.M., Sufian, M., Ambs, A.H., Goldstein, M.S., & Ballard-Barbash, R. 2008. Dietary supplement use in individuals living with cancer and other chronic conditions: A population-based study. *J Am Dietetic Assoc.* 108:483–494.

99. Murray, T.V., Dong, X., Sawyer, G.J., et al. 2015. NADPH oxidase 4 regulates homocysteine metabolism and protects against acetaminophen-induced liver damage in mice. *Free Radic Biol Med.* 89:918–930.

100. Myers, G.J., Davidson, P.W., & Strain, J.J. 2007. Nutrient and methyl mercury exposure from consuming fish. *J Nutr.* 137:280S–280S.

101. National Center for Complementary and Integrative Health. 2016. Autism. https://nccih.nih.gov/health/autism.

102. National Center for Complementary and Integrative Health. 2016. Chelation for Coronary Heart Disease. https://nccih.nih.gov/health/chelation.

103. National Environmental Education Foundation. 2005. *Environmental Management of Pediatric Asthma: Guidelines for Health Care Providers.* http://www.niehs.nih.gov/health/assets/docs_a_e/environmental_management_of_pediatric_asthma_guidelines_for_health_care_providers_508.pdf.

104. National Environmental Education Foundation. 2015. *Environmental Intervention Guidelines and Patient Handouts.* http://64.130.52.13/health/asthma/intervention_guidelines.htm.

105. National Institute of Environmental Health Sciences. 2016. *Perfluorinated Chemicals (PFCs).* http://www.niehs.nih.gov/health/topics/agents/pfc/index.cfm.

106. Nehlig, A. 2016. Effects of coffee/caffeine on brain health and disease: What should I tell my patients? *Pract Neurol.* 16:89–95.

107. Oosterveld, F.G., Rasker, J.J., Floors, M., et al. 2009. Infrared sauna in patients with rheumatoid arthritis and ankylosing spondylitis: A pilot study showing good tolerance, short-term improvement of pain and stiffness, and a trend towards long-term beneficial effects. *Clin Rheumatol.* 28:29–34.

108. Pak, V.M., Nailon, R.E., & McCauley, L.A. 2007. Controversy: Neonatal exposure to plasticizers in the NICU. *Am J Matern Child Nurs.* 32:244–249.

109. Phipps-Nelson, J., Redman, J.R., Dijk, D.J., & Rajaratnam, S.M. 2003. Daytime exposure to bright light, as compared to dim light, decreases sleepiness and improves psychomotor vigilance performance. *Sleep.* 26:695–700.

110. Physicians for Social Responsibility. *Hazardous Chemicals in Health Care: A Shapshot of Chemicals in Doctors and Nurses.* http://www.psr.org/assets/pdfs/hazardous-chemicals-in-health-care.pdf.

111. Pizzorno, J.E., & Murray, M.T. 2012. *Textbook of Natural Medicine*, 4th ed, p 480. London: Churchill Livingstone.

112. Popkin, B.M., Adair, L.S., & Ng, S.W. 2012. Global nutrition transition and the pandemic of obesity in developing countries. *Nutr Rev.* 70:3–21.

113. Posadzki, P., Watson, L., & Ernst, E. 2013. Contamination and adulteration of herbal medicinal products (HMPs): An overview of systematic reviews. *Eur J Clin Pharmacol.* 69:295–307.

114. Rago, R., Salacone, P., Caponecchia, L., et al. 2013. The semen quality of the mobile phone users. *J Endocrinol Invest.* 36:970–974.

115. Rahman, Q., Abidi, P., Afaq, F., et al. 1999. Glutathione redox system in oxidative lung injury. *Criti Rev Toxicol.* 29:543–568.

116. Rambaldi, A., Jacobs, B.P., & Gluud, C. 2007. Milk thistle for alcoholic and/or hepatitis B or C virus liver diseases. *Cochrane Database syst rev.* (4):CD003620.

117. Rauber, F., Campagnolo, P.D., Hoffman, D.J., & Vitolo, M.R. 2015. Consumption of ultra-processed food products and its effects on children's lipid profiles: A longitudinal study. *Nutr Metab Cardiovasc Dis.* 25:116–122.

118. Rice, D.C. 2008. Overview of modifiers of methylmercury neurotoxicity: Chemicals, nutrients, and the social environment. *Neurotoxicology.* 29:761–766.

119. Roberts, J.R., & Karr, C.J. 2012. Pesticide exposure in children. *Pediatrics.* 130:e1757–e1763.

120. Rocha de Oliveira, C., Ceolin, J., Rocha de Oliveira, R., et al. 2014. Effects of quercetin on polychlorinated biphenyls-induced liver injury in rats. *Nutr Hosp.* 29:1141–1148.

121. Rogan, W.J., Paulson, J.A., Baum, C., et al. 2014. Iodine deficiency, pollutant chemicals, and the thyroid: New information on an old problem. *Pediatrics.* 133:1163–1166.

122. Rogers, B. 2004. Environmental health hazards and health care professional education. *AAOHN J.* 52:154–155.

123. Ross, G.H., & Sternquist, M.C. 2012. Methamphetamine exposure and chronic illness in police officers: Significant improvement with sauna-based detoxification therapy. *Toxicol Indus Health.* 28:758–768.

124. Sandstrom, B. 2001. Micronutrient interactions: Effects on absorption and bioavailability. *Br J Nutr.* 85(Suppl 2):S181–S185.

125. Sathyanarayana, S., Calafat, A.M., Liu, F., & Swan, S.H. 2008. Maternal and infant urinary phthalate metabolite concentrations: Are they related? *Environ Res.* 108:413–418.

126. Sattler, B., Randall, K.S., & Choiniere, D. 2012. Reducing hazardous chemical exposures in the neonatal intensive care unit: A new role for nurses. *Crit Care Nurs Q* 35:102–112.

127. Sawa, T., Naito, Y., Katoh, H., & Amaya, F. 2016. Cellular Stress Responses and Monitored Cellular Activities. *Shock (Augusta, Ga.).* doi: 10.1097/SHK.0000000000000603.

128. Schnare, D.W., Denk, G., Shields, M., & Brunton, S. 1982. Evaluation of a detoxification regimen for fat stored xenobiotics. *Med Hypoth.* 9:265–282.

129. Schnare, D.W., & Robinson, P.C. 1986. Reduction of the human body burdens of hexachlorobenzene and polychlorinated biphenyls. *IARC Sci Publ.*(77):597–603.

130. Sears, M.E., Kerr, K.J., & Bray, R.I. 2012. Arsenic, cadmium, lead, and mercury in sweat: A systematic review. *J Environ Public Health.* 2012:184745.

131. Shabbir, M.A., Raza, A., Anjum, F.M., Khan, M.R., & Suleria, H.A. 2015. Effect of thermal treatment on meat proteins with special reference to heterocyclic aromatic amines (HAAs). *Crit Rev Food Sci Nutr.* 55:82–93.

132. Silver, M.K., Lozoff, B., & Meeker, J.D. 2013. Blood cadmium is elevated in iron deficient U.S. children: A cross-sectional study. *Environ Health.* 12:117.

133. Simmons, A.L., Schlezinger, J.J., & Corkey, B.E. 2014. What are we putting in our food that is making us fat? Food additives, contaminants, and other putative contributors to obesity. *Cur Obes Rep.* 3:273–285.

134. Singh, S., Mani, K.V., & Kapoor, N. 2015. Effect of occupational EMF exposure from radar at two different frequency bands on plasma melatonin and serotonin levels. *Int J Radiat Biol.* 91:426–434.

135. Solenkova, N.V., Newman, J.D., Berger, J.S., Thurston, G., Hochman, J.S., & Lamas, G.A. 2014. Metal pollutants and cardiovascular disease: Mechanisms and consequences of exposure. *Am Heart J.* 168:812–822.

136. Song, M., & Giovannucci, E. 2016. Preventable incidence and mortality of carcinoma associated with lifestyle factors among white adults in the United States. *JAMA Oncol.* 2:1154–1161.

137. Srinivasan, P., Suchalatha, S., Babu, P.V., et al. 2008. Chemopreventive and therapeutic modulation of green tea polyphenols on drug metabolizing enzymes in 4-nitroquinoline 1-oxide induced oral cancer. *Chem Biol Interact.* 172:224–234.

138. Stein-Behrens, B.A., & Sapolsky, R.M. 1992. Stress, glucocorticoids, and aging. *Aging (Milan, Italy).* 4:197–210.

139. Suarez-Ortegon, M.F., Mosquera, M., Caicedo, D.M., De Plata, C.A., & Mendez, F. 2013. Nutrients intake as determinants of blood lead and cadmium levels in Colombian pregnant women. *Am J Hum Biol.* 25:344–350.

140. Suh, Y.J., Lee, J.E., Lee, D.H., et al. 2016. Prevalence and relationships of iron deficiency anemia with blood cadmium and vitamin D levels in Korean women. *J Korean Med Sci.* 31:25–32.

141. Szilard, S., Szentgyorgyi, D., & Demeter, I. 1988. Protective effect of Legalon in workers exposed to organic solvents. *Acta Med Hung.* 45:249–256.

142. Tei, C., Orihara, F.K., & Fukudome, T. 2007. Remarkable efficacy of thermal therapy for Sjogren syndrome. *J Cardiol.* 49:217–219.

143. U. S. Agency for Toxic Substances and Disease Registry (ATSDR). 2015. Priority List of Hazardous Substances That Will Be the Candidates for Toxicological Profiles. https://www.atsdr.cdc.gov/spl/.

144. U. S. Consumer Product Safety Commission. 2015. Phthalates.

145. U. S. Consumer Product Safety Commission. 2016. Total Lead Content. https://www.cpsc.gov/Business--Manufacturing/Business-Education/Lead/Total-Lead-Content.

146. U. S. Environmental Protection Agency. 2016. Drinking Water Requirements for Lead. https://www.epa.gov/ground-water-and-drinking-water/basic-information-about-lead-drinking-water.

147. U. S. Environmental Protection Agency. 2016. Table of Regulated Drinking Water Contaminants. https://www.epa.gov/ground-water-and-drinking-water/table-regulated-drinking-water-contaminants.

148. van Praag, H., Fleshner, M., Schwartz, M.W., & Mattson, M.P. 2014. Exercise, energy intake, glucose homeostasis, and the brain. *J Neurosci.* 34:15139–15149.

149. Vatansever, F., & Hamblin, M.R. 2012. Far infrared radiation (FIR): Its biological effects and medical applications. *Photonics Lasers Med.* 4:255–266.

150. Vojdani, A. 2009. Detection of IgE, IgG, IgA and IgM antibodies against raw and processed food antigens. *Nutr Metab.* 6:22.

151. Vojdani, A. 2014. A potential link between environmental triggers and autoimmunity. *Autoimmune Dis.* 2014:437231.

152. Ward, J., Kapadia, K., Brush, E., & Salhanick, S.D. 2013. Amatoxin poisoning: Case reports and review of current therapies. *J Emerg Med.* 44:116–121.

153. White, C.P., Hirsch, G., Patel, S., Adams, F., & Peltekian, K.M. 2007. Complementary and alternative medicine use by patients chronically infected with hepatitis C virus. *Can J Gastroenterol.* 21:589–595.

154. Wolff, M.S., Engel, S.M., Berkowitz, G.S., et al. 2008. Prenatal phenol and phthalate exposures and birth outcomes. *Environ Health Perspect.* 116:1092–1097.

155. World Health Organization and United Nations Environment Programme. 2012. *State of the Science of Endocrine Disrupting Chemicals—2012.* 289 pp. http://unep.org/pdf/9789241505031_eng.pdf.

156. Xie, L., Kang, H., Xu, Q., et al. 2013. Sleep drives metabolite clearance from the adult brain. *Science.* 342:373–377.

157. Yiamouyiannis, C.A., Sanders, R.A., Watkins, J.B. 3rd, & Martin, B.J. 1992. Chronic physical activity: Hepatic hypertrophy and increased total biotransformation enzyme activity. *Biochem Pharmacol.* 44:121–127.

158. Zalata, A., El-Samanoudy, A.Z., Shaalan, D., El-Baiomy, Y., & Mostafa, T. 2015. In vitro effect of cell phone radiation on motility, DNA fragmentation and clusterin gene expression in human sperm. *Int J Fertil Steril.* 9:129–136.

159. Zentner, L.E., Rondo, P.H., Duran, M.C., & Oliveira, J.M. 2008. Relationships of blood lead to calcium, iron, and vitamin C intakes in Brazilian pregnant women. *Clin Nutr (Edinb.)* 27:100–104.

160. Zilberlicht, A., Wiener-Megnazi, Z., Sheinfeld, Y., Grach, B., Lahav-Baratz, S., & Dirnfeld, M. 2015. Habits of cell phone usage and sperm quality: Does it warrant attention? *Reprod Biomed Online.* 31:421–426.

INDEX

Page references for figures are indicated by *f*, for tables by *t*, and for boxes by *b*.

Absorption, distribution, metabolism, and
    excretion (ADME), 289–290
Acetaminophen (APAP)
    biomonitoring studies of, 147–149, 148*t*
    characteristics of, 145*t*
    developmental exposure to, male
        reproductive disorders and, 150,
        151*t*–157*t*, 158–160
    maternal exposure to, male genital
        outcomes, 160, 161*t*–162*t*, 163–164
    mechanisms of action of, 143–146, 144*t*
    pregnancy use and effects of, 142–143,
        144*t*, 146–147
    sources of exposure to, 149–150
    therapeutic and toxic responses to, 144*t*,
        146–147
Acetyl-salicylic acid (ASA)
    characteristics of, 145*t*
    developmental exposure to, male
        reproductive disorders and, 150,
        151*t*–153*t*, 155*t*–156*t*, 158–159
    maternal exposure to, male genital
        outcomes, 160–163, 161*t*
    mechanisms of action of, 143–146,
        144*t*, 146
    pregnancy use of, 143, 144*t*, 146
    therapeutic and toxic responses to,
        144*t*, 146
Activational effects, 291
Additives. *See also specific types*
    food, 255–273
    plastic, 35–39

Adolescents, 61–62
Adverse outcome pathways, 16
Agent Orange, 322
Agriculture. *See also specific chemicals*
    chemicals in, water pollution from, 102
    wastewater and biosolids use by, 91–92
Air, clean, 353–355, 362
Air fresheners, 74, 355
Air pollution, 355
Air purifiers, free-standing, 78
Air quality, indoor, 67–82. *See also* Indoor
    air quality
Albumin, 54
Aldrin, in amyotrophic lateral
    sclerosis, 185
Allergy
    incidence of, 67
    indoor air quality in, 69–70
Alzheimer disease, 181–184
    epidemiology of, 181
    genetics of, 182
    pesticides and, 182–183
    pesticide toxicity mechanisms
        in, 183–184
    vascular dementia *vs.*, 181–182
Ammonium chloride (ADBAC), 210–213.
    See also Quaternary ammonium
    compounds (QACs)
Ammonium nitrate explosion, on water
    supply, 92–93
Amyloid plaques, 182
Amyotrophic lateral sclerosis, 184–185

Analgesics, mild, 142–164. *See also*
  specific types
  developmental exposure to, male
    reproductive disorders from, 150–160,
    151*t*–157*t*
  maternal exposure to, male genital
    outcomes with, 160–164, 161*t*–162*t*
  mechanisms of action of, 143, 144*t*–145*t*
  pregnancy use of, 142–150, 144*t*–145*t*
  prevalence of use of, 142–143
Anastas and Warner's *Principles of Green*
    Chemistry, 315, 316*b*, 328*b*
Antibiotics, 125–126
Antimicrobials, 7*t*, 15
Antimony, 39, 41
Antiseptics, 198
Apolipoprotein E-4 (*APOE**E4) allele, 182
Aquaculture, 91
Arsenic, in water, 119
Artificial flavors, 271
Artificial sweeteners, 125
Asthma, 67, 68, 70
Atrazine, in water, 102
Autism
  chelation therapy for, 369
  glyphosate and, 122
  gut-brain axis and, 133
  gut microbiome and, 118*b*, 132
  prevalence of, 135
  radiofrequency radiation and, 232
  testing and, 287

Baby formula, 4
Benzene, 7*t*, 9–10
Betaproteobacteria, 129
Binding affinity, 293
Binding proteins, 53–55, 54*f*
Biocides, 199–213. *See also specific types*
  definition of, 198
  endo-disrupting, 199
  parabens, 199–203
  quaternary ammonium compounds,
    210–213
  triclocarban, 207–209
  triclosan, 203–207
Biomonitoring, human. *See also* Monitoring
  of acetaminophen, 147–149, 148*t*
  for antimony, 41
  for bisphenol A, 41
  of breast milk, 4, 40, 40*f* (*See also*
    Breast milk)
  for ethylbenzene, 41

for PBDEs, 41
for phthalates, 41–42
of placenta/cord blood, 4, 40 (*See also*
    Cord blood)
for plastics, 39–42, 40*f*
for polybrominated diphenyl ethers, 41
for styrene, 42
of tissues, 40–41
U.S. Centers for Disease Control
    and Prevention (CDC) National
    Biomonitoring Program on, 4
Biosolids, 91–92
Bioterrorism Act of 2002, 95
Bisphenol A (BPA), 7*t*, 13, 31–34, 323
  biomonitoring for, 41
  diabetes and, 130
  as endocrine disruptor and hormone
    mimic, 32–33
  on endocrine system, 55–56
  folic acid for, 341
  on gut microbiome, 130
  hazardous health effects of, 33–34, 43–44
  in healthcare setting, 364
  indoor air pollution from, 74–75
  limiting exposure to, 342–343
  multigenerational effects of, 33
  in thermal paper receipts, 32
  weak properties *vs.* potency of, 293
Bisphenol F (BPF), 13–14, 75, 130
Bisphenol S (BPS), 13–14, 75, 130
Boric acid (borate), 188
Brain cancer, radiofrequency radiation in,
    235–237, 236*f*
Breast cancer, 202–203, 237
Breast milk
  biomonitoring of, 4, 40, 40*f*
  BPA in, 41
  chemicals in, 4, 40, 40*f*
  DDE in, 129
  industrial chemicals and plastics in, 39–40
  PBA in, 40
  PDBEs in, 40, 41
  PFOA and PFOS in, 12
  phthalates in, 42, 44
  as prebiotic, 359, 360*t*
  triclosan in, 15, 205
Broman, Göran, 325. *See also Chemistry and*
    Sustainability (C&S) Bookcase
Brundtland Commission, 307
BTEX, 7*t*, 9–10, 75
Butyrate, 119
Byproducts, industrial, 7*t*, 10–11

C8, 80
Cadmium, in water, 120
Cancer
    brain, radiofrequency radiation in,
        235–237, 236f
    breast, 202–203, 237
    colon, 133
    epigenome in, 132
    gut microbiome and, 132–133
    probiotics on, 133
    salivary gland, 237
    testicular, 237
Candles, synthetic, 355
Carbamates, neurotoxicity of, 183–184
Carboxymethylcellulose, 124
Carpet padding, flame retardants in, 78
Carpets, chemicals and off-gassing from, 72,
    73f, 74, 78
Carrageenan, 124–125
Carson, Rachel, *Silent Spring*, 6, 186, 280–282
Cell phone radiation, 223–243. *See also*
    Radiofrequency radiation
    in pregnancy, 363
Charleston, West Virginia,
    4-methylcyclohexanemethanol spill,
    93–94, 94f
Chelation therapy, 367–369
Chemical exposures, 3–17. *See also specific
    chemicals*
    adverse outcome pathways for, 16
    in baby formula, 4
    body burden in, 27
    in breast milk, 4
    in children *vs.* adults, 4
    in development, lasting effects
        of, 5–6
    in disease, 5–6
    documentation of, research for, 4
    effects of, evidence on, 16–17
    endocrine disruptors in, 4–5
    exposome in, 16
    green chemistry in, 16
    low concentrations of, 4
    monitoring of, 105
    in newborns, 4
    precautionary approach to, 17
    public awareness of, 4
    safety testing deficiencies for, 5
    in socioeconomically stressed
        communities, 4
    in utero, 4–5
    warning signs of, 4

Chemical regulation industry, deficiencies
    in, 75–76, 289, 298
Chemicals, 6–16, 7t. *See also specific types*
    categories of, 6, 7t
    cumulative health effects of, 266–268
    dioxins, 7t, 10–11
    flame retardants, 7t, 12–13
    lead, 7t, 9
    perfluorinated compounds, 11–12
    pesticides, 6–9, 7t, 8f
    phthalates, 7t, 14–15
    solvents, BTEX, 7t, 9–10
    synthetic, growth in, 5, 5f
    triclosan, 7t, 15
*Chemistry and Sustainability (C&S)
    Bookcase*, 313–323, 314f, 328
    endocrine disruptors in, 322–323
    green synthesis in, 315–317, 316b
    persistent molecular compounds in,
        320–322
    renewable feedstocks in, 317, 317b
    safe energy in, 317–319
    structure and functions of, 314–315, 314f
    toxic elements in, 319–320
Children
    chemical exposures on, 4
    chemical vulnerability in, 61–62
    proactive approach to, 361
Chloracne, 11
Chlordane, 129
Chlorinated water, 120–121, 206
5-Chloro-2-(2, 4-dichlorophenoxy)-phenol.
    See Triclosan
Chloroform, from triclosan and chlorine/
    chloramine, 206
Chlorpyrifos, 6–8
Chronic obstructive pulmonary disease
    (COPD), 70
9-*cis* retinoic acid receptor, 288
Clean air, 353–355, 362
Cleaning products, 79
    on air quality, 355
    do-it-yourself, 352b–353b
    safe, 352
    toxins in, 352
Cleanliness, 198
Clean Production Act, 330
Cleanses, 367
Clean Technica, 324
Clean Water Act of 1972, 88–89, 103
Climate, earth, 28
Coagulation, 90

Codons, 57
Colborn, Theo, 281–282
Collaborative of Health and the
    Environment (CHE), 324
Colon cancer, gut microbiome and, 133
Complex 1, 180
Cookware, 80
Copper
    dietary, 356, 357
    in plating wastewater, 95
Cord blood
    biomonitoring of, 4, 40
    BPA in, 40, 41
    chemicals in, 361
    industrial chemicals and plastics in, 39–40
    PBA in, 40
    PFOA and PFOS in, 12
    triclocarbon in, 208
Cruciferous vegetables, 341–342
Cryptorchidism, from maternal analgesics,
    160–164, 161t–162t. *See also specific*
    analgesics

10-DAB, 318b
Dairy products, 125–126
DDT, 6–8, 7t, 99, 185, 186
Detox protocols, 366–369
    chelation therapy in, 367–369
    cleanses and fasting in, 367
Development, chemical exposure on,
    5, 61–62
Developmental origins of health and disease
    (DOHaD), 61–62, 295
Di-2-ethylhexyl phthalate (DEHP), 75,
    166–167
Diabetes, 130–131
Diabetogens, 129–131
Diatomaceous earth, 188, 189
Diazinon, 79
Dichlorodiphenyldichloroethylene
    (DDE), 129
Dichlorodiphenyltrichloroethane (DDT),
    6–8, 7t, 99, 185, 186, 321
2,4-Dichlorphenoxyacetic acid (2,4-D), 123,
    185, 186
Didecyl dimethyl ammonium chloride
    (DDAC), 210–213. *See also* Quaternary
    ammonium compounds (QACs)
Dieldrin, 185
Diet, 340–346. *See also* Drinking water; Gut
    microbiome
    artificial sweeteners in, 125

cruciferous vegetables, 341–342
    Dirty Dozen in, 189, 322, 343, 344t
    emulsifiers in, 124–125
    on endotoxin absorption, 115
    fertilizers and pesticides in, 121–123
    fish in, 344–345
    food chemicals on, 122–127
    glyphosate in, 122–123
    on gut microbiome, 115, 116–120
    irradiated foods in, 126–127
    microwaved foods in, 127–128
    pesticides in produce in, 342, 344t
    phone apps for, 346b
    phytonutrients in, 118–119
    potassium bromate in, 124
    in pregnancy, 361–362
    recommendations for, 342–343
Dietary supplements, 356–360
    calcium, 356
    glutathione and N-acetyl-cysteine, 359
    milk thistle, 358
    niacin, 356
    prebiotics and probiotics, 359–360, 360t
    selenium, 356
    vitamin C, 356
    vitamin E, 356
    vitamin excess, 357
    zinc, copper, and manganese, 356
Diethylhexyl phthalate (DEHP), 99f, 261,
    364–365
Diethylstilbestrol (DES), 61, 98, 141–142,
    202–203, 295–296
Differentiation, gamete, 57
Di-isononyl phthalate (DINP), 75
Dimercaptosuccinic acid (DMSA), 367–368
Dimethylamine epichlorohydrin
    copolymer, 270
Dioxins, 10–11, 129, 321–322
Dipyrone, 143
Direct food additives, 257, 259, 262
Direct potable reuse (DPR), 108
Dirty Dozen, 189, 322, 343, 344t
Disinfection, 197–215. *See also specific agents*
    addendum to, 215
    antiseptics in, 198
    biocides in, 198, 199–213 (*See also* Biocides)
    cleanliness and, 198
    disinfectants in, 199
    disinfecting agents in, 198
    of drinking water, 90
    future directions in, 213–215
    microorganism control in, 198–199

sanitizers in, 199
sterilants in, 199
Dithiocarbamate, 185
DNA methylation, 134
Docosahexaenoic acid (DHA), 345
Dopamine metabolism, reactive oxygen species from, 178
Dose, 105
    effect and, 289
Dose responses
    linear and sigmoidal, 294, 294*f*
    nonlinear and nonmonotonic, 291, 294–295, 294*f*
Drinking water, 89–92, 346–347
    agriculture wastewater and biosolids use and, 91–92
    arsenic in, 120
    cadmium in, 120
    chlorination of, 120–121
    contamination of, 120–122
    filtration of, 90, 347
    indirect potable use of, 96
    metropolitan water supplies in, 89–91, 100, 347
    National Primary Drinking Water Regulations on, 90–91
    in pregnancy, 361–362
    well water in, residential, 91, 346, 347
Dust, 71
Dust, natural insecticidal, 188
Dust control, 71–75
    dusting products for, 79
    for endocrine-disrupting chemicals, 72–74, 73*f*
    for flame retardants, 72–74, 73*f*
    importance of, 71–72
Dye industry, 311
Dysbiosis, 116, 117*t*, 123. *See also* Gut microbiome

Economic performance, 311–312, 312*f*
Eicosapentaenoic acid (EPA), 345
Electromagnetically hypersensitive individuals, 239–241
Electromagnetics, 226–227, 226*f*
Emerging chemical, 11
Emulsifiers, 124–125
Endocrine-disrupting chemicals (EDCs), 4–5, 97–100, 279–298, 322–323. *See also* *specific types*
    actions of, 97, 98
    adverse effects of, 282–283

biocides, 199–213 (*See also* Biocides)
    categories of, 98–99
    chemical structures and properties of, 98, 99*f*
    cost-benefit analyses for, 297–298
    definitions of, 32, 97, 199, 282–283
    on development, 98
    in dust, 72–74, 73*f*
    early history of, 280–282
    endocrine principles in, 290–291
    endocrinology *vs.* toxicology approaches to, 291–296, 294*f*
    epidemiological studies of, 288
    Federation of Gynecology and Obstetrics on, 46
    on gut microbiome, 130
    harm of, evidence of, 295
    identification challenges for, 285–288
    legacy contaminants in, 99
    less-persistent, chronic exposure to, 100
    manufactured doubt about, 284–285
    parabens, 199–203
    in pharmaceuticals, 100
    potential, 282
    prioritizing, by exposure level, 292–293
    prioritizing, by relative potency *vs.* weak properties, 293
    quaternary ammonium compounds, 210–213
    research on, 97–98, 142
    risks of, 98
    safe doses of, predicting, 294–295, 294*f*
    science of, 283–284
    scientific disciplines in study of, 288–289
    Stevia rebaudiana, 125
    studies of, good, 292
    systematic review and integrated assessment of, 330
    tier1 and 2 assays of, 285–288
    tiered protocol for endocrine disruption (TIPED) for, 296–297, 309, 313, 329, 329*b*
    toxicology on, 289–290
    triclocarban, 207–209
    triclosan, 7*t*, 15, 130, 203–207
    Wingspread Conference statement on, 281–282, 322, 340
Endocrine-disrupting diseases, 280
Endocrine Disruption Exchange (TEDX), 4–5, 324
Endocrine principles, 290–291
Environmental performance, 311–313, 312*f*

Environmental Working Group (EWG), 40, 330
  Dirty Dozen of, 189, 322, 343, 344*t*
Epigenetic changes, 57–60
  gene silencing in, 58
  to gut microbiome, 116
  histones and nucleosomes in, 58, 59*f*
  inheritance of, 60–61
  mother-fetal transference of, 58
  probiotics in, 133
  sources of, 58–60
  timing and effects of, 58
Epigenome, in cancer, 132
Estrogen, in milk, 126
Ethinyl estradiol (EE2), 100, 101
Ethylbenzene biomonitoring, 41
Ethylene, 7*t*, 9–10
Ethylene bisdithiocarbamates (EDBCs), 181
Ethylenediaminetetraacetic acid (EDTA), 367–368
Eugenol, 119
Exercise, 350
Exogenous semiotic entropy, 122
Exposome, 16, 214
Exposure, 105, 289. *See also specific types*
Extremely low frequency (ELF), 226f, 227

Fasting, 367
Feedstocks, renewable, 317, 317*b*
Female reproductive disorders. *See*
  Reproductive disorders, female
Fenoprofen, 145*t*
Fertility, proactive approaches to, 361–363
Fertilizers. *See also specific types*
  ammonium nitrate, 92–93
  in diet, 121–123
Fetus, 61–62
Fibers, plastic waste, 28
Filtration
  drinking water, 90, 347
  HVAC, 76–77
  technologies for, 108
Firmicutes, 129
Fish
  consumption advisories and legacy
    contaminants in, 99
  in diet, 344–345
  ethinyl estradiol on, 100, 101
  plastic waste in, 28
  in pregnancy, 362
Flame retardants
  chemicals in, 7*t*, 12–13

diabetes and, 130–131
  on indoor air quality, 72–74, 73*f*
  TB-117, 12–13, 72–74
  tetrabromobisphenol A, 55
Flavors and flavoring agents, 270–271
Flint, Michigan drinking water, 68, 94–95, 346
Flocculation, 90
Folic acid, for bisphenol A effects, 341
Food Additive Amendment, 256, 259
Food additives, 255–273
  cumulative health effects of, 266–268
  decision-making process for, 257, 258*f*
  definition of, 256–257
  direct *vs.* indirect, 257
  flavors and flavoring agents, 270–271
  food-contact chemicals, 270
  GRAS exemption of, 257–259, 258*f*
  on gut microbiome, 122–127
  history of, 255–256
  incidental additives, 269–270
  increase in, 259
  labeling exceptions for, 269–272
  limiting exposure to, 272–273
  prior sanctioned process for, 258–259
  recommendations on, actionable, 273
  safety determination for, 262–266, 263*f*, 264*f*
  safety of, 259–262
  spices, 271
  voluntary submission of, 257–258
Food allergies, 70
Food chemicals. *See* Food additives
Food-contact chemicals, 270
Food processing, 255–256
Food sensitivities, 70
Formaldehyde off-gassing, 74
Fracking, 10, 103–104
Framework for strategic sustainable development (FSSD), 325–332
  assessment in, 327–330
  education in, 327
  origins and overview of, 325, 326*b*
  participants' role in, 327
  for regulatory agency deliberations, 325
  sibling sustainability field collaborations in, 327, 328*b*–329*b*
  social sustainability principles of, 325, 326*b*
  stewardship in, 330–332
Frank R. Lautenberg Chemical Safety for the 21st Century Act, 330

Fruit, pesticides in, 342, 344*t*
Fungicides, 79
Furnishings, 79, 354–355

Generally Recognized as Safe (GRAS), 74,
    215, 257
    flavors as, 271
    food additives as, 257–259, 258*f*
Gene silencing, 58
Genetically modified organisms (GMOs), 123
Genitals, male, maternal analgesic exposure
    on, 160–164, 161*t*–162*t*. *See also specific*
    analgesics
Globulins, 54
Glutamine, for gut health, 357
Glutathione, 359
Gluten intolerance (sensitivity), 70
Glycoproteins, 54
Glyphosate, 122–124, 320
Gonadotropes, triclosan on, 204, 206
Good laboratory practices (GLPs), 292
Granulated activated carbon (GAC), 108
Green chemistry, 16
    Anastas and Warner's principles of, 315,
        316*b*, 328*b*
    definition of, 305–306, 309
    EPA on, 305–306
Green science, 309, 313
GreenScreen for Safer Chemical, 330
Green stewardship, 310
Green synthesis, 315–317, 316*b*
Ground water, 102–104
Gut-brain axis, 133–134
Gut microbiome, 115–136
    antibiotics on, 125–126
    artificial sweeteners on, 125
    autism and, 132
    bisphenol A on, 130
    brain axis to, 133–134
    cancer and, 132–133
    changes to, on disease, 116
    diet on, 115, 116–120 (*See also* Diet)
    disease and dysbiosis in, 116, 117*t*
    dynamic, 119
    emulsifiers on, 124–125
    endocrine disruptors on, 130
    environmental chemicals in, 128, 129*f*
    environmental factors on, 115–116
    epigenetic changes to, 116
    flame retardants on, 130–131
    food additives on, 122–127
    future of, 134

    glyphosate on, 122–124
    hormones on, 126
    importance of, 115, 120
    irradiated foods on, 126–127
    Lactobacillus on, 119
    in metabolism and sequestration, 128
    microwaved foods on, 127–128
    obesogens and diabetogens on, 129–131
    organotins on, 130
    pesticides on, 116
    phthalates on, 131
    phytonutrients on, 118–119
    potassium bromate on, 124
    seasonal changes on, 116
    synbiotics on, 119
    in systemic nickel allergy syndrome, 131
    tributyltin on, 130
    triclosan on, 130
    vaginal *vs.* cesarean delivery on, 119
    xenobiotics on, 128
Gyres, 28, 30

Harm, defined, 260
Hazardous substance, 306
Healthcare settings, hazardous chemicals in,
    364–366
Health performance, 311–313, 312*f*
Heating, ventilation, and air conditioning
    (HVAC), on indoor air quality, 76–77
Herbicides. *See also specific types*
    glyphosate, 122–124, 320
    Parkinson disease and, 179–181
    reducing exposure to, 190
    water pollution from, 102
Heritable changes, 60
Heterocyclic aromatic amines (HCAs), 342
Hexachlorobenzene (HCB), 129
High-density polyethylene (HDPE), 29
High-efficiency particulate arrestance
    (HEPA) filter, 77
Histone modification, 58, 59*f*
Home furnishings, 79, 354–355
Homeostasis, 52–53
Hops, 349
Hormone-binding proteins
    (HBPs), 54, 54*f*
Hormone mimics, 32–33. *See also* Endocrine-
    disrupting chemicals (EDCs)
Hormones, 126, 290–291
Hospitals, hazardous chemicals in, 364–366
Human biomonitoring. *See*
    Biomonitoring, human

Human health studies, of plastics, 42–45
  bisphenol A, 43–44
  epidemiology limitations in, 42–43
  phthalates, 44–45
Humidity control, 77–78
Hydraulic fracturing, 10
4-Hydroxyphenyl 4-isoprooxyphenylsulfone
  (BPSIP), 13–14
Hygrometer, 77
Hypervitaminosis A, 357

Ibuprofen (IBP)
  developmental exposures to, male repro-
    ductive disorders, 151*t*, 154*t*, 158–159
  endocrine and reproductive effects of,
    151*t*, 154*t*
  environmental chemical interactions
    with, 165
  maternal exposure to, male genital
    outcomes, 160, 161*t*
  mechanisms of action of, 143–146, 144*t*
  pregnancy use of, 143, 144*t*
  therapeutic and toxic responses to,
    144*t*, 146
Immunoglobulin E (IgE), 70
Incidental additives, 269–270
Indirect food additives, 257, 259–262, 267, 270
Indirect potable reuse (IPR), 108, 109*t*–110*t*
Indirect potable use (IPR), 96
Indole3-carbinol (I3C), 342
Indomethacin, 150
  characteristics of, 144*t*
  developmental exposures to, male
    reproductive disorders, 150, 151*t*–153*t*,
    155*t*–156*t*, 158–159
  pregnancy use of, 143, 144*t*
Indoor air quality, 67–82
  air fresheners on, 74
  on allergic symptoms, 80–82, 81*f*
  on asthma, allergy, and sinusitis, 67
  bisphenol A on, 74–75
  clean house for, 76–80
  dust control in, 71–75
  flame retardants on, 72–74, 73*f*
  formaldehyde on, 74
  heating, ventilation, and air conditioning
    on, 76–77
  humidity control on, 77–78
  mites on, 77
  mold on, 77–78
  phthalates and polyvinyl chloride on, 75
  regulations on, 75–76

in respiratory diseases, 68–70 (*See also*
    Respiratory diseases, indoor air
    quality in)
Industrial byproducts, 7*t*, 10–11
Infants, 61–62
Insecticidal soap, 188
Insecticides, 79. *See also* Pesticides;
    specific types
  diazinon, 79
  organophosphate, 79
  Parkinson disease and, 179–181
  reducing exposure to, 190
Institute for Green Science, 306, 313
  *Chemistry and Sustainability (C&S)
    Bookcase* of, 313–323, 314*f*, 328 (*See also*
    *Chemistry and Sustainability (C&S)
    Bookcase*)
  oxidation catalysis program of, 321
  TAML activators of, 331–332
Integrated pest management (IPM), 186–189
  key points of, 186–187
  origins and history, 186
  urban, 187–189
In utero chemical exposures, 4–5
Iodine supplementation, in pregnancy, 341
Irradiated foods, 126–127
Irrigation water, 91–92

Ketoprofen, 143, 145*t*
Klimisch score, 292

Lactobacillus, 119
Lactobacillus reuteri, for systemic nickel
    allergy syndrome, 131
Lead, 7*t*, 9
  in drinking water, 346
  in Flint, Michigan drinking water, 68,
    94–95, 346
  in glazed pottery, non-U.S., 343
  in paint, 80
Leading from behind, 34
Legacy contaminants, 9, 99
Limonene, 355
Lindane, 99
Linear dose responses, 294, 294*f*
Lipoproteins, 54
Livestock, water for, 91

Male reproductive disorders. *See*
    Reproductive disorders, male
Maneb (manganese ethylene
    bisdithiocarbamate), 180–181

Manganese, 181, 356
Manganism, 181
Manufactured doubt, 284–285
Mauveine, 311
Meat irradiation, 126
MEHP, with analgesics, fetal effects of, 166–167
Melamine-formaldehyde plastic tableware, microwaving on, 127
Melatonin, 349
Mercury, in fish, 344–345
Messenger molecules, 53–57
 binding proteins for, 53–55, 54*f*
 environmental chemicals as, 54*f*, 55
 origins of, 53
 receptors and effects of, 55–57, 56*f*
 second messengers in, 55, 56*f*
 transport of, 54–55, 54*f*
Metals
 chelation therapy for, 367–369
 lead, 7*t*, 9
1-Methy-4-phenyl-1, 2, 3, 6-tetrahydropyridine (MPTP), 178
Methylation, 59*f*, 134
Methyl bromide, 185
4-Methylcyclohexanemethanol (MCHM) spill, 93–94, 94*f*
Microbiome, gut, 115–136. *See also* Gut microbiome
Microorganisms, 198
Microwaved foods, 127–128
Microwave-emitting devices, 226f, 227
Microwave radiation, 223–243
 bioeffects of, 228
 cardiovascular effects of, 233
 clinical approaches and public policy on, 238
 electromagnetics of, 226–227, 226*f*
 genetic damage from, 229
 studies of, human, 231–234, 234*f*
 studies of, *in vitro* and *in vivo*, 228–231
Milk, 125–126
Milk thistle, 358
Minimum efficiency reporting value (MERV), 76–77
Mites, 77
Mold, 77–78
Monitoring. *See also* Biomonitoring, human
 of chemical exposures, 105
 of water quality, 105–106
Monomers, plastic, 31
MPTP, 178
Mushroom irradiation, 126–127

N-acetyl-cysteine (NAC), 359
N acetyl-p-aminophenol (APAP). *See* Acetaminophen (APAP)
Naproxen, 143, 145*t*
National Biomonitoring Program, CDC, 4
National Institute of Environmental Health Sciences (NIEHS), 32, 199, 324
National Pollutant Discharge Elimination System (NPDES), 92, 103
National Primary Drinking Water Regulations (NPDWRs), 90–91
Natural flavors, 271
Neem oil, 188
Neonatal intensive care unit, 364–365
Neurodegenerative disorders, pesticides and, 175–190
 Alzheimer disease, 181–184
 amyotrophic lateral sclerosis, 184–185
 definition of, 177
 Parkinson disease, 176–181
Neurofibrillary tangles, 182
Newborns, 4–5, 365
Niacin, dietary, 356
Nickel allergy syndrome, systemic, 131
N-(4-chlorophenyl)-N-(3,4-dichlorophenyl) urea. *See* Triclocarban
Nonlinear dose responses, 291, 294–295, 294*f*
Nonmonotonic dose responses, 291, 294–295, 294*f*
Nonsteroidal anti-inflammatory drugs (NSAIDs), 142–143, 144*t*–145*t*, 146. *See also* Analgesics, mild; *specific types*
Nonylphenols, 39
Nucleosomes, 58, 59*f*
Nutrition labeling, 268–269, 269*f*
Nutrition Labeling and Education Act of 1990, 268–269, 269*f*

Obesogens, 129–131
Ocean, plastic waste in, 26–28, 27*f*
Omega-3 fatty acids, 341, 345
Organic foods, 343
Organizational effects, 291
Organochlorines, 185
Organophosphates, 79, 183–184
Organotins, 38–39, 130
"Our Common Future," 307
"Our Stolen Future," 97, 322

Pacific yew tree, 317, 318*b*
Paclitaxel, 317, 318*b*
Paint, lead, 73*f*, 80

Parabens, 199–203
  breast cancer and, 202–203
  definition and use of, 199
  endocrine-disrupting properties of, 200
  exposure to, 200–201
  persistence of, 201
  reproductive effects of, 201–202
  take-home message on, 203
  types and metabolites of, 200
Paracetamol. *See* Acetaminophen (APAP)
Paraquat, 180, 181
Parkinson disease, 176–181
  epidemiology, 177
  genetics of, 177–178
  history and prevalence of, 176
  insecticides, herbicides and, 179–181
  maneb and, 180–181
  MTPT mechanisms and, 178–179
  paraquat and, 180, 181
  pathophysiology of, 176
  permethrin and, 179–180
  rotenone and, 179
  substantia nigra dopaminergic neuron
    vulnerability in, 178
Paroxenase1 (PON1), 183
Perfluorinated acids, in fish, 344
Perfluorinated compounds (PFCs), 11–12
Perfluoroalkyls (PFAs), 92
Perfluorooctane sulfonic acid (PFOS), 12, 74
Perfluorooctanoic acid (PFOA), 12, 74,
    80, 105
Performances, four, 310–313, 312f, 328b
Permeability transition pore (PTP), 180
Permethrin, 179–180
Peroxidase enzymes, 331
Peroxisome proliferator–activated receptor-
    γ (PPARγ), 158, 200, 283–284, 288
Persistent bioaccumulative toxic compounds
    (PBTs), 321–322
Persistent molecular compounds, 320–322.
    See also specific types
Persistent organic pollutants (POPs), 11,
    320–321, 367
Personal care products, 351–352, 361
Pest, 186
Pest control, non-pesticide, 185–189. *See also*
    Integrated pest management (IPM)
Pesticides, 6–9, 7t, 8f. *See also specific types*
  definition and use of, 177
  in diet, 121–123
  on gut microbiome, 116
  in produce, 342, 344t

  reducing exposure to, 189–190
  Silent Spring on, 281
  transgenerational effects of, 8–9
  water pollution from, 102
Pesticides, neurodegenerative disorders
    from, 175–190
  Alzheimer disease, 181–184
  amyotrophic lateral sclerosis, 184–185
  Parkinson disease, 176–181
Pet allergens, 73f, 80, 81f
PET plastics, 39
Pharmaceuticals, 141–169. *See also*
    specific types
  analgesics, mild, 142–164 (*See also*
    Analgesics, mild; *specific types*)
  drug and environmental chemical inter-
    actions in, 164–168, 167f
  endocrine-disrupting, 100
  water pollution from, 101
Phosphorylation, 56–57
Phthalates, 7t, 14–15, 36–37
  in air fresheners, 74
  biomonitoring for, 41–42
  in breast milk, 42, 44
  in cleaning materials, 79
  diabetes and, 131
  environmental chemical interactions
    with, 164–165
  fetal effects of, 164–165, 167f
  fetal effects of, with mild analgesics,
    165–167, 167f
  on gut microbiome, 131
  human health studies of, 44–45
  indoor air pollution from, 75
Phthalate syndrome, 164–165
p-hydroxybenzoic acid (PHBA), 200
Physiology, environmental chemicals
    on, 51–62
  childhood and adolescent, 61–62
  epigenetic changes in, 57–60, 59f
  epigenetic changes in, inheritance
    of, 60–61
  fetal and infant, 61–62
  homeostasis in, 52–53
  messenger molecules in, 53–57 (*See also*
    Messenger molecules)
Phytonutrients, dietary, 118–119
Placenta blood, 40
Plant-based oils, insecticidal, 188
Plasma-binding proteins, 54, 54f
Plastic additives, 35–39. *See also specific types*
  antimony, 39

ethylbenzene, 39
nonylphenols, 39
organotins, 38–39
PET plastics, 39
phthalates, 36–37
polybrominated diphenyl ethers, 37–38
to polymers, 35–38
Plastic monomers, 14–15, 31, 34–35
Plastic polymers, 25–28. *See also specific constituents*
Plastics, 7*t*, 23–46. *See also specific types*
bioactivity of, 26
biodegradation of, 26
biomonitoring of, 39–42, 40*f*
bisphenol A, 7*t*, 13, 31–34, 43–44
debris and pollution from, 24–25, 25*f*
disposal and cleanup of, 30
history of, 24
human health studies on, 42–45
medical community on, 45–46
phthalates, 7*t*, 14–15, 36–37
production of, 24
recycling and reuse of, 29
seawater on, 26, 27, 27*f*
styrene, 35
thermoplastics, 26
thermoset, 26
ubiquity of, 24
ultraviolet radiation on, 26
Plastics, chemicals in, 30–35
permeability and, 31
plastic monomers, 31
variety of, 30
Plastic waste, 26–28
fibers in, 28
in fish, 28
in gyres, 28, 30
marine, 26–28, 27*f*
Plating operations, water pollution from, 95
Polybrominated diphenyl ethers (PBDEs), 37–38, 72, 129, 322
biomonitoring for, 41
diabetes and, 130–131
Polycarbonate, 31
Polychlorinated biphenyls (PCBs), 99, 321
contamination by, continuing, 129–130
diabetes and, 129
in fish, 344, 345
quercetin for, 341
Polychlorinated dibenzofurans (PCDFs), 344
Polychlorinated dibenzo-*p*-dioxins (PCDDs), 344

Polyethylene terephthalate (PET), 29
Polymers, plastic, 25–28
Polysorbate-80, 124
Polyvinyl chloride (PVC), 14–15, 34–35, 75
Potassium bromate, 124
Potassium ferricyanide terrorist attack, 95
Potency, 293
Prebiotics, 359–360, 360*t*
Precautionary principle (approach), x, 6, 17, 340, 370
Pregnancy
analgesic use in, mild, 142–150, 144*t*–145*t*
iodine supplementation in, 341
maternal abuse in, epigenetic effects of, 60–61
mobile phones and tablets in, 363 (*See also* Radiofrequency radiation)
personal care products in, 361
proactive approaches to, 361–363
seafood consumption in, 362
smoking in, 73*f*
toys and, 362–363
Presidential Green Chemistry Challenge Awards, 315, 317, 318*b*
Proactive approaches, 339–370
air in, clean, 353–355
in children, 361
cleaning products in, 352, 352*b*–353*b*
detox protocols in, 366–369
dietary supplements in, 356–360 (*See also* Dietary supplements)
diet in, 340–346 (*See also* Diet)
exercise in, 350
fertility and pregnancy in, 361–363
healthcare settings in, hazardous chemicals in, 364–366
personal care in, 351–352
vs. precautionary principle, 340, 370
radiofrequency radiation in, 369–370
sauna and sweating in, 350
sleep in, 347–349, 348*t*
stress reduction in, 355–356
tools for clinician in, 363–364
toxin testing in, 366
water in, 346–347
Probiotics, 133, 359–360, 360*t*
Processed foods, 340–341
Processing aids, 270
Prostaglandin D$_2$ (PGD$_2$), 150, 166
Pyrethroids, 185
Pyrethrum, 189

Quaternary ammonium compounds
(QACs), 210–213
chemistry and use of, 210
on cholesterol synthesis, 210–211
common forms of, 210
exposure to, 211
FDA ban of, 215
health concerns with, 212–213
persistence of, 211–212
personal protective equipment for, 210
take-home message on, 213
Quercetin, 341

Radiofrequency radiation, 223–243. *See also*
Microwave radiation
absorption of, 225, 225*f*
bioeffects of, 227–228
cancer and, 230–231, 235–238, 236*f*
carcinogenicity of, 235
cardiovascular effects of, 230, 233
cellular responses to, 228–229
clinical approaches to, 238
definition of, 224
developmental and neurological impacts
of, 230, 232
electromagnetically hypersensitive individuals and, 239–241
electromagnetics and, 226
exposure standards for, 224
genetic damage from, 229
natural experiments on, 231
ocular effects of, 225*f*, 233, 234*f*
proactive approach to, 369–370
public health recommendations on, 238–239
public policy on, 242–243
on reproduction, 229–230
studies of, human, 231–234, 234*f*
studies of, *in vitro* and *in vivo*, 228–231
toxicant synergism of, 228, 234–235
on voltage-gated calcium channels, 229
Reactive oxygen species (ROS), 178, 228
Receptors, 55–57, 56*f*
binding affinity to, 293
binding of, 290
Recycling, plastics, 29
Reference dose, 295
Regrettable substitution, 14
Renewable feedstocks, 317, 317*b*
Reproductive disorders, female
from parabens, 202
from radiofrequency radiation,
229–230, 232

Reproductive disorders, male
from acetaminophen, 150, 151*t*–157*t*,
158–160
from acetyl-salicylic acid, 150, 151*t*–153*t*,
155*t*–156*t*, 158–159
from analgesics, mild, 150–160, 151*t*–157*t*
from ibuprofen, 151*t*, 154*t*, 158–159
from indomethacin, 150, 151*t*–153*t*,
155*t*–156*t*, 158–159
from parabens, 201–202
from radiofrequency radiation,
229–230, 232
Respiratory diseases, indoor air quality
in, 68–70
allergy, 69–70
asthma, 70
diet and, 70
sinus inflammation, 68–69
Reversible electroporation, 229
Risk = hazard x exposure, 317–319
Robèrt, Karl-Henrik, 325
Rotenone, 179
Roxarsone, 320

Safe, 317
Safe energy, 317–319
Safety, 260
Safety testing. *See* Testing, safety
Safe Water Drinking Act (SWDA), U.S., 346
Salivary gland cancers, 237
Salmon, mackerel, anchovies, sardines, and
herring (SMASH), 345
Sanitizers, 199
Sauna, 350
Seafood, 344–345, 362
Second messengers, 55, 56*f*
Sedimentation, drinking water, 90
Selective serotonin reuptake inhibitors
(SSRIs), 57
Selenium, dietary, 356
Sensitivities, tissue-specific, 290
Set, 104, 107*f*
Setting, 104, 107*f*
Sex hormone–binding proteins (SHBG),
54–55, 54*f*
Sibling sustainability fields, 307–310
Brundtland Commission on, 307–308
collaborations in, 327, 328*b*–329*b*
qualities of, 308–310
Sigmoidal dose responses, 294, 294*f*
Silencing, gene, 58
Silent Spring (Carson), 6, 186, 280–282

Silica dusts, 188
Sinusitis, 67–69
Skin, 351
Sleep, 347–349, 348*t*
Sludge, treated, 92
Smoking, 73*f*, 354
Solvents, 7*t*, 9–10
Soy candles, 355
Specific absorption rate, 225, 225*f*
Spices, 271
Spinosad, 189
Starvation, transgenerational effects of, 60
Sterilants, 199
Stevia rebaudiana, 125
Stewardship, 330–332
Stress reduction, 355–356
Styrene, 35, 42
Substantia nigra, 178
Sulfiting agents, 270
Supplements, dietary, 356–360. *See also*
    Dietary supplements; *specific types*
Sustainable chemistry, 305–332
    challenges and solutions in, 323–324
    codifying and prioritizing challenges of,
        313–323, 314*f* (*See also Chemistry and
        Sustainability (C&S) Bookcase*)
    as communal effort, 310
    definitions of, 305–306
    framework for strategic sustainable
        development, 325–332, 326*b* (*See also
        Framework for strategic sustainable
        development (FSSD)*)
    green chemistry in, 305–306
    green stewardship in, 310
    importance and value of, 306–307
    performances in, 310–313, 312*f*, 328*b*
    sibling sustainability fields in, 307–310,
        327, 328*b*–329*b*
Sustainable development, 307–310
Sweating, 350
Sweeteners, artificial, 125
Synbiotics, 119
Synclein, 180
Systematic review and integrated assessment
    (SYRINA), 330
Systemic nickel allergy syndrome, 131

TAML activators, 331–332
TAML/peroxide, 331
Tamoxifen, 295
Tau aggregates, 182
Taxol, 317, 318*b*

Taxus brevifolia, 317, 318*b*
TB-117, 12–13, 72–74
TCDD, 10–11
Technical performance, 311–312, 312*f*
Technology sustainability compass, 328*b*
Teflon, 80
Terrorist threats, to water supplies, 95–96
Testicular cancer, 237
Testing, safety
    autism and, 287
    government, for chemical exposures, 5
    proactive approaches to, 366
    third-party, lack of, 340
    for toxins, 366
Testosterone, sex hormone–binding protein
    for, 54–55, 54*f*
Tetrabromobisphenol A (TBBPA), 55
2, 3, 7,8-Tetrachlorodibenzo-*p*-dioxin
    (TCDD), 10–11
The Endocrine Disruption Exchange
    (TEDX), 4–5
Theobromine, on dogs, 104–105
Thermoplastics, 26
Thermoset plastics, 26
Thompson, R. C., 27
Throw-away society, 27
Thyroid hormones, triclosan on, 204, 206
Tiered protocol for endocrine disruption
    (TiPED), 296–297, 309, 313, 329, 329*b*
Tight junctions, 116
Tissue-specific sensitivities, 290
Tolerable daily intake dose, 295
Toll-like receptors, 133
Toluene, 7*t*, 9–10
Total maximum daily loading (TMDL), 89
Tox21 assays, 287–288
Toxaphene, 185
ToxCast assays, 287–288
Toxic elements, 319–320. *See also
    specific types*
Toxicology, 289–290
Toys, 362–363
Tributyltin, 130
Triclocarban, 207–209, 215
Triclosan, 7*t*, 15, 203–207
    antimicrobial actions of, 204
    chemistry and uses of, 203
    chloroform from, 206
    diabetes and, 130
    endocrine-disrupting properties of,
        204–205
    exposure to, 205

Triclosan (*Cont.*)
  FDA ban of, 215
  health concerns with, 207–208
  persistence of, 206–207
  production of, 204
  take-home message on, 208
  on thyroid hormones and gonadotropes, 204, 206
  toxicity of, 204
Trimethylamine-*N*-oxide (TMAO), 118
2,4-Dichlorophenoxyacetic acid (2,4-D), 123, 185, 186

U.S. Centers for Disease Control and Prevention (CDC) National Biomonitoring Program, 4

Vacuum cleaners, 78–79
Valerian, 349
Value proposition, 310–313, 312*f*
Vascular dementia, *vs.* Alzheimer disease, 181–182
Vegetables, 341–342, 344*t*
VERIFIED mark, 330
Vinyl chloride, 34–35
Vitamin A, excess, 357
vom Saal, Frederick, 32

Waste, plastic, 26–28, 27*f*
Wastewater, agricultural use of, 91–92
Water
  drinking, 89–92, 346–347 (*See also* Drinking water)
  ground, 102–104
  monitoring quality of, 105–106
Water pollution, chemical, 87–114
  acute threats in, 92–96
  agricultural chemicals in, 102
  ammonium nitrate explosion on, 92–93
  chemical accidents on, 92–95
  chronic threats in, 96–97
  Clean Water Act of 1972 on, 88–89, 103
  clean water resources and, 110
  contaminant exposure in, 104–105, 107*f*
  direct potable reuse for, 108
  drinking water in, 89–92 (*See also* Drinking water)
  endocrine-disrupting chemicals in, 97–100, 99*f* (*See also* Endocrine-disrupting chemicals (EDCs))
  exposure pathways for, 100–110 (*See also specific pathways*)
  exposure to, reducing, 106–110
  filtering technologies for, 108
  Flint, Michigan drinking water, 68, 94–95, 346
  fracking chemicals in, 103–104
  indirect potable reuse for, 108, 109*t*–110*t*
  industrialization in, 100, 102
  man-made toxicants in, 96
  4-methylcyclohexanemethanol spill in, 93–94, 94*f*
  metropolitan water supplies in, 89–91, 100, 347
  from mining operations, 100–101
  monitoring water quality in, 105–106
  pharmaceuticals in, 101
  physicochemistry and toxicology of, 105
  plating operations on, 95
  terrorist threats to, 95–96
  wastewater and biosolids in, agricultural, 91–92
  water quality and, U.S., 88–89
  well water in, individual, 91, 346, 347
Water safety, 119–121
  arsenic in, 119
  cadmium in, 120
  chlorination and, 120–121
Well water, individual, 91, 346, 347
WiFi signals, 226*f*, 230, 232, 235, 370. *See also* Radiofrequency radiation
Wingspread Conference statement, 281–282, 322, 340

Xenobiotics, 128
Xylene isomers, 7*t*, 9–10

Zinc, 95, 356

Printed in the USA/Agawam, MA
June 9, 2021

776041.013